THE ECONOMICS OF MENTAL HEALTH CARE

For
Connie, Melanie, Annette (and RMGH),
Paul and John,
and others who provided
the *raison d'être*

The quality of mercy is not strain'd
It droppeth as the gentle rain from heaven
Upon the place beneath: it is twice blest;
It blesseth him that gives and him that takes...

Portia in *The Merchant of Venice*

The Economics of Mental Health Care

Industry, government and community issues

RUTH F.G. WILLIAMS
School of Applied Economics
Victoria University of Technology, Australia

D.P. DOESSEL
Department of Economics
The University of Queensland, Australia

Routledge
Taylor & Francis Group
LONDON AND NEW YORK

First published 2001 by Ashgate Publishing

Reissued 2018 by Routledge
2 Park Square, Milton Park, Abingdon, Oxon OX14 4RN
711 Third Avenue, New York, NY 10017, USA

Routledge is an imprint of the Taylor & Francis Group, an informa business

Publisher's Note
The publisher has gone to great lengths to ensure the quality of this reprint but points out that some imperfections in the original copies may be apparent.

A Library of Congress record exists under LC control number: 2001089074

ISBN 13: 978-1-138-73487-6 (hbk)
ISBN 13: 978-1-315-18690-0 (ebk)

Contents

List of Figures

List of Tables

Foreword

I re-commenced academic life in 1998 when our daughter was two-and-a-half years old, having suspended my academic role shortly before she was born. The combination of the demands of this project and my other academic responsibilities with my domestic commitments made life quite demanding.

With the benefit of hindsight, I believe now that this mix of academic and domestic responsibilities involved unconscious applications of Grossman's household production theory and Becker's theory of the allocation of time. Since I restricted my absences from home predominantly to teaching and student consultation (with the remainder of my academic responsibilities undertaken at home), most of the week involved allocating, and constantly re-allocating, time inputs at home between academic and domestic responsibilities. Some parts of this manuscript were drafted under circumstances that were 'a little bit different'. On two afternoons a week, a very capable young lady with nanny skills came to our home; this was a lovely experience for our daughter, and usually a (little) friend or two. This young lady and I had a mutual preference, both being drawn to the idea that I should be home, not to be hovering but just for Mum to 'be around'. Hence, I worked nearby the fun, focussing upon this manuscript (well, ninety per cent). Books such as this are often written in the peace and quiet of a university library or in the time of reflection that often accompanies the still of the night. However, only parts of this book came into existence under such ideal conditions.

When, one day, it all seemed too hard, and I felt like giving the project away, my thoughts turned to the people about whom this book is written. I considered the lives that many lead and I thought about how so few of them enjoy complete cure, i.e. for many, whether or not to have their illness is not an option, and life is a daily struggle. With this in mind, I felt I could push on and complete the project.

Several months later, the project took another turn. I asked the person who had supervised my thesis, Darrel Doessel, to join me as the co-author. Darrel and I had maintained our communication over the conceptual work contained in this book for several years and, even during the period when I was the book's sole author, Darrel had kindly begun reading drafts. For Darrel's input, then, to be formalised and expanded was just a natural step (which he made somewhat reticently). Over the eighteen months of co-authorship that ensued, parts of the manuscript re-formed and it has become a joint piece. While some parts of the manuscript have still remained the work of one or the other of us, a large portion of the final draft became a joint output. Our inputs had become very entwined. I feel extremely appreciative of Darrel's contribution: it is one that is, as always, very scholarly and highly stimulating.

My joint role in family and academic life, over some years now, led me to some particular thoughts for the Acknowledgements of this book. Often in such Acknowledgements, there are words about the author's family that read something like this: 'without whom this book would not have been written'. Such words do not apply too well here. It is the stark truth that this book certainly would have happened considerably faster without them! Yet my household role, influenced by the nebulous boundaries of 'family life', involves very important work too; despite the book taking longer to complete than I had thought, there is one other stark truth: the wonderful presence and support of my family has been a great encouragement to me. And so it is that the preciousness of my husband and our daughter makes living, writing a book, being around for a small child, and even cleaning the fridge, worthwhile.

Ruth Williams
Kyneton, Australia

Acknowledgements

This project was partially funded by the Australian Government via a grant from the National Health and Medical Research Council, an organisation that seemed to have lost all trace of us. For this we are **truly grateful**.

We would now like to acknowledge with gratitude the assistance of many people. We are very grateful to Dianne Crowther whose interested, very meticulous and gentle ways made the proof-reading work pleasant. We are extremely grateful to Shirley Keun who, in the preparation of this piece for the publisher, exercised her skills with the utmost care and reliability. Shirley has, once more, weaved her magic on a final manuscript. We also greatly appreciate Ian Williams who, in drafting the diagrams, was always very gracious and applied his eye for detail to a somewhat different task from those he normally carries out. Over the years, we have been blessed with the assistance of four librarians, who have worked in the smallish, and intimate, Economics Library at The University of Queensland. The pleasant dispositions of Hazel Imison, Tanya Ziebell, Ros Roche and Fei Yu have been matched only by their continuing ability to find 'needles in haystacks'. At the Victoria University (Sunbury Campus) Library, Valerie Johnson and Catherine Sellwood have been most attentive and able in their assistance. Tom Bolton willingly assisted in physically locating some of the material for Chapter 4.

Anne Doessel gently guided our reading on some complex issues associated with disability; she also reminded us why the issues contained herein matter. Belinda Clatworthy excelled in being a somewhat different 'research assistant' for one of us. We would also like to thank the following people who have kindly assisted us in a range of specific ways: Peter Ascot, Dr Luke Connelly, Dr Geoff Dixon, Professor Cynthia Dixon, Dr Rhodes Hart, Dr John McGrath, Dr Ian Ring, Dr John Turner, Dr Christine Williams, Professor Ken Wilson, and Connie, Melanie, Annette and John W. Needless to say, the usual *caveat* applies.

Lastly, we would like to express our heartfelt acknowledgement of the patience and support of our spouses, Anne Doessel and Ian Williams.

Ruth Williams
and
Darrel Doessel

List of Keywords

mental disorders
rationality
inputs
outputs
mental health care
socially unacceptable preferences,
impaired preference capacity
role of government
the ‘imposed indifference curve’
deinstitutionalisation
institutional care
non-institutional care
social capital
co-production

Introduction

This book is a revised and extended version of a Master of Economic Studies thesis entitled *Economics and Mental Health Care: Outputs and Implications for Government* that was presented to The University of Queensland in 1989 (Hart, 1989). The purpose of that thesis was, and thus, the purpose of this present study is, to analyse and clarify some aspects of economic behaviour and policy arising from mental illnesses and disorders.

Issues associated with mental illnesses and disorders are glossed over by the economics profession generally. After all, how could conventional microeconomic theory, which involves theory about rational choice, preference ordering and individual optimising behaviour, possibly be relevant to the issue of mental illness, other than for topics like insurance and (general) funding? This book is an economic study that treats seriously the preferences, or to use colloquial language, the needs and the wants, of people with mental illness, and also those of their care-givers. There is evidence (e.g. Jablensky, McGrath *et al.*, 1999) that the majority of those with mental illness live years of life in social isolation, with multiple handicaps that may not be dramatic, but are remarkably disabling. These are resilient people surviving rather rationally, i.e. optimising, in a society where prejudice, and both financial insufficiency and economic inefficiency in service provision, make life unnecessarily hard.

This study uses the tools of conventional economic theory to approach the issue of where the preferences of individuals need to be over-ridden for legal or medical reasons. It then integrates this issue of intervention with an analysis addressing another aspect of the issue. The second dimension is that when no legal or medical reason exists to intervene in preferences, the needs and the wants of people with mental illness and their care-givers in our contemporary society are being neglected.

Although the focus is on mental health care, the approach of this book is unambiguously economic. Some readers may not think of the production of mental health services as occurring in an industry, but there is no reason to think of such services as being any different from other services in the economy. An industry-wide focus is a **common** procedure in economics, a discipline with an historic concern for the material well-being of people. The mental health care industry is a different and difficult industry, and yet many knotty issues about this industry can be unravelled under the light that is shed by economic theory. The difficulty of that task, though, is considerable: topics normally found in textbooks on Industrial Economics are noticeably absent from this study. A reader scanning the Contents pages of this book finds few hints about any Industrial Economics herein. Absent are chapters on such conventional issues in Industrial Economics as market structure, barriers to entry, collusion, strategic behaviour, mergers and joint ventures, innovation, and so forth. Present in this book, though, are chapters concerned with another issue, a prior issue, that of defining the outputs of mental health care. The definition of output is an issue that is seldom studied in the analysis of industries that are typically the focus of Industrial Economics. The output of, say, the car industry is not difficult to define, relatively speaking. Topics conventionally studied in Industrial Economics, such as those just mentioned, may well be proven relevant to the economics of mental health care. But this book does not undertake to debate that concern.

Here, then, is a study that explores the economic nature of the outputs of mental health care, in an era of history where, despite propitious comparisons with the state of knowledge in previous centuries, very little is known about the medical treatment of mental illness. The particular focus is on theoretical matters relating to the outputs of mental health care. Other relevant issues are then addressed: the role of government; and the economic behaviour arising from care in the community, i.e. non-institutional care. Although the focus of attention is on the welfare of the people who are afflicted with mental disorders, there are implications in this analysis for the welfare of others, such as family members and carers generally.

Chapter 1 addresses the broad issue of why economists would want to take an interest in mental illnesses and disorders.

The purpose of Chapter 2 is to address some methodological issues that are of special significance in mental health care. For example, consideration is given to the relevance of the rationality assumption in the economics literature to a study concerned with mental illnesses.

Issues pertinent to economic method are discussed also in Chapter 3. This Chapter considers the Theorems of Welfare Economics, and attention is then directed to the degree to which the Theorems are useful when *Homo Economicus* has a mental disorder.

In Chapter 4 , the survey of the literature addresses the recent, burgeoning and mainly North American literature on the economics of mental health care. It should be noted that there is a convention in the literature in the United States (US) to link 'mental illness' and 'substance abuse'. The position taken in this study is that the two diagnoses involve overlapping sets. The focus in this study is specifically on the care arising with mental illnesses. The survey of the literature here indicates important cost studies and demand studies that dominate the literature. The literature survey also reveals that, perhaps due to a focus on currently pressing policy matters (relevant to domestic institutions in the US), some fundamental conceptual issues relating to the outputs of the mental health care sector have not yet been addressed. However, there is now a literature addressing highly inter-related issues in regard to the output, including expenditure trends in mental health care, input prices and productivity.

The perspective provided here contrasts with the US literature just mentioned, which is discussed in Chapter 4 and Chapter 5. That literature has arisen out of a recent concern with accurately monitoring price changes and expenditure trends in the health sector. It is impossible to provide meaningful information about price changes if price data are collected in the absence of information about changes to the quantity and the quality of life achieved from purchasing a health output. This US literature recognises the importance of conceptualising health output that is health-related. Two studies, one concerned with ischaemic heart disease and the other with depression, are discussed.

Chapters 5 and 6 outline the new perspective being presented in this study. The perspective of this present study is different from that recent literature. Generally, a theoretical *lacunae* on the outputs of mental health care exists, and this gap is addressed by casting the outputs in multi-dimensional space, wherein preferences are expressed. Chapters 5 and 6 suggest that it is helpful to think of mental health care as entering a household production function as a commodity vector; and that it is possible to apply household production theory (Grossman 1972a, 1972b) to describe and give meaning to 'the outputs' of mental health care. Such an analysis presents a theoretical problem of whether, or how, individual preferences can count with respect to mental health services. The use of indifference curves enables an explanation of the relationship between mental health care inputs and the outputs of the mental health care sector. It also enables us to provide an explanation of what it means, in an economic sense, when an individual is committed, involuntarily, to in-patient care.

In the conceptual framework of the 'new' characteristics theory of consumer demand, associated with Lancaster (1966a, 1966b) and Ironmonger (1972), the outputs of mental health care can be understood in terms of (at least) five phenomena or characteristics: treatment, accommodation, medical/nursing care, familial/personal support, and deprivation of liberty. In Chapter 7 government intervention into the (joint) production of these characteristics is examined in terms of the desires of society for a particular level of quality of care and treatment. The interests and concerns of other people, often relatives and friends, are also considered. In other words, externalities are all-pervasive in mental health care. It is argued that these externalities can manifest themselves in a variety of ways although they reduce to two types. First, externalities arise because the preference functioning capacity of the individual is impaired so that preferences cannot be expressed or exercised successfully. Society cares that the individual, or the care-giving family, suffers as a result of this impairment in the ability to form preferences. (The meaning intended here is that 'care' exists. It is not intended to judge whether the care is either enough or appropriate. Rather, it is just to note the presence of the externality.) Second, externalities arise because the individual's utility function itself conflicts with society's norms. In this regard, it is a matter of whose rights prevail. Society, or its agents who are providers of health and/or support, may believe that what is best for others is best for the individual, since he or she exhibits irrationality. But this explanation of government intervention fits better into the organic view of the state: it sits uncomfortably with the individualistic and/or liberal conception of the state that is the standard fare of Welfare Economics. Currently, the medical profession, perhaps unwittingly, is playing a significant economic function of government intervention, in its capacity as 'agent' or 'gatekeeper' of care or treatment. Whether this significant role is desirable is not considered in this study.

Thus, Chapters 5, 6 and 7 together elaborate a conceptual foundation or framework for the economic analysis of the multi-dimensional, and multiple, services that comprise the outputs of the mental health care sector involving the government. While no empirical application of the conceptual framework provided in Chapters 5, 6 and 7 is undertaken in this study, an approach is suggested. The relevant approach to empirical studies of heterogeneous goods or services (like mental health care) is the estimation of hedonic prices. See the Section on 'Future Research' in Chapter 11 for a discussion of empirical issues.

The focus of the book then turns to deinstitutionalisation and community-based, or non-institutional, care.

The literature on deinstitutionalisation is voluminous. It is not our wish in this study to survey that literature, nor to duplicate descriptions of the issue or the accounts of failure.[1] Rather, the purpose here is to bring an economic perspective to bear on the issue. A brief introduction to that literature is useful, however, because the deinstitutionalisation literature is not generally the subject of study by economists.

The concept, 'deinstitutionalisation', has institutional origins as well as conceptual origins. Its institutional origins are generally regarded to be in

---

1 People with mental illnesses are not the only ones vulnerable to the failures of deinstitutionalisation. A moving, though confronting, account of how deinstitutionalisation can fail is depicted in a partly autobiographical film about the experiences of a woman with severe cerebral palsy, Heather Rose. The film, 'Dance Me to My Song' (1998), is co-written by Heather Rose with the film's director, Rolf De Heer, and Frederick Stahl. It is a story about the infringements upon the 'personhood' of a very vulnerable individual who is now living in, and receiving care from, 'the community'; it is about abuses of power. Abuses of power can most certainly arise in large institutions, as graphically described in *One Flew Over the Cuckoo's Nest* (Kesey, 1973), but 'deinstitutionalisation' does not guarantee the absence of the abuse of power. Deinstitutionalisation is no guarantee that the trust that vulnerable people must place in others is not abused. Benevolent or malevolent people can fill the power vacuum that arises from disability, whatever the origin of the disability. Changing the location of where services are provided (e.g. from institutions to 'the community') does not guarantee the integrity, disposition or personal attributes of service providers. That is, no one-to-one correspondence exists between service location and the ethical behaviour of people providing the service.

Denmark's *Mental Retardation Act*, 1959. However, the conceptual origins of deinstitutionalisation are taken to be Nirje's concept of normalisation (Nirje, 1969). Subsequently, Nirje defined this concept (a concept that simultaneously was an objective) as 'making available to all mentally retarded people patterns of life and conditions of everyday living which are as close as possible to the regular circumstances and ways of life of society' (Nirje, 1980, p. 33). Nirje regards the key aspects of such a lifestyle to be the following: the rhythm of the day, week, year; progression through the stages of the life cycle; self-determination, involving choice of actions; the development of heterosexual relationships; and economic rights and access rights, with the latter involving the absence of physical and environmental barriers. This conception was Scandinavian. A North American conception followed with Wolfensberger and Nirje (1972) who also used the term 'normalisation', although he – Wolfensberger – subsequently employed another term, 'social role valorisation' (Wolfensberger, 1983). See also Wolfensberger (1998).

It is relevant to ask what lies behind the concept, normalisation. Put otherwise, why should we be concerned with normalisation? A brief discussion of 'personhood' gives a way of providing an answer. The notion of personhood involves 'a standing or status that is bestowed upon one human being, by others, in the context of relationship and social being. It implies recognition, respect and trust' (Kitwood, 1997, p. 8). Kitwood argues that personhood resides conceptually in a number of literatures: psychology, particularly social psychology, employs the notion; 'personhood' is present also in western philosophy in the theme, 'each person has absolute value'; and both theistic and non-theistic discourses about transcendence draw upon the notion of personhood.

Consider, now, the multi-faceted nature of the vast literature on deinstitutionalisation which has arisen from these roots just outlined. The literature covers various conditions, e.g. mental illness (Horsfall, 1987; Barham, 1992; Prior, 1993), intellectual disability (Taylor, Bogdan and Racino, 1991; Young, Sigafoos, Suttie, Ashman and Grevell, 1998), physical disability (Joint, 1996; Means and Smith, 1998) and multiple disability (Cocks, 1993). It also covers various countries, *inter alia*, the United Kingdom (Malin, 1994; Mansell and Ericsson, 1996) and Australia (Fine and Thompson, 1995; Maddison, 1998); different issues, such as housing (Racino, 1993), the provision of services (Malin, 1994) and ethics (Peele and Chodoff, 1999); and different disciplines, for example, social work (Payne, 1995) and psychology (Carling, 1995).

To an economist, care should be taken in the use of 'deinstitutionalisation' and 'non-institutional care'. While there is a common attitude about humanity implied in both words, 'deinstitutionalisation' has come to represent the political and bureaucratic processes that have brought about the present changes to ways of delivering care. The emphasis in the present day is on 'non-institutional care', or 'community-based care'. Economically speaking, non-institutional care differs from institutional care in both its input combinations and outputs.

Chapter 8 presents some descriptive information about care undertaken in the community by households, and attention turns briefly to some aspects of how economics conceptualises household care-giving. Chapters 9 and 10 then address the phenomenon that multiple inputs into mental health care are flowing from various channels, i.e. within government and 'the community'. In Chapter 9, the conceptual foundation for these multiple inputs is drawn from recent theories of social capital. Attention turns in Chapter 10 to the concept of co-production and the 'synergy hypothesis'. Two questions arise. First, what is the relationship between social capital and government? A second, more specific question is this: does government action or expenditure increase or decrease private action or expenditure? In other words, is social capital from a government source a substitute for, or a complement to, social capital from non-government or community sources? The answers to these two questions are empirical. In order to shed light on the issues relevant to empirical work, a general theory of co-production is given, in which inputs from government and inputs from citizens are employed. Therein an important research agendum is suggested: a new conceptual approach to the evaluation of non-institutional care and the processes of deinstitutionalisation that brought about such care.

Chapter 11 summarises the contributions of the book and suggests four areas for further research. First, a Section on Baumol's cost disease provides an analysis of the rising real costs that are found in particular types of economic activities. It is likely that the cost disease is present in mental health care. Second, a Section on estimating hedonic functions is concerned with empirical work on the demand for commodities which have multiple attributes or characteristics, such a mental health care. This Section provides an approach to the empirical application of the three Chapters on the outputs of mental health care, Chapters 5, 6 and 7. Third, the issue is raised of whether new pharmaceuticals are employed as substitutes for existing therapies and treatments, or as complements. One important determinant of the outcome of this issue is the relative price of labour (e.g. medical practitioners, providers of domestic support, and so forth) compared with the relative prices of pharmaceuticals. Fourth, a Section on uncertainty in mental health care considers two approaches to filling the gaps in medical knowledge which affect the mental health production function: studies about variations in practice style, referred to in the literature as the 'small area variation' phenomenon; and 'evidence-based medicine' with its concern that the relationship between therapies (inputs) and outcomes (outputs) is a positive one. Attention is drawn to these four issues in the final Chapter because, for the economics of mental health care, each issue is an important area of study in its own right; and together these issues should be regarded as four important building blocks to be incorporated in future empirical work.

Matters about readership are now addressed. A relevant question is this: for whom has this book been written? There is a 'readership dilemma' in writing any book, but in this case, the authors' dilemma has been most severe. Both authors are economists working in an academic environment, and typically they write with their peers in mind. However, in this case, we have kept others in our focus, *viz.*, professionals (psychiatrists, nurses, social workers, etc.) and volunteers (family members etc.) who provide services to people subject to the impairments of mental illness. Members of such groups frequently have a 'narrow' conception of economics: they may conceive of the discipline as being synonymous with 'cost cutting', 'economic rationalism' or some such term. Caricatures of economics are widespread. One of our objectives is to indicate that economics is not concerned with reducing inputs. At a very general level, economics is concerned with people's living standards and this concept involves, among many matters, the investigation of the important relationship between inputs and outputs. In economics, this relationship can be investigated in reference to physical goods (like cars) or services (such as those provided by banks) or services involving the provision of personal care services to people with mental illness.

There is another readership matter. Readers with a background in economics will notice that the amount of descriptive material about mental illness contained herein is unusually large, relatively speaking. Mostly, economic studies of mental illness, particularly those involving empirical work, discuss the illness and its implications in a matter of several sentences. However, various factors have convinced us of the value of incorporating description and discussion of mental illness, and about people with mental illness. First, as opposed to being an empirical piece, this study is conceptual in nature; putting it another way, having the concepts 'right' matters in this study. Second, it is apparent that the amount of misinformation and stigma associated with mental illness is not a trivial issue for our society. Third, there is generally a lack of study of the economic behaviour of people with mental illness within our own profession. These three factors influenced us in our decision to include descriptive material about mental illness, alongside text that is strictly of an economic nature. We trust that our readers are not bemused by this: those with an economic background may not be happy that we have digressed into non-economic material; and those who are involved directly with mental illness, either professionally, or as carers, or people with mental illness themselves, may wonder why the book contains text that is so self-evident to them. Pointing out here these dilemmas in writing for multiple groups of readers may help to address some possible reactions felt across the potential breadth of readership of this study.

Essentially, this book is an industry study of the mental health care sector. More specifically, it is about some aspects of the economic behaviour of consumers, producers and funding agencies with respect to mental disorders.

In a climate of stigma and consumer ignorance (apart from 'clear-cut' cases wherein society ought to impose its preferences upon individuals), there is little opportunity for exercising consumer preferences. In this regard, special attention is warranted to the meaning of the outputs, and to the role of government and the community.

1 Economics and Mental Health Care

Introduction

The major mental illnesses and disorders cause suffering world-wide, regardless of socioeconomic group. Of a population of 19 million in Australia, around 500,000 people are thought to be sufferers of major mental illnesses and disorders. Schizophrenia, for example, affects more Australians than many other better-known illnesses and conditions, around one per cent of the population. The World Health Organization reports that the prevalence rate, that is, the frequency of cases of all mental illnesses and disorders present at any one time in populations world-wide, is remarkably high: one person in every five.

The nature and impact of expenditures upon services and support for mental illnesses is something of an enigma. The 1993 *Report of the National Inquiry into the Human Rights of People with Mental Illness* (commonly called 'The Burdekin Report')(Human Rights and Equal Opportunity Commission, 1993) indicates that the annual outlays by governments throughout Australia is some $3.45 billion each year on 'services and income support' for people with mental illnesses and disorders. Another estimate of the level of spending on mental health and related services is provided by the 1996 *National Mental Health Report* (Mental Health Branch Commonwealth Department of Health and Aged Care, 1998, p.15). This is a lower estimate, which excludes income support, of $2.07 billion, and it totals spending on 'mental health and related services' in 1996-97 by Commonwealth, state and territory Governments and by private hospitals. For an overview of the Australian mental health system, see Whiteford, Thompson and Casey (2000). The entire expenditure in Australia arising from mental illnesses and disorders is yet unknown: it includes Commonwealth, state and territory Government funding; voluntary agency funding; and an unknown level of support from family and friends. But the standard of living and the level of well-being of people with mental illness, especially the serious conditions, is known to be far from satisfactory.

This study is undertaken for the purpose of clarifying economic behaviour arising from mental illnesses and disorders. This economic behaviour relates both to individuals themselves, whose well-being is impaired and whose standard of living is deplorable in many instances, and to other people and institutions. In elaborating this purpose, a description is given of some of the forces behind both private sector activity, including voluntary support, and government involvement in this area of the health sector. In particular, a conceptual approach is taken towards describing various aspects of current trends in levels of funding, as well as the composition of services consumed by the mental health care sector. In such a conceptual work as this, model-building is involved. Model-building is a first step in giving answers to questions such as this one: what can society look to purchase from its services and strategies for people with mental disorders and illnesses? This study gives an economic framework for examining **what is being produced** in this sector. In taking a conceptual approach, this study is not involved, for example, in cost-effectiveness analysis or collection of data for statistical analyses. Before any evaluation study or statistical/econometric analysis of costs is undertaken, it is best to ask, 'What is produced? What is being evaluated? What economic arrangements create well-being in the mental health sector?'

Economic concepts are involved in examinations of expenditures in mental health care. There is, however, little economic understanding of the mental health sector, and some of the theoretical and empirical problems posed by this sector challenge the frontiers of economic understanding. Hoary problems seem to beset anyone who is involved with this sector: those who suffer from a condition; those who provide services to them; and economists too.

Mental Illnesses and Disorders

For an economist to attempt to define mental disorder would be to step into a minefield of medical, legal, social and ethical judgements that change with time and context. Yet it is initially adequate to state that mental disorder is a state of disarray in the functioning of the mind or psyche, and that it is a very general term referring to a diverse group of conditions or illnesses.[1] Disagreement in the mental health literature arises over what the mind is, or the psyche; over how to explain and investigate personality and to treat aberrations; and over which professions are best at performing which tasks (Spitzer and Klein, 1978; Reich, 1981).

Some Basic Points [2]

Mental illnesses are very disabling. Although all humans experience deep, uncontrollable and exaggerated feelings of tension, fear, depression or sadness,

1 The terms, 'condition', 'illness' and 'disorder', will be largely used in this study. Sometimes, the term, 'disease', is appropriate for an organic brain change due to infections of the brain tissue. This is one sub-group of all mental disorders.

2 The account that follows is drawn from various sources. For further references, see American Psychiatric Association (1994); Rosenhan and Seligman (1984); Kenny and Whitehead (1973).

for a variety of reasons such feelings can become so distressing for some individuals that they cannot cope with day-to-day activities such as going to work, preparing meals, enjoying leisure time, or relating to others. Individuals suffering these states are given a diagnosis from one of the neurotic disorder groups that include anxiety, obsessional states, neurotic depression and phobias. See also American Psychiatric Association (1994). A hallmark of neurosis is that the individual is aware that his or her distress is out of proportion to reality (Rosenhan and Seligman, 1984, p. 192).

There are more serious disorders, the psychotic disturbances. Individuals may suffer disturbances of their higher mental processes, particularly thinking, speaking, feeling and testing reality. They are out of touch with a real world that people generally seem able to experience. If a person is unable to sense and test reality, this causes confusion and an inability to make sense of one's surroundings. This can be so real to many such individuals that they may explain their surroundings or cope with themselves by developing false ideas, ideas of persecution, of grandeur or of guilt, or they may see, hear, taste, smell or feel things which are not present. In the most severe cases, individuals may behave in ways that appear strange and disturbing to others. In less severe cases, individuals seem just to be different, as if somehow they are 'marching to a different drum'.

These 'more serious' conditions are the psychotic disorders. The distinction between psychosis and neurosis is not always clear. In the absence of complete understanding of mental illnesses and their causes, this is not unexpected. Historically, the use of these terms has changed quite considerably since 'psychosis' was coined in 1845. The distinction, although generalised (and perhaps blurred), is useful (Beer, 1990).

Most sufferers of psychotic disorders are afflicted with one of four conditions: schizophrenia, bipolar affective disorder, psychotic depression and dementia.[3] The schizophrenias are a group of conditions where a person's feelings, thoughts and behaviour become fragmented, disorganised, no longer integrated (Kenny and Whitehead, 1973, p. 50). Some people think a common feature of schizophrenia is the problem of 'split personality', that is, of one person leading two lives. This is a misunderstanding of schizophrenia. More commonly, the symptoms may involve an individual's speech becoming illogical; he or she may face an inability to experience emotions; initiative can become blunted; decision making and planning often is a burden; and 'withdrawal' may be experienced. With schizophrenia, particular behaviour and emotions seem inappropriate to an onlooker, especially in instances when some individuals suffer delusions and hallucinations. Table 1 gives an example of the diagnostic criteria for schizophrenia from the *Diagnostic and Statistical Manual of Mental Disorders*, fourth edition, (DSM-IV).

---

3 Rosenhan and Seligman (1984, ch. 17) argue that there is only one psychosis, schizophrenia.

Table 1.1 Diagnostic criteria for schizophrenia

A. Presence of characteristic psychotic symptoms in the active phase: either (1), (2) or (3) for at least one week (unless the symptoms are successfully treated);
   1. two of the following:
      a. delusions
      b. prominent hallucinations (throughout the day for several days for several times a week for several weeks, each hallucinatory experience not being limited to a few brief moments)
      c. incoherent or marked loosening of associations
      d. catatonic behaviour
      e. flat or grossly inappropriate affect
   2. bizarre delusions (i.e. involving a phenomenon that the person's culture would regard as totally implausible, e.g. thought broadcasting, being controlled by a dead person)
   3. prominent hallucinations [as defined in (1)(b) above] of a voice with content having no apparent relation to depression or elation, or a voice keeping up a running commentary of the person's behaviour or thoughts, or two or more voices conversing with each other.

B. During the course of the disturbance, functioning in such areas as work, social relations, and self-care is markedly below the highest level achieved before the onset of the disturbance (or, when the onset is in childhood or adolescence, failure to achieve expected level of social development).

C. Schizoaffective Disorder and Mood Disorder with Psychotic Features have been ruled out, i.e. if a Major Depressive or Manic Syndrome has been ever present during an active phase of the disturbance, the total duration of all episodes of a mood syndrome has been brief relative to the total duration of the active and residual phases of the disturbance.

D. Continuous signs of the disturbance for at least six months. The six-month period must include an active phase (of at least one week, or less if symptoms have been successfully treated) during which there were psychotic symptoms characteristic of schizophrenia (symptoms in A), with or without prodromal or residual phase, as defined below.

   Prodromal phase: A clear deterioration in functioning before active phase of the disturbance that is not due to disturbance of mood or to Psychoactive Substance Use Disorder and that involves at least two of the symptoms listed below.

   Residual phase: Following the active phase of the disturbance, persistence of at least two of the symptoms noted below, these not being due to a disturbance in mood or to a Psychoactive Substance Use Disorder.

   Prodromal or Residual Symptoms:
   1. marked social isolation or withdrawal
   2. marked impairment in role functioning as wage-earner, student, or home-maker
   3. markedly peculiar behaviour (e.g. collecting garbage, talking to self in public, hoarding food)
   4. marked impairment in personal hygiene and grooming
   5. blunted or inappropriate affect
   6. digressive, vague, overelaborate, or circumstantial speech, or poverty of speech, or poverty of content of speech
   7. odd beliefs or magical thinking, influencing behaviour and inconsistent with cultural norms, e.g. superstitiousness, belief in clairvoyance, telepathy, 'sixth sense', 'others can feel my feelings', overvalued ideas, ideas of reference
   8. unusual perceptual experiences, e.g. recurrent delusions, sensing the presence of a force or person not actually present
   9. marked lack of initiative, interests, or energy
      Examples: Six months of prodromal symptoms with one week of symptoms from A; no prodromal symptoms with six months of symptoms from A; no prodromal symptoms with one week of symptoms from A and six months of residual symptoms.

E. It cannot be established that an organic factor initiated and maintained the disturbance.

F. If there is a history of Autistic Disorder, the additional diagnosis of Schizophrenia is made only if prominent delusions or hallucinations are also present.

Source: American Psychiatric Association (1994, pp. 194-95).

A disorder in which the person suffers extreme disturbances of mood is currently called bipolar affective disorder, to replace the more pejorative term, manic-depression. There are two mood states, the manic state in which the individual's behavioural state is elated far more than what could be warranted, and the depressed state where the individual experiences exaggerated feelings of pessimism, becoming withdrawn and under-active. Episodes of illness may be mild or severe, may vary in their duration and may involve one or both of the mood states. In between episodes, the person can be free of symptoms.

Psychotic depression, or unipolar affective depression, is a mood (affective) disorder that may be differentiated from neurotic depression. That is, there is an **internal** stress or disease (as opposed to stresses external to the person) which results in deep misery and overwhelmingly unrealistic feelings of personal worthlessness. With everything seeming hopeless, individuals dread the future and death often seems the only solution. Psychotic depression is one of the more successfully treated mental disorders (Kenny and Whitehead, 1973, p. 57; Rosenhan and Seligman, 1984, p. 325).

The dementias are a grouping of conditions and they can arise from a number of causes, including head injury, various medical conditions and the ageing process (though it is not an inevitable consequence of ageing). Dementia is a failure of the brain function and involves intellectual and memory problems, confusion and changes in personality.

Most individuals would prefer to be without the suffering that accompanies mental disorder. They cannot just 'pull themselves together', just as will-power alone cannot cure diabetes or a broken wrist. Mostly, people are treated effectively outside hospital and never need to be admitted. Many people experience just one episode of a mental disorder; a small percentage of people suffer recurrent episodes; a smaller percentage face mental illness all their lives. In some cases, symptoms are so disturbing to the sufferer or to others that treatment is undertaken in a health establishment that also provides residential facilities, often only for a limited term. Most wards in psychiatric hospitals are not locked since most mentally ill individuals are no more dangerous or violent than other members of the community. In fact, they are more likely to be vulnerable and afraid. However, recent findings would indicate a sub-group that is more dangerous than the rest of the general population, and that usually the diagnosis of psychiatric illness involves substance abuse as well (Torrey, 1994). This sub-group is subject to addiction as well as mental disorder.

Relating to people who have a mental illness is most difficult when unpleasant behaviour is occurring. Either the symptoms of mental illnesses or the individual's own adaptations to the symptoms they suffer,[4] or both together,

4 Some evocative accounts describing remarkable adaptations in seven patients suffering from various neurological diseases have been written by Oliver Sacks. These accounts may offer readers insight into the types of adaptations that are likely to be made by individuals with psychiatric conditions (Sacks, 1995).

can result in undesirable, at times obnoxious, behaviour. Such behaviour may not occur continually with mental illnesses but, unfortunately, it is the behaviour that is most often remembered by members of the general public and is, therefore, regularly associated with mental illness. To assume that unpleasant behaviour is the norm with mental illness is a misconception. Indeed, it may do the 'normal' population well to remember that obnoxious behaviour and obnoxious people are numbered within the 'normal' population too.

In an Appendix attached to this Chapter, accounts are presented which describe the course of illness of five individuals. Some of the accounts are about fictitious people, although the ideas/concepts/behaviours are factual. These accounts together provide a construction of stories of a random selection of experiences. Although the accounts do not provide representative data about people with psychotic disorders, even with the broad spectrum reflected in the descriptions, important differences among the descriptions nevertheless reflect various insights and perspectives. These five accounts have been written by different authors from different perspectives.

The first account is by a family member. The second is written by an individual suffering with a disorder. The third, another from the perspective of a family member, is about an individual who lives more or less outside of the treatment system. The fourth account, written by a psychiatrist, reflects an individual's encounters with the treatment system. Finally, the fifth is written by a journalist about a person who has been, but is no longer, institutionalised.

The accounts indicate the responses of individuals, of family, friends, government, professionals. In selecting the accounts, our preference is not to include stories of people whose illnesses are cured. Nor have accounts been included where the outcome is suicide. While both those outcomes (cure and death) are pertinent to this study, perhaps the stories of people who live a long-term struggle to survive with a mental illness have special significance here. Thus, the accounts in this Appendix broadly indicate some of the economic issues of chronic psychiatric illness.

Other descriptions of the problems of people with chronic mental illness can be found in Schwartz and Goldfinger (1981), Freedman and Moran (1984a, 1984b) and Peterson (1982).

Reported Prevalence

In Australia, the reports of the National Survey of Mental Health and Wellbeing provide thorough, recent information about several aspects of the health status of people with mental illness. The *Fourth Report*, entitled *People living with Psychotic Illness: An Australian Study 1997-98* (Jablensky, McGrath *et al.*, 1999), provides both an estimated point prevalence (one month) of psychotic disorder and detailed descriptions of the disabilities, as well as of the symptoms, the quality of life and the side effects of medication of the sample group. Jablensky, McGrath and colleagues find that between four and seven persons per 1,000 adult population living in urban areas are in contact with mental health care due to symptoms and disabilities of psychoses. Data concerning the range of 'multiple handicaps' suffered by these people, which were described in an anecdotal fashion in the previous Sub-section, and detailed in that *Report*, will not be given here. These data, presented fully in the *Fourth Report*, as mentioned above, are summarised on pages *xvi-xvii* and Chapter 21 of that *Report*.

Another approach to describing 'the consumers of mental health services' is that of two brief surveys that are contained in the *Annual Report* of the National Mental Health Strategy, and titled 'Profile of Mental Health Consumers' and 'Consumers with Special Needs' (Mental Health Branch, Commonwealth Department of Health and Family Services, 1997, pp. 91-97).

The Diagnostic Spectrum

The previous Sub-sections outlined the broad nature of conventionally defined mental disorder.[5] Many people with these conditions seek professional help at some time, although they are not the only ones who do so.[6] Others within the population perceive themselves to be at 'less than potential' and, though not ill, wish to function at a higher level of self-fulfilment or achievement in personal life and relationships, at work, in sport and so forth. Such individuals are not classed as suffering a mental disorder.

In between mental disorder and the quest for achievement or self-fulfilment is a group of people in a grey area of emotional and mental health problems. This group, often referred to as 'the worried well', arises because of problems due to psychological and emotional distress caused by the stresses of daily life, and are not within the conventional criteria of mental disorder.

A stylisation of these groups of individuals is given in Figure 1.1, indicating states along the diagnostic spectrum, between mental illness and mental health, although the populations within the boundaries are not always readily defined. For example, the Commonwealth Government reports in two separate publications the prevalence of mental disorders in adults in Australia. There is a study reporting low prevalence of psychotic disorders, such as schizophrenia, which are thought to have high use of services; and a separate study of high

---

5 For example, in the ICD-10 Classification of Mental and Behavioural Disorders a mental disorder refers to 'the existence of a clinically recognisable set of symptoms or behaviour associated in most cases with distress and interference with personal functions' (World Health Organization, 1992, p. 5). Most diagnoses require criteria to be met in regard to duration and severity of symptoms (Australian Bureau of Statistics, 1998, p. 58).

6 Another category, the 'undiagnosed', presents significant issues. Some are hidden by themselves or by family. Others are unaware of their state or just try quietly to cope. Some are in prison. Others have 'fallen through the cracks' of the systems of treatment and support.

prevalence disorders ranging across anxiety disorders, affective disorders, alcohol use disorders and drug use disorders.[7]

The distinctions between the various areas in Figure 1.1 are not a trivial concern, particularly when choices have to be made about which groups are to be granted subsidised access to government-financed or -provided services.

Figure 1.1 The diagnostic spectrum

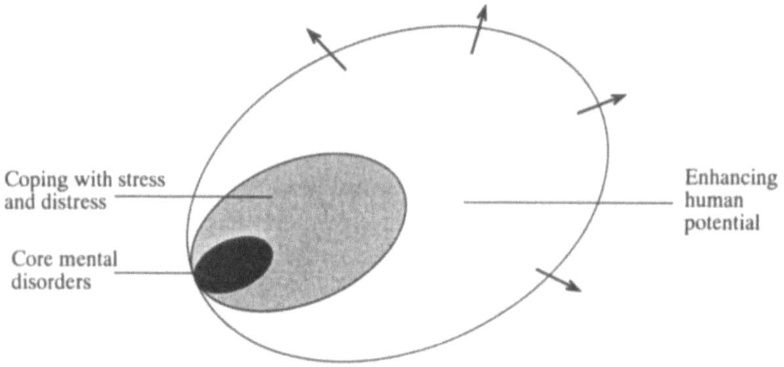

Source: Klerman and Schechter (1981, p. 122), by permission of Oxford University Press.

A Qualification: Two Confusing Issues

It is useful to draw readers' attention now to two issues of confusion regarding mental illness, **where the confusion has an economic dimension**. First, confusion is likely to arise over the existence of a range of **causes** of inappropriate behaviours. Not all 'inappropriate behaviour', a term used in the vernacular, is within the purview of this study. Only the behaviours caused by mental illness are under investigation here. Another area of confusion arises where inadequacies in the services for mental illnesses exist. Both sources of confusion have an economic dimension and both sources of confusion will now be introduced.

Odd behaviour, which is one of a range of socially difficult and/or unacceptable behaviours, is often associated with mental illness. It can be due

7 The following disorders are reported in the 'high prevalence' study: Panic Disorder, Agoraphobia, Social Phobia, Generalised Anxiety Disorder, Obsessive-Compulsive Disorder, Post-Traumatic Stress Disorder; Depression, Dysthymia, Mania, Hypomania, Bipolar Affective Disorder; Alcohol Use Disorders and Drug Use Disorders which include both Harmful Use and Dependence (Australian Bureau of Statistics, 1998, p. 3).

also to factors other than mental illness, such as a drug episode, drunkenness, involvement with the occult, intellectual disability, loneliness and neglect, and so on. The implication of the range of factors just acknowledged is that confusion can arise for the general population (and economists are not immune to this confusion) in interpreting the origins of bizarre or adverse behaviour.

Before addressing the matter of the economic implications, let us consider an illustration of a type of behaviour that seems to be relatively well understood, in terms of how people interpret the origin or motive. Take murder, for example. The general population recognises that an act of murder could be due, say, to intoxication or to drugs or jealousy or Satanism. In such cases, it is classed as a criminal act. A criminal act is generally understood to be a different case from an act of murder by a person who is found to be insane. While it seems that the possible factors that can lead to an act of murder are relatively well understood in the general population, there is confusion with respect to less serious behaviour.

Consider, by way of contrast, a man who spends his day digging up his yard with a shovel, yelling abuse or blasphemy at anyone who talks to him, whose house resembles a pig's sty and who has antagonised his family to the point that he has lost contact with them. Neglect, criticism, provocation and ridicule are not appropriate forms of response to such a person. Depending on the cause of his behaviour, some possible types of help are treatment, general counselling, spiritual counselling, domestic help and general friendship and support. Neighbours are likely to be concerned with the issue of whether or not the man is institutionalised.

Many other individual stories of socially unacceptable behaviour could be told. Some stories would bring to the fore the group of people with mental disorders whose illnesses cause different symptoms from those in the instance above. Such people may be extremely withdrawn, depressed, unmotivated, inactive and unkempt, perhaps a little strange in habits or behaviour, and so forth. These are people whose lives are awful struggles too, and whose symptoms can be extremely difficult for others to live with and deal with, difficult in another way from the story in the previous paragraph.

This book seeks to ascribe to mental illness only the behaviour and the consequences of that behaviour which are due to mental illness. It is very important to be quite clear that bizarre behaviour might have origins in mental illness, or it might have sources in factors other than mental illness, or there might be a mix of origins. This is not a trite matter when odd, adverse or socially unacceptable behaviours are misinterpreted, and when there are economic implications of both the behaviours and the misinterpretations.

Attention now turns to the other area of confusion, related closely to the first. The other source of confusion arises where inadequacies in the services for mental illnesses exist. The individuals just described live in a range of inadequate circumstances. Some are homeless. Others live in rented hovels. Some live in prison, where the problems of their health status exclude them from the benefit of sufficient treatment. Others are living in the kinds of hostels periodically under investigation by the press. A recent Australian example of a press *exposé* of scandalous neglect in Brisbane was Smith and Wenham's account of hostel residents forced out of government institutions (*The Courier-Mail*, 1 April, 2000, p. 26). Others yet again live at home, with either ageing parents or worn-out spouses struggling to address compounding needs. When the struggles faced by carers exhaust them or are insurmountable, as is not infrequently the case, some carers become very ill themselves.

This book is not a study that decides on the kinds of intervention and care that are best in any of these situations. While socially unacceptable behaviour creates a reasonably obvious need for appropriate intervention and treatment, general members of the community understand the medical and legal dimensions better than they do the economic dimension. The concern of this book is with addressing confusion associated with the economic dimension. This concern is all the more important if it is recognised that, historically, considerable haphazardness has occurred over the lot of persons like those just described. In some eras of history, virtually nothing was done to help such people; another era put them in asylums; some eras put many in gaol; and some eras 'treat' and 'support' them 'in the community'. Some eras exercise relatively more care, other eras more neglect. Some eras shut such individuals away. In an era of non-institutional care, there are family members and neighbours who are indignant to have contact with such people. There are other family members or neighbours who express concern for, and exercise responsibility towards, such people.

A key purpose of this book is to recognise and understand the **economic forces**, i.e. not just medical, legal or social forces, **at play in deciding the outcomes** of the lives of people affected by mental illness, the people themselves, and their carers. The outcomes relate to whether such people are institutionalised or placed in the community, to what therapies are provided, to whether they are neglected or instead are cared for appropriately, and so forth. Hence, the previous paragraphs raised some important issues of confusion. The issues were as follows. Difficult or affronting behaviour has consequences that have an economic dimension that is not well understood. When such behaviour affects others, treatment or other intervention results, often, though not always. The services provided may vary both in appropriateness and efficiency. (It would seem that the greater are the consequences from the behaviour, the greater is the amount of intervention.) Both the degree and the type of treatment and intervention available have an economic dimension, and therein lies a further *raison d'être* for a study such as this.

The Standard of Living and Mental Health Care

The standard of living, defined most simply, is the level of material well-being of an individual or household (Pearce, 1986, p. 400). This study, in addressing the outputs of mental health care, is concerned, in part, with examining some aspects of the association between goods and services and the standard of living of people with mental illnesses and disorders, as well as of others, such as family members and carers. To that end, the technical concern of Chapters 5, 6 and 7 of the study is to give an economic account of the outputs of mental health care. In Chapters 8, 9 and 10 an economic approach to mental health care in the community is developed. In the present Section it is useful, therefore, to examine briefly the notion of the standard of living, and how it relates to people with mental illnesses. Attention will turn in the next Section to some basic points about economics and mental health care. This Chapter then concludes with further comments about the scope and purpose of this study.

The standard of living, also called 'economic welfare', 'prosperity', 'utility' or 'level of living', is increased by the satisfaction derived from the consumption of economic goods and services. One of the great scholars of Welfare Economics, I.M.D. Little, explains economic welfare in the following manner:

> There is no part of well-being called 'economic well-being'. The word 'economic' qualifies not well-being, but the causes of well-being ... Thus the sentence 'I am interested in the economic welfare of Smith' is to be translated as 'I am interested in the economic causes of (changes in) Smith's happiness' (Little, 1957, p. 6).

An individual's standard of living is not depicted completely by the bundle of goods and services in the possession of the individual. Knowing about the well-being of individuals involves knowing also about the varying abilities among people to conduct their lives. Moreover, a 'thriving' human life usually involves consideration of a range of matters: issues about education, for example, not only its availability but also its nature and quality; health care; labour issues, and the quality of the workplace; issues concerning the political privileges allowed in the society; issues regarding social and personal relationships, and family relations; also, how these relations support or inhibit other areas of living; and so on. For an account of the complexity involved in knowing about prosperity, see Nussbaum and Sen (1993).

The relationships between goods and services and satisfaction or well-being are not simple in all instances. It is likely that this is more so with individuals who have a mental illness. Hence, an understanding of the nature of the relationship between goods and services and satisfaction is pertinent in regard to people with mental illnesses for whom their standard of living is far from adequate, at least anecdotally speaking, if not empirically established.

In the Sub-section that follows, attention is directed to an approach to the standard of living given by Sen (1987a; 1987b). Sen (1987a) acknowledges the existence of many competing approaches to the standard of living and he gives a thorough critique of each of these. Initially in the next Sub-section, an overview of his critiques is presented. The focus then turns to Sen's conception of the standard of living.

Sen's Approach to the Standard of Living: Lives and Capabilities

Traditional approaches to the living standard conceptualise it in several ways which, according to Sen (1985; 1987a; 1987b), involve either a subjective, or objective, interpretation of the notion of the living standard.

Subjective interpretations perceive utility itself to be the object of value. In other words, particular mental states are seen as valuable, e.g. happiness or the fulfilment of desire. Sen points out that the limitation of interpreting the living standard in this manner is that being satisfied with one's lot may not be real, psychologically speaking, but rather the result of social conditioning or some other factor, like mental illness where, for example, both depression and mania can cause a person to be 'satisfied' with his or her lot. Both happiness and the fulfilment of desire are relevant to the standard of living but are not sufficient in explaining the notion.

Another traditional conception of utility involves the individual's 'choice' behaviour. For example, if a person chooses x when y is available, then x must have a higher utility for the person than has y. The difficulty with this interpretation is that 'choice' is confused with the notion of benefiting. Sen argues that while the notions of choice and benefit are close, they are not substitutable ideas. A further difficulty is, according to Sen, that what a person chooses depends on his or her motivation. The choice which benefits one's own well-being is only one aspect of achieving a good outcome, and a beneficial outcome is not always ensured. It could well be argued, for example, that not enough altruism from other people in society is directed towards people with mental illnesses. Again, choice is relevant to standard of living but is not sufficient in explaining the notion.

A third traditional approach is the popular approach to the standard of living where the living standard is described in terms of a person's possession of commodities. This approach involves an objective interpretation of the standard of living. In economic language this is the notion of real income. A further development of this third notion can be found in the quest for a definition of the minimum living standard. The minimum standard or 'poverty line' or 'the basic needs' approach is variously defined but, commonly, reference is made to some defined quantity and quality of accommodation, food, medical care, education, safety, leisure and so forth. Now, while any practical analysis of the living standard must pay some attention to these features, the limitation is that commodity possession reflects little about the quality of the life being lived. Deeper questions exist.

A full account of the limitations of this so-called 'opulence' conception of living standard is found in Sen (1987a; 1987b, pp. 24-26). Sen's argument can be summarised here by way of a quip made in his Tanner Lectures, that '[a]s a direction to go, concentration on the possession of vital commodities seems fair enough. ... The more exacting question is not whether this is the right direction to go, but whether taking stock of commodity possession is the place to stop. Opulence in the form of commodity possession is undoubtedly important in enhancing the standard of living, but is the standard of living best seen as *opulence* itself?' (Sen, 1987a, p. 15).

The overview of Sen's critiques given above does not, of course, present Sen's case fully. The full arguments can be found by referring to Sen (1985, 1987a). Essentially, Sen seeks to make sense of the following types of paradoxes, many of which are pertinent to the paradoxes that arise when mulling over the living standard of people who suffer with mental illnesses:

> You could be *well off*, without being *well*. You could be *well*, without being able to lead the life you *wanted*. You could have got the life you *wanted*, without being *happy*. You could be *happy*, without having much *freedom*. You could have a good deal of *freedom*, without *achieving* much. We can go on (Sen, 1987a, p. 1).

Attention now turns to Sen's approach which, he argues, is not just another competing definition of the standard of living but another conceptual approach.

Sen's approach (1985, 1987b) is about the role of human functionings and capabilities in the concept of the living standard. He argues that an important distinction ought to be made between the various living conditions which a person can or cannot achieve (his or her 'functionings') and the ability to achieve these living conditions (the person's 'capabilities'). A 'functioning' is an achievement, whereas a 'capability' is the ability to achieve. In other words, Sen's conception of the standard of living is more a matter of the relationships between functionings and capabilities than just about competing claims concerning whether opulence, commodities, utility or something else is the correct emphasis.

Sen's 'capability approach' can be summarised in another way, using a depiction by Muellbauer (1987, p.40). It is given below in Figure 1.2. Muellbauer's depiction shows the factors other than goods, as emphasised by Sen, that affect the generation of utility. The right-hand side of Figure 1.2 shows the 'environment' as well as market 'goods' determining how many 'material characteristics' can be achieved by a person's consumption.[8] The environment involves not only physical features but also public goods, such as

---

[8] Sen's use here of the term, characteristics, is in the stream of economic literature called characteristics theory (Lancaster, 1966(a)) which, most simply, describes the household as producing, out of market goods, more fundamental commodities or 'characteristics', e.g. from purchases of food, households produce nutrition. This conception is applied in some detail in Chapters 5 and 6 to analyse specific issues associated with mental illness.

clean air, the absence of crime, and individual liberty. Next are the individual's 'personal characteristics' ('Capability of a person to function' in Figure 1.2) like his or her metabolism which, together with 'Material characteristics', such as nutrition, determine in varying dimensions a person's capabilities to function. Finally, a person's 'psychic state', and his or her capacities to function (Functionings), together determine the levels of achievement within the various types of functionings. While 'functionings' are mostly related closely with actual living, Sen suggests many examples where capabilities have a greater bearing on a person's standard of living. Sen also points out that the relations between functionings and capabilities are much more complex than they might at first appear.

Figure 1.2 Utility, functionings, capabilities and their sources

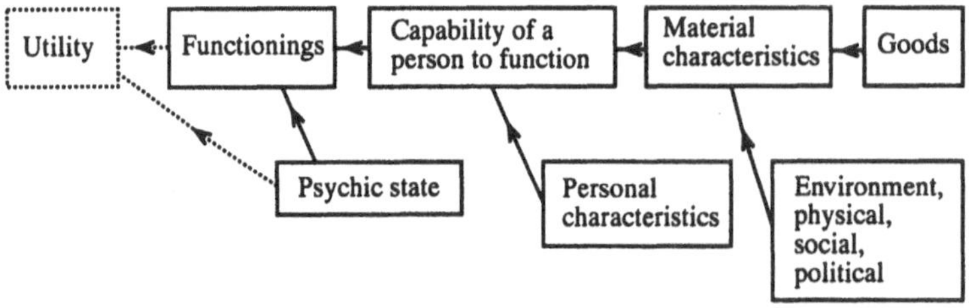

Source: Muellbauer (1987, p. 40).

In Sen's approach, the set of available capabilities of a person to function is multi-dimensional; also the **extent** of a person's opportunity set of basic capabilities largely determines the individual's standard of living. This set represents the person's real opportunities available for the life he or she may lead. As explained in the previous paragraph, the set of capabilities available to a person is determined by environmental factors and personal characteristics, not just by goods and services.

Sen argues that the freedom to choose is an important ingredient in the standard of living. 'Freedom to choose' is, according to Sen, the extent of the opportunity set. Put otherwise, the **extent** of the opportunity set is important to a person's living standard, **not just a point** in the opportunity set that happens to be chosen. Any chosen point merely indicates a bundle of goods and services chosen. For a person with a mental illness, an alternative bundle of goods and services that serves his or her preference set better would be chosen, if it were available, and if the individual's environment and personal characteristics enabled him or her to consume it.

From Figure 1.2, it is clear that the Sen conception incorporates two pathways in which a person's 'psychic state' (or mental illness) may affect utility. An indirect effect occurs when a person's psychic state affects his or her 'functionings'. For example, studies by Clark and Oswald (1994) and by Flatau *et al.* (1998) find that unemployment, rather than loss of income, has a statistically significant adverse effect on mental well-being. The implication is that people with mental illness who are unable to find, or sustain, a job are likely to find that unemployment itself then triggers further mental ill-health, due to this indirect 'unemployment effect' upon well-being. A second direct effect occurs via the 'psychic state' to 'utility' pathway in so far as mental illness directly affects a person's ability to enjoy life.

In essence Figure 1.2 shows clearly Sen's intent: he prefers to focus attention upon capabilities and functionings, two of the intermediate stages between goods and utility, and the dotted line leading to utility in Figure 1.2 indicates the weakness of the final link in the chain to utility. A final point about the approach to standard of living suggested here is contained in the following comment by Geoffrey Hawthorn in regard to Sen's approach:

> 'The value of the living standard', as he [Sen] puts it, 'lies in the living'. And if that means, against some prevailing academic fashions, that we have to reject being precisely wrong in favour of being vaguely right, so be it. But this is not to say that one can be cheerily – or in the popular conception of economists and what they do, even gloomily – loose. Much of what falls within 'the standard of living', like much of living itself, may not admit much empirical precision. And even if it did, such precision would usually have little point for those in government, who act with instruments that are blunt in conditions which they only fitfully control. Conceptual precision, however, is quite a different matter and is in this issue as important for citizens as it is for social scientists. It is Sen's first concern (Hawthorn, 1987, p. *viii*).

Economics and Mental Health Care

The previous Section introduced conceptual matters that are likely to arise in considering the living standards of people with mental illnesses. Such conceptually precise approaches are ultimately very important in evaluating the standard of living of this sub-set of the population. Abundant anecdotal and other evidence is available in health care journals about the lives of people with mental illnesses and disorders, evidence that generally provides support for the approach advocated by Sen, although those accounts have been written in ignorance of Sen's conceptual framework. This evidence suggests that the living standards of people with mental illnesses and disorders are very low in most instances. In the present era, the collection of empirically precise data that illustrate the notions of the previous Section unfortunately is not possible.

The work of this study is not to conduct exercises evaluating living standards. This study focuses on a narrower issue, on just one aspect of the factors associated with the living standard, on mental health care itself. More precisely, in later chapters an economic study is presented of the economic dimensions of mental health care outputs. The outputs are a phenomenon about which little is known. The present Section seeks to present some introductory principles of economics relating to mental health care, in order to prepare for the study of the conceptual nature of the outputs of mental health care in later chapters.

An understanding of the economic nature of mental health care outputs is useful, among other reasons, for evaluating mental health care. The economic evaluation of mental health outputs is not simply an accounting balance of the arguments for and against pursuing an action. Rather, an outcome, in its economic sense, is more like a coin having two sides: an outcome embraces value (that is, the valuation of individual and social preferences over an outcome) and costs (in terms of resources foregone in achieving that outcome). For some goods and services, both the value gained and the cost borne (in terms in resources foregone) can be quite difficult to determine, and yet, when the nature of mental health care outputs is not understood, the supply of economic meaning arising from evaluation studies is next-to-nothing.

A basic economic principle is that the provision of goods and services (or the lack of their provision, as in many instances in regard to mental health care) is borne at an economic cost. 'Economic' is an adjective. Economics, the discipline, studies phenomena that are economic. The conventional explanation in modern economics texts of the adjective, economic, is as follows: Any good or service that is scarce, in other words not free, is classified as an economic good. Also, the adjective, economic, can be usefully employed to qualify 'welfare' because it addresses that aspect of life where something has to be given up in order for welfare to be attained. (Both the welfare of the individual and the welfare of groupings of individuals can be analysed economically.)

Now economists are meticulous over the meaning of the word 'free'. Neither goods that have a zero charge, such as those provided by governments or benefactors, nor goods which have the appearance or even a sensation of being free, such as property owned and enjoyed in common, like a park or a clean environment or happy family relations, are 'free' in an economic sense. Only a good or service which, in becoming available for consumption, does not cause fewer resources to be available for other goods and services, is classified as being 'free', economically speaking. (In that sense, 'nothingness' may be the one phenomenon that is free, economically speaking.)

The nature of all economic goods is that their provision comes at an economic, or opportunity, cost. Resources are foregone in order for an economic good to be provided. If someone quips that there is little in life that is free, the implication is not that an imperative exists to be stingy or selfish. Even freeness is scarce. The word, economic, is meant as a descriptive term of the phenomenon of scarcity that is a narrow, but very influential, aspect of human existence.

The catalysts are diverse that move human endeavour to live life given the set of constraints uniquely faced by each individual. The diversity encompasses selfishness and selflessness, ardour and obsession, jealousy and anxiety, vulnerability and whimsy, to name just a few. In economic studies, motivations and catalysts in the human psyche are normally not examined, but rather taken as given. This is an acceptable working rule but is, of course, tenable only to the extent that the revealed preferences of the individual reflect adequately the person's wishes.

By convention, the economic side of human nature is delimited by the following statement: Individuals exhibit optimising behaviours when pursuing their living standard. In order to depict the individual's economising behaviours, economics sometimes employs a simple 'construct' of the mind (Pearce, 1986) called *Homo Economicus*. This construct, *Homo Economicus,* serves to delimit cognitively the economising side of human nature, in an elementary way at least. It represents that side of the human personality which chooses how to employ one's endowments, technologies and information in order to be as well-off as possible.

When the best possible action from the point of view of the chooser is undertaken then, in economics, choice is said to be rational. Hence, economic rationality is defined as being present when *Homo Economicus* pursues an economic objective, say, maximum utility in the face of the constraints. Put otherwise, if the optimising behaviour of *Homo Economicus* is observed, the only observable phenomenon when an individual is maximising his or her utility in the face of constraints is the outcome of the process. While income is a very familiar constraint, it is just one aspect by which the endowment set of an individual is constrained. For example, the absence of full information is a persistent impediment in virtually all optimising activity.

In Chapter 2, attention is directed to the implications of the following question, 'What if *Homo Economicus* has a serious mental illness?'. To address this matter is an important step in the process of depicting the nature of the outputs of mental health care. The presence of mental illness poses a fundamental problem for economic methodology, specifically, for the assumption about the economising behaviour (i.e. rational optimisation) present across the human race.

In the next Section, some matters concerning the scope and purpose of the study are presented.

Scope and Purpose

For readers with a background in economics, it may seem at first glance to some as if there is little that economic theory can contribute to the issues associated with mental health care. Mental disorders frequently are understood in terms of a loss of individual preferences which arises from the nature of the illness itself or else, in serious cases, because society has deemed it preferable to take away some individuals' rights to liberty and decision-making.

To desire to know where theory can be applied, and where it cannot, to the issue of economic behaviour arising from mental disorder is a task that could appear deceptively simple. Unless thought is given to these matters, though, it is impossible to inquire into inefficiencies in present ways, albeit scantily funded in the public sector, of matching services to individual wants.

This work is the product of thinking about the demand for services by, and for, people suffering mental disorders, and the supply of services to these people. Such thinking arises because of the consequences of the ways individuals, and societies, make choices (or choices made by not consciously choosing). The choices which are of interest here are those over the allocation of resources, the scarcity of which is relative only to unlimited ends.

One criterion used to assess the efficacy of resource allocation is to ask whether it is efficient. The popular meaning frequently given to the word, 'efficiency', noticeably in the psychiatry and mental health care literatures, refers to what economists may call cost-effectiveness. Cost-effectiveness usually means that a given activity is being performed at a given rate *at least cost.* This may be what Eisen and Wolfenden (1988) had in mind in the consultancy in Australia on mental health services, in their reference to utilisation efficiency (p. 52).

The economic concept of efficiency, or allocative efficiency, is both broader and more precise than this. One aspect of allocative efficiency is exchange efficiency. Exchange efficiency exists only when the marginal valuations by each individual over his or her own shares in the allocation of goods and services, i.e. each person's budget, are equal. Only then is there no further scope for mutually beneficial reallocation of each person's budget – one person may gain but only at the expense of another. Each consumer has the best possible allocation of his or her budget.

Another aspect of allocative efficiency is productive efficiency or technological efficiency. This exists when the costs of producing a given output are as low as possible. Economic efficiency occurs when no resources are wasted either in a productive sense or in respect of consumer budget allocation.

To imbue services for mental illness (a condition which, at its worst, is tragic enough in its impact) with desires for allocative efficiency (a concept which is not always recognised beyond the economics profession for its precise definition) is not hearkening to the more ruthless aspects of efficiency. Nor is it a personal indictment of highly dedicated people who work in various services, or who give care in their home, and who face critical, 'coal-face' decisions affecting disadvantaged and vulnerable individuals. Neither is it to discount other economic or societal goals, such as economic justice, as causes that were overlooked in the authors' personal trade-off over goals that ought to be pursued in a study such as this.[9] Trade-offs between allocative efficiency

---

9 An account of the trade-off between efficiency and equity can be found in Okun (1975).

and economic justice do occur frequently in some aspects of economic policy, but if approaches taken in this study were to be considered seriously at the level of policy, significant Pareto improvements would result in the level of welfare and these would occur well before the need for trade-offs arises (Culyer, 1980, p. 22*ff*). Blinder (1987) takes a similar approach with respect to some other social problems. A similar argument is presented by Olson (1996) in the context of the development of low-income countries. See also Olson and Kähkönen (2000).

Appendix 1.1

Accounts of Five Persons with Very Disabling, Chronic Mental Disorders[10]

The following accounts are presented to describe the course of illness of five individuals. As explained previously in Chapter One, some are about fictitious persons. Whether a story is entirely factual or whether it is based on facts with some details hidden to disguise identity, the important similarities and differences between the stories provide useful data about people with mental illnesses, and about the outcomes of the treatment system which they experience.

The authorship of each account differs, with contrasts in authorship representing differing perspectives. The accounts also contrast in the descriptions of the responses of family, friends, government and professionals. The first account is of a person in a family context. It is a true account. The second account is one written by an individual who has a mental illness, in this instance, bipolar disorder. The third account, written from a family member's perspective, is a story about a person living mostly apart from the system of treatment, including psychiatry and medication. The fourth account, created by a psychiatrist, is fictionalised, but written with a view to reflecting 'typical' encounters with the treatment system from the psychiatrist's perspective. The fifth account, by a journalist, is about a person who has been, but is no longer, institutionalised. It is not fictitious. (Note that none of the stories has been created by the authors of this study; nor is any story about a friend or a relative of the authors.)

As has been said previously in Chapter One, our preference is not, in selecting the accounts, to include stories of people whose illnesses are cured. Nor have accounts been included where the outcome is suicide. While both those outcomes are pertinent to this study, perhaps the stories of people who live a long-term struggle to survive with a mental illness have special significance in this study.

The accounts in this Appendix broadly indicate some of the economic issues of chronic psychiatric illness.

10 It is irregular to give detailed individual case studies in economics. Indeed, an economist has to be careful, for methodological reasons, in doing so. Economics, being a social science, is concerned ultimately with populations. A reader who is not well-versed in how economists think about the individual case could usefully read Chapter 5 of Little (1957), particularly pages 71-75, in conjunction with these accounts.

Account One: This account is written by a person whose husband was diagnosed with bipolar disorder. The account tells of the sorts of experiences that occur and of encounters, and of encounters lacking, with mental health, and other, services.

Connie's story

My husband is a fifty-seven year old Anglo-Saxon. We have three sons and three daughters. He lives at home with me and one daughter. He has been retired for the past twelve years because of his illness. When he became ill, he held a senior administrative position with the public service. He now receives a Disability Support Pension.

He was diagnosed as having Manic Depression over eighteen years ago. He does not agree that he has been manic but he admits that he suffers from severe depression. However, there have been times when both medical staff and I have witnessed episodes of mania. He has displayed grandiose ideas, overspending, reckless elation and supreme confidence. But, on the whole, it would be accurate to say that he is severely depressed much more often which is demonstrated by periods of morbid despair, loss of interest, guilt and a slowing down of mental and physical functioning.

By the mid seventies he consulted his General Practitioner (GP) about problems he was experiencing, e.g. insomnia, memory loss, lack of energy and interest in everyday activities. He had a complete neurological examination for his symptoms. Basically, he was told to slow down. (At the time he had a full-time job and two part-time jobs.) His depression was overlooked. This outcome leads me still to question: was overlooking his illness due to the way he presented, i.e. a highly functioning person, or was it that at times major psychiatric disorders are poorly recognised and, consequently, inadequately treated in adults?

By 1980 he was having even greater difficulty coping with everyday functions, both at home and at work. Again, he sought medical advice and this time his GP referred him to a psychiatrist who hospitalised him for two weeks. The diagnosis was pre-senile dementia. The whole family was devastated. The psychiatrist suggested to me that it would be best (for both my young family and for me) if I were to divorce my husband. With the long-term prognosis of this incorrect diagnosis in the back of my mind, when my husband became aggressive and physically violent towards the family, I took out a restraining order and had him put out of our home by the police. However, he consulted another psychiatrist who diagnosed him as having manic depression.

Although he still lives in the family home with one of my daughters and me, he isolates himself from the family. He eats his meals in his bedroom and not with us. He tries to avoid attending and participating in family functions and activities. In addition, he has severed contact with his friends, and he is reluctant to participate in social activities because maintaining conversation is difficult, even with people he knows well. Because of the anxiety created by these situations, he does not like to leave his own home where he can retreat to his bedroom. He does not like to discuss the home situation with his psychiatrist and over the years I have become somewhat excluded from the consultations. I consider this to be a detrimental aspect of the treatment, as it is recognised that the family's attitude can be crucial in meeting the needs of people with mental illness.

My husband, on the other hand, feels he has been treated fairly well by the health system, but he has said, 'Possibly, if I couldn't explain myself verbally and in a far more coherent manner than many sufferers of mental illness, my treatment could have been different.' He also added that 'from my observation they appear to treat those with lower intelligence less decisively and with less professionalism.' Nonetheless, he has become a passive recipient of treatment, not wanting any information and/or education about his illness in case such knowledge 'clouds or influences how I explain myself and to prevent my explanations being tainted by commonalities.' He also accepts that there will be no reduction in the amount of medication he takes. It is as if he has lost any hope in recovery or improvement in lifestyle.

When asked about how the illness affected his ability to function physically, he answered, 'I lack the capacity to function. At the end of last year I accepted I had to live with it. I can work everything out but can't carry it through. You get an elevated feeling of frustration when you can't accomplish what you like to do. I express myself verbally with confidence but can't apply myself to follow through.' When asked about the adjustment mechanisms he has used, he replied, 'I put my mind in neutral and do simple chores like mowing the lawn. I keep jobs isolated. I can't do things to a plan. I'm doing them by instinct. Finding motivation is a problem so, when I can't do something I would like to do, I find some simple thing I can do and I do that.'

Furthermore, he can be described as a passive recipient because he happily changes his medication when requested without question. These changes have been occurring over the years as he is prescribed every new anti-depressant as it comes onto the market. I often wonder if this is a trial-and-error exercise with him being used as a guinea pig rather than justifiable health care.

What is it like for the family? Mental illness is responsible for taking away the man whom I married and the father our six children knew in their earlier years.

This loss has had far-reaching consequences and has affected me in many ways. It has not been just an isolated crisis. We all encounter that in life. This is a prolonged crisis. The chronicity of my husband's illness has left me living with uncertainty for the past twenty years. It is something one needs to get used to, but the demands of coping and adapting can, at times, be extremely arduous. I have never been able to dispel the uncertainty entirely.

When my husband was diagnosed as mentally ill, I baulked at the diagnosis and clung to other explanations. The reason for this may have been the severity of the mental illness, the stigma and ignorance attached to it in our society, and the anxiety caused by the genetic basis of such a disease. A period of denial followed. However, denial did not last forever. I realised that it is our brain that makes us distinctly human and that when someone's brain malfunctions, as opposed to other illnesses, it is difficult to recognise the human being within. When I worked this out, the realisation that my husband had a serious mental illness registered with me. This was an extremely painful and difficult experience, and it was only the beginning of a long, lonely and sad journey. The pain and isolation I felt may well have equalled that felt by my husband. Thus, although it would become vital for me to begin the process of retreating from my husband before my own emotional pain became so intense that it made living problematic for my young family and me, I was not able to retreat initially. Consequently, I was pulled down to the depth of depression myself.

I remember a few days after my husband had been removed from our home and how I was completely shocked and amazed by the deterioration in his general appearance, emotional state and self esteem. It made me realise that I could not turn my back on this man. It was a combination of loving him and feeling bound to take care of him. I was not sure he could survive on his own. I convinced myself that there had to be an alternative for coping with this situation and we, as a family, had to adapt to the changed living circumstances.

Life has not been easy, though. My husband had stopped working. In addition to being a mother to my children, I soon found that caring for my husband took up a lot of time and energy. Initially, I became his twenty-four hours on-call nurse, with him spending most of his time in bed. The only breaks were when he needed hospitalisation. Although my husband is more active now, there are still many ways in which he needs assistance.

I have developed and grown as a person and have gained a university education. I am extremely proud of my children and what they have achieved. When I look back, though, the thing that stands out most for me is that although I went to every psychiatrist's consultation with my husband during the early years of his illness, I never received any guidance about my mentally ill soul-mate. I feel every family needs counselling and support from the day mental illness is diagnosed. Families need to understand and deal with the effects of the illness, and they have to deal with their own fluctuating emotions.

Account Two: This account is written by Melanie. Melanie was diagnosed with bi-polar disorder at 21 years of age. It tells of her encounters with mental health services and of her effort to live life in spite of a serious mental illness.

Melanie's story

In my youth I thought I was incredibly broad-minded. I always had friends who were a bit left of centre and, much to my father's dismay, was constantly bringing home people who definitely did not fit into the status quo. My focus in high school centred on the arts, and I was always testing boundaries of what was considered acceptable and normal. I was fascinated with people, music, film and theatre that challenged society's 'normal' boundaries. I believed in the unconditional acceptance of people and believed I held no prejudices.

Yet, when I had my first psychotic episode, my initial judgements and prejudices about myself were incredible. I had always been a logical thinker and people used to comment that I 'had my head screwed on right'. The worst thing that mental illness affected were my thoughts, the essential 'me'. That is what I had lost control of. The internal confusion, guilt and shame were huge. The things I had said and done while ill were not 'me'. Yet they were. It was this **self**-stigma that I had to overcome, not only to accept, and to deal positively with, my illness but also to be able to accept and feel comfortable again with myself.

It was this loss of me, the grief, internal confusion, guilt and shame that the system didn't, wouldn't, couldn't acknowledge because at that point, I had instead become a diagnosis. I was given some information about my disorder but, in terms of treatment, I became the illness. All that was really acknowledged, worked with, spoken to, was this new illness. While the wider issues of external stigma are often cited, it was never conceded that this self-stigma even existed. Who I was, everything I was, became relative to my illness. All my emotions became symptomatic of my condition.

There is much literature around at the moment about the lowered life expectations that so often accompany a diagnosis of mental illness. We are encouraged to be more modest in our aspirations. The world that was our oyster becomes our shell. In my case, after my second serious psychotic episode, the consultant psychiatrist and the registrar sat down with my parents and me, and calmly told them my future did not look good. They wanted to put me on a Disability Support Pension and, sensing the concealed outrage in the room, suggested that maybe I could, perhaps maybe, aspire to work part-time, one day, when my condition was under control.

I was totally devastated, disbelieving. I was still intensely shell-shocked and vulnerable, and I still had all the self-stigma to work through too.

I am intensely fortunate, however, that I had a mother who wasn't so vulnerable and accepting. She knew me, the 'me' that I had lost touch with, the 'me' that had been kidnapped and replaced with this awful illness. Early on in the piece, she had a clear distinction between Melanie, and 'Melanie-when-she-is-sick'. My mother would constantly reinforce this distinction. She had a firm belief that I would get better and that I could still achieve something with my life.

As I recovered from that second severe episode, I learnt all I could about my illness, about theories and about the treatments. I was overawed with how 'hit and miss' it all was. And yet it was these experts who had enormous power to determine my future.

Instead of a Disability Support Pension, I ventured back into the workforce and, shortly thereafter, started my business. I ran my business quite successfully until recently when I commenced working, firstly, being offered a position convening an international mental health conference and, next, working with other people in hope and recovery.

I get goose bumps sometimes when I think where I could have so easily ended up. I am intensely scared by how much power the system has in determining outcomes for the lives of people. And how completely it does. These feelings are partly due to the sorts of stories like the one I will now tell. When I was in hospital, there was a girl there who was in Year 10 at school and, admittedly, quite ill at the time. She desperately wanted to study while in hospital, and be able to sit the end-of-year exams with the rest of her class. Yet it was determined that she had to have low stimulus and her mother was asked not to bring in her books. The distress and mental stress this caused her was enormous, yet it was deemed that her health was the most important thing. What health? And by whose definition? But her mother complied, as she believed she was doing the best thing for her daughter under the direction of the mental health staff. Eighteen months later when I was back in hospital again, this same girl was there. She had never gone back to school, and had been distanced from her friends. Her hopes for the future were non-existent. She had embarked on the roller-coaster ride of the system.

I have come across a view of treatment that is, in my opinion, a commonsense approach when looking for good outcomes and quality of life. Professor Charles Rapp's 'Strengths Model of Case Management' focuses on the strengths of people.[11] It looks at the key elements to success in living, rather than in existing. Existing is what so many people are encouraged to believe is all they are capable of under the traditional system of treatment.

According to Rapp, people who are successful in living have goals and dreams. The diagnosis and the prognosis of mental illness can blow your goals and dreams out of the water. How often are you encouraged to dive back in and find them again? When I was told by two psychiatrists that I would not be able to have a career, a part of me died inside. My mother held on to my goals and dreams for me, and used them to revive me.

People who are successful in living use their strengths to attain their aspirations. People with mental illness often lose touch with their strengths. Their strengths become secondary. They pale in comparison to where the spotlight is on, on the disorder. It was determined in my diagnosis that stress was a factor in the illness. It was deduced by those treating the illness that I must avoid stress but the career I wanted involved stress. My strengths were never figured into the equation.

People who are successful in living have the confidence to take the next step towards their goal. With the diagnosis of mental illness, when adding up

---

11 A possible reference here is C.A. Rapp (1998), *The Strengths Model: Case Management with People Suffering from Severe and Persistent Mental Illness*, Oxford University Press, New York.

the weight of self-stigma, generalised lowered expectations, and the old cliche that 'If you tell someone something long enough, they'll believe it', where does confidence come into it? In my personal experience, and from so many stories I've heard and seen, the mental health system inadvertently works to undermine self-confidence rather than encourage it.

People who are successful in living have a meaningful relationship with at least one other person. This should never mean a case-manager or a mental health worker. How often does a mental health service become a central point in a person's life. How real a situation is that, but how often does it occur? Even outside of family and friends, the mental health system often unquestionably becomes central to a person's entire being.

People who are successful in living have access to opportunities relevant to their goals. With mental illness, it may be harder and may take longer, and involve risks. But no-one should be discouraged from fulfilling their ambitions. I knew I was taking a risk when I started. (Anyone starting a business does!) But life does not come with guarantees for anyone. Starting a business may have had a possible detrimental effect on my mental health. But living the life that had been prescribed to me was not, in my eyes, a life. I still get upset about the young girl in the next bed to me in hospital whose studies were not seen as important.

The quality of niches that people inhabit determines their achievement, quality of life and success in living. When the niche you fall in is completely submerged in illness, it is not good.

I hate to consider where I would be if my illness had manifested itself a few years earlier. Would I have had enough strength and confidence then to challenge my prognosis? Would I have had a strong enough perception of the real 'me' to differentiate it from the ill 'me'? How different would my outcome have been? Mental health professionals have to acknowledge the influence they have over people's lives, and on the outcomes.

Account Three: Here is another story from the perspective of a family member. It is an attempt to depict the life of someone diagnosed with a psychiatric disorder. Again, the focus is upon the sorts of experiences that occur and of encounters, or the lack thereof, with mental health, and other, services.

Annette's story

Annette, my sister, is 40 years of age. She lives alone in a small city flat in Sydney. At the age of 19, she was diagnosed with schizophrenia.

As a child, Annette had few friends. She was strongly introverted, and often seemed to me, to our parents and to classmates to be in a world of her own. Throughout school she was at the top of her class, and passed University entrance exams with the highest possible score. The future lay at her feet.

Mum and Dad were delighted with these results but were increasingly concerned that she had little social life. However, most of Mum and Dad's attempts to change this ended up in big fights, and home life was often tense. Annette was well aware of her brilliance and could argue her case powerfully if she had to.

At University, Annette enrolled in medicine. However, she never seemed to settle into life there. She couldn't get assignments in, often because she put excessive time into refining one small part. This also happened in exams so that she barely passed. She was involved in student life only peripherally.

By the end of her second year, the difficulties with study were escalating. She started paying noticeably less attention to dress and personal hygiene. She was becoming increasingly withdrawn and suspicious. She was taking no part now in student life, and she kept to herself.

Mum and Dad were so worried. They finally managed to get her to see a doctor who referred Annette to a psychiatrist. It turned out that Annette had been hearing voices warning her about her classmates, her lecturers, Mum and Dad, and even me, even though we got on quite well, or as closely as anyone could. After a period of time, a diagnosis of schizophrenia was made.

Annette was then hospitalised for six weeks, on medication. The voices disappeared over time, and the suspicions eased but the side-effects from the medication were very annoying for Annette. With few friends, Annette felt very much alone, especially when she came home.

I remember how excluded Mum and Dad and I felt from the treatment. We found it hard to get information about what was happening and how to help. This made Mum and Dad feel they were being blamed for Annette's sickness.

After a year Annette was able to return to University part-time, and complete a Science degree, majoring in Biology. Most of her peers and lecturers had little idea about mental illness. However, upon graduating one sympathetic lecturer found her a part-time position as a research assistant. She was able to contribute some episodes of brilliant work but all in all she found working too stressful. Although her contributions were brilliant, the little she did made it difficult for her boss because she would have trouble completing enough to get the project done. Her position was not renewed when the research grant finished.

Some months later, Mum and Dad found some part-time work for Annette, through our neighbour. It involved shipping parcels in a warehouse. She loathed the warehouse as a workplace. Things remained tense with Mum and Dad and she finally moved out of home. After a while, Annette stopped taking her medication. This was partly because of the side effects of the medication and partly in response to increasing interest in alternative medicine.

She eventually disconnected from psychiatrists and the formal treatment system entirely.

The severe symptoms have never returned but, in many ways, my sister is quite disabled. She had to stop working because she was increasingly irregular in attendance and her performance at work was poor. These days she lives on social security.

Annette manages to keep her flat in an acceptable state but it takes her a tremendous effort to do so. No-one who has had little contact with someone like Annette is likely to believe how hard it is for her because if I say anything, most people just think that they find it an effort to keep their own place clean and tidy too. But with Annette, by 'tremendous effort', I mean tremendous. Like, even the most basic task can take her all day. Bills frequently remain unpaid. She needs to rest a lot.

It's hard to describe Annette. She's my sister and I love her. Mostly, I like her and she's quite likeable really, although I find her quite frustrating too, in extreme ways. She is exceptionally oblivious to anyone else's needs and I know this is the illness but I do have needs too, you know, although I try awfully hard to help Annette.

Annette finds it extraordinarily hard to keep commitments, like appointments because she says how she feels and what she feels she can cope with is so unpredictable. At times, she has periods of depression when doing anything seems impossible and hopeless.

A few friends have tried to help, but often nothing gets done because negotiation is so difficult. People are attracted by the strength of her intellect, but friends tend to come and go because they find her difficult to relate to.

Mum and Dad continue to try to help of course, but they find Annette's blame towards them difficult, and there have been some blazing rows. In frustration, Mum and Dad try to push things along faster than she wants, well we all do because what else can you do?

In my opinion my sister is heavily disabled but Mum and Dad and I all have great trouble getting government help for her. This is partly because services are so stretched that there is only enough for crises. There seems never enough for chronic, lower intensity illnesses. There are just not enough services for people like Annette. Annette seems to frustrate initiatives one way or another, needing to have things done her way or not at all. The system seems to focus on the medical side too much, rather than finding ways to help Annette with her daily living.

My sister lives in a bind. She is disempowered by her illness and isolated in the community; my family does not have the skills needed to help; and society is unwilling or unable to find the necessary resources to help.

Account Four: This account is written by a medical practitioner. Though fictitious, it tells of the experiences that regularly occur and of various encounters with mental health, and other, services.

Paul's story

Paul is a thirty-three year old single man, currently an inpatient of a large, metropolitan chronic psychiatric hospital. This account will describe, in brief, the course of his illness and the consequences to Paul and to his family. The case is fictitious but broadly representative of people with chronic psychiatric conditions.

Paul was born in Brisbane, the second of three siblings. His father is an accountant and his mother, a trained nurse, has not worked since starting their family. Paul was an alert, bright child who performed in the top ten per cent of his class at school. In Grade 12 his results were sufficient for him to enter teachers training college. At college, he initially enjoyed his study and had a wide network of friends, including a steady girlfriend.

In his second year Paul's college results declined and he found it increasingly difficult to organise his time and concentrate on his study. At this time his girlfriend left him because she could not agree with his increasingly fanatical beliefs about vegetarianism. At home his parents tolerated his diet as best they could. At one stage Paul emptied his parents' refrigerator and forbade them ever to bring meat into the house again.

Paul's parents spoke to their local GP but Paul refused to attend the surgery. Later that year Paul withdrew from college because he wanted to spend more time reading the Bible. His behaviour at home became increasingly bizarre. On one occasion he covered up every mirror in the house to avoid seeing his own reflection. He began to neglect his personal hygiene, often failing to wash for days at a time. He lost weight because of his increasingly restrictive diet. His friends no longer visited, and Paul made no efforts to meet people or to maintain his social contacts.

Despite his parents' begging, he refused to see his local GP. He did however agree to talk to his local priest. He told the priest and his parents that he was hearing voices from the devil giving him commands. He also believed that all the mirrors had been replaced by two-way mirrors for some of his college-mates to spy on him.

The priest advised the parents to contact a self-help group comprising friends and relatives of the mentally ill. Eventually, after much anguish, Paul's parents called to the house the local community psychiatry team, which diagnosed Paul as having schizophrenia. He was admitted as an involuntary patient to a psychiatric unit of a general hospital.

His first admission lasted three months. During this time Paul was prescribed anti-psychotic medication. This suppressed the auditory hallucinations, and his diet and personal hygiene improved considerably. His family visited the unit almost daily, however none of his ex-college friends bothered to visit. After discharge, Paul was placed on Sickness Benefit and returned home with weekly visits to a day-hospital for rehabilitation.

Six months later, Paul's mental state deteriorated: his medication was causing him troublesome side-effects and he ceased the medication. Despite ceasing the medication, Paul spent most of the day in bed. He rarely initiated conversation with his family, and showed little enjoyment for living.

After a psychotic episode, Paul attempted to commit suicide by slashing his wrists. He was readmitted to a psychiatric unit where he stayed for five months. During this time his father had been dismissed from work because of his repeated absences to visit his son. Paul's fifteen-year old sister became increasingly argumentative at home. She demanded to move out into a flat because she felt her parents did not care about her, and she felt her family life had been wrecked by her brother's psychiatric illness.

Over the next seven years Paul spent almost half the time in psychiatric hospitals around Australia. He had taken to travelling without any warning. Often for the parents, first news of their son's whereabouts was from staff at a southern psychiatric hospital where Paul had been admitted, or from police who had picked Paul up for vagrancy. The family always flew down to collect Paul and escort him back to their home.

At age 27 Paul was escorted from a short-stay unit to a long-stay psychiatric hospital. He was now chronically psychotic. Medication was having no positive effect on his health status. He made several more suicide attempts. At the hospital he managed a regular routine and some low level occupational therapy.

Paul receives the Disability Support Pension, most of which pays for his board in hospital, his cigarettes and occasional outings. His family has him home for regular weekends, on leave, but he has developed delusions that his father had harmed him as a child and, as a consequence, he is hostile and suspicious around his father.

Paul has been a patient at the long-stay psychiatric hospital for five years. It is expected that he may settle down slowly in the years to come. He may be able to return to life in the community in one of the privately run supervised hostels in Brisbane. A community psychiatry team will be able to monitor his mental state and help protect his interests in the community, and ensure prompt hospitalisation if his mental state worsens.

Paul falls into the one-third of patients with schizophrenia who have an unremitting, chronic pattern of illness. He will never be able to join the work force, and is expected to require regular re-admissions and constant support in the community.

Account Five: This account by the journalist, Peter Ascot, is a true story of John W. who was institutionalised for over 30 years and is now living in the community. The story appeared in The Big Issue *which is a magazine sold on the street by unemployed people. The vendor is paid a portion of the selling price per sale. This story, called a 'Vendor Portrait' by the magazine, is used here with permission.*

John's story

Thirty-two years can be a long, frustrating time. Just ask any long-in-the-tooth Collingwood fan who lived through the torture of the Magpies premiership drought between 1958 and 1990. But let's not talk of Collingwood. John is an

Essendon supporter, and has been ever since he grew up just a few blocks away from Windy Hill in Melbourne's North.

He's now a member, and sees all the Bombers' home games. High on his list of ambitions is to save enough for a holiday to Perth – to see Essendon play Freemantle, of course. But for 32 years, he couldn't even get to a home game.

'I was institutionalised when I was only 16,' he says without a trace of bitterness. 'Teenager problems – I was a bit rebellious. But people over-reacted. I still think to this day it was a drastic step to put me in Caloola, a psych place. Once in there, it was hard to get out. I was more a victim of the system and caught up.'

John was caught up from 1959 until 1991.

Caloola, outside Melbourne in Sunbury, is now part of a University.[12] But that's the closest John got to further education. The only course he ever went on was a course of sedatives. But it wasn't all bad. 'I've got a girlfriend I met there,' he says. 'They had dances and that; it was a solid community of its own. I've been out in the community for six years now, and I think I've done pretty well.'

Part of John's reintegration has been with *The Big Issue*. After seeing vendors around the city, John took the step himself in July last year. 'I was initially reluctant,' he recalls, 'because I wasn't sure about counting out the change, and meeting people was a bit intimidating at first. It's not a problem now.'

It seems there's a regular parade of high-profile politicians and sportspeople at John's regular pitch at Collins Place in Melbourne. 'I met Mrs Kirner this morning,' he reports, 'and Mr Kirner bought a magazine. And I spoke to Jeff Kennett yesterday morning. He was polite and said 'Good morning', but he didn't buy a magazine.'

Of course, it's the regular buyers who are making the real difference to vendors' lives, and John is grateful for their support: 'There's one lady buys it off me every time, she's so loyal,' he says. 'I believe that I am leading a better life than I was before. More active and involved, as well as more income. I feel I am doing something worthwhile and being a worthy part of the community.'

With 85 per cent of his income going toward his supported accommodation, John is glad of a bit of extra money. 'It helps me with things like buying clothes and going to pictures occasionally, things I couldn't otherwise do.'

'I've been saving a bit of money, but to be honest, some of it goes on smokes,' he adds a little guiltily. After all that's happened, I think we can overlook that, John.

12 It is now the Victoria University of Technology, Sunbury Campus (RFGW and DPD).

2 Some Methodological Issues

Introduction

Because this study is fundamentally concerned with economic welfare, a framework is needed for examining those mental health care problems that have an economic dimension. The appropriate framework is one that sheds light upon economic welfare and in the next Chapter, the conventional framework is considered (that of Welfare Economics).

Prior to that task, this Chapter examines various issues pertinent to economic method: the relevance of the rationality assumption of economic method for studies of mental health care; the importance of distinguishing positive from normative method in economics; the relevance of the individualistic framework of conventional economics; the economic meaning of so-called 'consumer ignorance' in mental health care; and, finally, the role of social investment appraisal. Attention then turns to a definitional Section on the economics of mental health care. The Chapter concludes with a Section dealing with the complicated nature of mental illness and its treatment.

With the Welfare Economics of mental health care considered in the next Chapter, Chapters 2 and 3 together lay further foundations for the material presented in later Chapters of this study.

Some Issues in Economic Method

Rationality

In what sense is it meaningful to employ the concept 'rationality' in a study that relates to individuals' irrational behaviour? Some clear distinctions of meaning will be made initially, in order to clarify the concepts relevant to the task.

Rationality has clinical and economic meanings, since a clinically irrational person can, conceivably, be economically rational. Rationality can be understood in clinical parlance to mean having full possession of one's reason, i.e. being sane. Clinically, the types of conditions affecting a person's rationality are exemplified in delusional thinking, in affective disorders like depression, or in subjective thought disorders, where thoughts are believed to be inserted into the mind by an external agency or one's own thoughts are believed to be directly accessible to others.

Rationality in economic theory (i.e. theory concerned with people's economic behaviour) is a term with specialised meanings. According to Sen (1987c), economists sometimes use the concept in a **prescriptive** sense, such as when it is useful to know how one should behave in a particular situation, ethical considerations assumed. A different application of the concept arises with **model-building,** where rational behaviour is assumed so that **actual** behaviour can be explained and predicted. The idea is that, although people's actual behaviour can range across a spectrum of possibilities, it is reasonable to assume that people's behaviour generally is of the kind that could be called 'rational'.

In both uses just mentioned, economists adhere in practice to a rather simplistic notion, indeed, an axiom, of rationality with respect to economic behaviour: due to rational choice, general well-being can be maximised because individuals maximise their objective functions, subject to constraints. It is axiomatic that people optimise. Technically, this implies that well-being is maximised for a consumer in so far as a basket of commodities is chosen in which the marginal utility of the last dollar spent on all commodities is equal.

Having recalled here these general notions of rationality, it is important to note that a spectrum of understanding exists across economics generally. The rationality hypothesis behaves rather like a wolf in sheep's clothing: the notion looks innocent enough but this is a somewhat dangerous understanding. Though economists generally would say that there is common understanding in the profession as to what 'rationality' means, this understanding is probably not as clear-cut as is thought. Economists are dealing with a multi-dimensional phenomenon, drawn to our attention by Arrow (1986) and by Sen (1987c).

A pithy sentence by Arrow which opens a paper entitled 'Economic Theory and the Hypothesis of Rationality' captures the issue:

> In this paper, I want to disentangle some of the senses in which the hypothesis of rationality is used in economic theory. In particular, I want to stress that rationality is not a property of the individual alone, although it is usually presented that way. Rather, it gathers not only its force but also its very meaning from the social context in which it is embedded. It is mostly plausible under very ideal conditions. When these conditions cease to hold, the rationality assumption becomes strained and possibly self-contradictory. They certainly imply an ability at information processing and calculation that is far beyond the feasible and that cannot well be justified as the result of learning and adaptation (Arrow, 1986).

Arrow's paper is an important elaboration of these issues.

Another approach to the multi-dimensionality of this issue is taken by Sen (1987c). He begins by emphasising that economists define rationality in two different, though inextricably bound, ways. One of these relates to the optimising behaviour of individuals. The other, a more modern view, considers rationality as choosing consistently. Sen also points out that maximising behaviour does not relate specifically to the maximisation of self-interest, as people 'may truly want to promote causes that are not identical to their own welfare' and that can be incorporated into an objective function (cited in Klamer, 1989, p. 142*ff.*).

Both Arrow and Sen re-address the arguments that show rationality to be an imperfect assumption. While it is not necessary to repeat the imperfections here, note that Sen concludes his seven-page entry about 'Rational Behaviour' in *The New Palgrave Dictionary of Economics* with the following:

> ... [T]he existing literature is indeed deeply incomplete in that real difficulties have been identified [with the rationality assumption] without providing an adequate structure for solutions. The need to go beyond the existing literature is apparent enough, but where to go to is less clear (Sen, 1987c, p. 74).

The point so far is this: rationality is a multi-dimensional phenomenon. This is not a trivial matter. It has been drawn to our attention by Arrow (1986) and also by Sen (1987c). The key point in both of these contrasting accounts of rationality is that the tendency exists in economics for the rationality assumption to be permitted **too much** unquestioning assent.

And yet, in applications of economics to mental health care, rationality has been dismissed, i.e. given **too little** assent. This is paradoxical. Indeed, to see that a paradox might exist is probably very helpful in understanding the economics of the mental health care industry. What is intended fully by the three preceding sentences cannot be explained in a few sentences; it is the work of much of this entire study. Attention turns now, however, to consider some dimensions of these matters just mentioned.

Important distinctions at the margin should be noted. For example, highly distressed individuals may volunteer to spend time, and even money, to be in a psychiatric unit or hospital. They judge that to be 'inside' at least makes them feel able to cope, to be safer, at ease, i.e. they prefer to be 'in' rather than 'out'. Such individuals gain utility from the consumption of inpatient services, and would normally consume such services at zero charge to themselves, if it is tax-financed, or with their bills paid by a private health fund. In this instance, such individuals are choosing consistently as well as maximising their objective function subject to constraints.

On the other hand, society may impose standards of behaviour on clinically irrational people. Such standards may well interfere with their economic rationality, e.g. a person with alcoholic psychosis may be committed involuntarily to a rehabilitation unit for treatment, during which time the purchase of alcohol is not possible. In this instance, the individual may continue to choose consistently by still wishing to consume alcohol, and may arrange to smuggle in alcohol, although the choice itself is personally destructive. As such, the individual's objective function is maximised in the presence of a constraint, the constraint being treatment that bans the person's means to personal well-being, indeed their own definition of well-being, in terms of excessive alcohol consumption. Additionally, treatment actually re-conditions desire itself, the desire for alcohol, that is.

Another distinction is pertinent to the rationality issue. In making another distinction, it is necessary first to consider, by way of contrast, some aspects of the economic issues of people with physical disabilities. Consider a physical disability that creates additional costs in daily living that people without that physical disability do not incur. People with profound hearing impairment, for example, need hearing aids, special telecommunications devices and interpreters; and they have to learn 'Sign Language', as well as overcome the obstacles of being proficient in English, requiring special forms of schooling. Another example is that people with severed spines need special (expensive) alterations to their homes and to their cars, and they cannot travel on most forms of public transport (thereby benefiting from those economies of scale). Now consider in contrast an everyday task like grocery shopping at a supermarket for some people with chronic mental illness. Supermarket shopping involves a concentrated period of decision-making and of filtering many stimuli, of relating with people and of dealing with stress. In the absence of assistance for people with mental illness, these features of supermarkets make this the **type of experience** that, for people with some of the diagnoses of mental illnesses, can be virtually impossible. Shopping may instead happen at a small (expensive) convenience store, or not at all.

The point is this. Many people who are diagnosed with mental illness are actually disabled people, and mental illness can be viewed as a special case within a grouping of phenomena classified as 'disability', and can therefore be examined as such. See, for example, Doessel and Marshall (1983) who argue that issues of ageing or senescence are not unique, but involve problems of disability.

Consider another distinction. People with mental illnesses suffer acute episodes of illness, maybe only once, sometimes more. In many instances acute episodes call for extreme forms of medical and even legal intervention in a person's life, an intervention that may over-ride a person's preferences. However, in between, or else after, the acute phase(s) of illness, for those 60 to 70 per cent who do not make a good recovery, often years of life are lived with impairment, disability and handicaps. Attention so often focuses on the acute episode. Perhaps the symptoms of chronic illness are not as threatening as those of acute illness, but they are hardly less disabling, disabling partly because care and support are mostly less than adequate.

For economists in particular, there is a challenging thought: when economists and others think about the economics of the issues in mental health care, they probably think about those whose illness is briefly visible. For example, 'visibility' could involve someone subject to delusion in a public place, or someone who attempts suicide publicly in a dramatic way, requiring dramatic forms of police or medical intervention, or someone we come across when we have been 'minding our own business' whose illness has intruded through an odd or unpleasant encounter.

Indeed, it takes deliberate thought by economists not to focus on such partial data in these personal backgrounds and experiences. The evidence (e.g. Jablensky, McGrath *et al.*, 1999) is that the majority of those with mental illness live years of life in social isolation, with multiple handicaps that may not be dramatic, but are remarkably disabling; and that they are resilient people surviving rather rationally, i.e. optimising, in a society when prejudice, and both financial insufficiency and economic inefficiency in service provision make life unnecessarily hard.

In view of the discussion in this Sub-section, the conventional rationality assumption has a useful application in model-building in mental health care. It is, therefore, applied in this study. Nevertheless, whether rationality is defined in terms of objective maximisation or in the more modern view of choosing consistently, and while it is likely to be useful as an assumption even in the presence of mental disorders, it is a blunt instrument. Where employed, it ought not to be without qualification: the phenomenon with which we are dealing is multi-dimensional.

Positive and Normative Science

Important distinctions ought to be made between the positive or descriptive aspects of scientific method and the normative aspects that arise out of a need for policy. This distinction, so fundamental to economic method, is no less vital to the topic at hand. The notions of positive and normative science will be cast within the context of the medical task.

Part of the task of the medical practitioner is to diagnose precisely the nature of an individual's medical condition. As such, it is an act of positive scientific method. Additionally, medical practitioners make decisions regarding a sick individual, in terms of what is in the best interests of the individual (Arrow, 1963b; McGuire, Henderson and Mooney, 1988, p. 154*ff.*), or in the case of problems involving more people, then in terms of what is in the best interests of everyone. This is a normative decision. While it may not always be a straightforward clinical matter to commit an individual to a psychiatric institution, or to have an individual detained under the relevant Act of a Parliament, nevertheless such decisions are made. Furthermore, these decisions are recognised as a responsibility of members of the clinical and legal professions, who are expected to act as agents of the legal and social norms of a society.

A strong case can be made, on the other hand, that advice relating to resource allocation, that is, regarding individuals' claims on health care resources, requires a framework of thought **different** from that of the medical profession. Resource allocation decisions initially need to determine the outcome for which the system is designed but, after that step, the methods of positive and normative science are applicable. Normative economic method is 'the study of criteria for ranking alternative economic situations on a scale of better or worse' (Mishan, 1981, p. 3). See also a later Sub-section on Social Investment Appraisal in this Chapter. Mishan adds that deciding what ought to be done in matters of resource allocation does not require us to neglect an ethical foundation. See Mishan (1981). Nor is the 'categorical imperative' to be imposed.[1] The nature, priorities and objectives of health care delivery should be the province of societal decision making (either within an individualistic or an organic framework),[2] and both positive and normative economics have a special contribution to make. In this precise aspect in the delivery of mental health care, due regard for the place of economics is a helpful attitude (Culyer, 1975; Mooney, 1986).

The Individualistic Framework

Given the nature of mental disorder and the need, at times, to override individual preferences, can an individualistic framework from economic methodology be validly applied to economic studies about these disorders? This question also invites consideration of the corollary, namely, whether mental health problems can be analysed in terms of another type of framework which would describe the institutions in which some psychiatric patients find themselves, that is, the psychiatric hospital (public or private), the nursing home or the prison. Is it preferable perhaps to analyse such systems from an altogether different conceptual stance, e.g. in terms of the degree of public good characteristics provided by these services; or in terms of 'merit good' characteristics associated with these services; or through an entire application of the organic framework?

The position taken in this study, and in Chapters 5, 6 and 7 especially, is to ask first where the individualistic framework of understanding **offers light** on the subject of how a society provides for individuals with a mental disorder. Chapters 8, 9 and 10 then relax that position, namely, of applying the individualistic framework, by examining the role of social interaction in the context of community-based care-giving.

Finally, consider another aspect of the role of the individualistic framework. Part of the outcome of treatment which psychiatrists and psychologists offer is surely the restoration of an individual's ability to have, and to express, his or her preferences. See Knesper, Belcher and Cross (1989, p. 305). Simultaneously, psychiatric hospitals (at least in the form in which they functioned until a

---

1 The categorical (or Kantian) imperative is the unconditional 'ought' statement, like 'You should not murder' rather than a statement, like 'If you murder, you will lose your own life' which is in the conditional imperative. Further discussion can be found in Mishan (1981), pp. 15-16.

2 For a statement of an organic conception, see Ritschl (1931).

decade or two ago) exist in order that they offer individuals sanctuary and respite from the need for exercising the choice-making function so essential to survival in society.

Consumer Ignorance

The economics of mental health care needs to take cognisance of consumer ignorance. It is true that people with less serious mental disorders (neuroses and mild psychoses) probably are functionally able to express preferences in the 'market place' of mental health services, but still may lack the knowledge to do so. The reason for this is that individuals are frequently making their consumption decisions in a world of uncertainty about the future and of elusive product or service information, including such questions as whether to see a psychologist, a social worker or a psychiatric nurse as opposed to a psychiatrist. Furthermore, informed decision making is difficult for an individual, in view of the various 'brands' amongst the professions, the Jungian product range as against the Freudian product range or the cognitive behavioural range, for example. In such an environment, it is frequently the general practitioner (GP) who operates as an agent of the ill-informed patient (Mooney, 1986, p. 85), and who delivers a decision to a patient in the form of a referral to a psychiatrist, or not. In Australia, the patient can claim visits to GPs and psychiatrists under the post-1984 universal (compulsory) national health insurance scheme (Medicare), whereas the services provided by other health professionals are not covered by this societal system of health insurance. The implications of the agency problems will be elaborated in Chapters 5 and 6.

Social Investment Appraisal

Social investment appraisal is an important part of economic research in health care. Most simply, social investment appraisal is concerned with evaluating government projects and programs. In mental health care, there are many examples of various evaluation studies of services and it is a natural question to wonder if the present study is going to be one of those types of evaluation studies. If it is not (and indeed it is not), then why are the authors not doing evaluation work, given that mental health care professionals and government officers from various academic backgrounds, and economists as well, all can be found undertaking evaluation? Is evaluation work not urgently important? Or perhaps some differences exist in the evaluations being done across the range of professions? This Sub-section considers answers to these questions.

According to Doessel (1994), the answer to the last question above is found by looking for differences in the nature of the question being addressed, rather than in the profession of the person doing the work or even in what a person asserts is the nature of the study being done. In this Section, the essential elements of social investment appraisal are briefly re-stated. While, in

Chapter 4, the literature survey will consider the contribution of economic evaluation of mental health care, the purpose of this Sub-section differs from that of Chapter 4. Here, a technical matter is addressed, namely, the standard issues that can be recognised as being undertaken in social investment appraisal.

At this juncture, it ought to be clear that this study does not report empirical results of any type of economic evaluation of an aspect of mental health care. For an economist to put aside such a task may confuse some readers. Is not appraisal work the role of economists in health care? The answer to this question is affirmative, but it reveals a limited understanding of the role of economists. It will be helpful to such a reader if it is explained that, compared with evaluation work, this study is different and more essential. However, the prior matter for attention here is that of the elements of social investment appraisal.

Recall in Chapter 1 in the Section entitled 'Economics and Mental Health Care', the point was made that social investment appraisal, sometimes loosely referred to as economic evaluation, is not simply an accounting balance of the arguments for and against pursuing an action. Rather, an outcome, in an economic sense, is more like a coin having two sides, embracing notions of value and costs. For some goods and services, including mental health care, both the value gained and the cost borne can be quite difficult to determine.

Social investment appraisal is, by nature, a normative task. It is an aspect of Welfare Economics. In the field of economics, the generic term used for the normative aspects of economics is Welfare Economics, and refers to 'that branch of economics that has for its agenda the study of criteria for ranking alternative economic situations on the scale of better or worse' (Mishan, 1982, p. 27). Welfare Economics is a vast body of economic literature and provides, among other things, the conceptual basis for evaluating the social desirability of alternative arrangements of economic activities and resources. The survey by Mishan (1960) gives an introduction to this part of the economic literature.

Now in the health sector, different types of health, medical, hospital or related services may undergo social investment appraisal of possible techniques, programs, projects, innovations, technologies, etc. Economists are more concerned about the precision of the methods in economics for dealing with the value judgements that necessarily arise with social investment appraisal of health services than they are in the actual technique/program that delivers a health service. Put otherwise, economists are concerned with the **technique of social investment appraisal** itself. Indeed, social investment appraisal is just one of many elements of a welfare economist's tool-kit.

Perhaps the one major concern of an economist is that social investment appraisal must be seen to be different from financial investment appraisal for the private sector. Three techniques of social investment appraisal exist: cost-benefit analysis, cost-effectiveness analysis and cost-utility analysis. Three techniques exist because each provides answers to different questions and the techniques must address the issues. In an overview of the techniques, Doessel

(1994) gives standard explanations of the conventional issues in the Welfare Economics literature. The main issues, listed as follows, are not discussed here since they should not be treated superficially and explanation of them is not the purpose of this study. The issues are: the difference between private investment appraisal and social investment appraisal, and the role that externalities play in the distinction; the necessary conditions for a welfare optimum and the debate about partial welfare criteria; matters concerning the appropriate rate of discount, and alternative rules for financial and economic viability; the problems arising with assigning distributional weights; and lastly, the limitations of accounting prices.

Now, the statement just given of the issues involved in social investment appraisal is an attempt to remind the reader of possible pitfalls in undertaking such work. Doessel (1994) expresses two of these pitfalls. First, he warns that social investment appraisal is 'not an area of work that the uninitiated should be undertaking' (p. 24). To put this otherwise, the imprecise judgements and rough estimates required of social investment appraisal are a far more difficult task to get right than the arithmetic. Second, many people in the health field may find they have never before heard the concepts, such as those above, in which the Welfare Economics literature is replete. Doessel's comment is that this can be taken as 'a manifestation of the deplorable state of welfare economic discourse' (p. 24). The present study is placed firmly within the framework offered by Welfare Economics. This is done in spite of theoretical problems in Welfare Economics, which are also well-expounded in the literature. That such problems exist reflects only the need for progress of knowledge in Welfare Economics itself. In other words, that such limitations exist is not an excuse for the authors to escape the discipline of grappling with the meaning of Welfare Economics for mental health care, and its limitations (which is the purpose of the following Chapter).

The final pitfall of undertaking social investment appraisal is related to a problem raised earlier in this Section, as well as in Chapter 1. The pitfall is related to an earlier point that social investment appraisal is not just adding up the 'pros' and 'cons' of an activity. The pitfall is that little economic meaning arises from social investment appraisal or economic evaluation in mental health care if the nature of the outputs of mental health care is not understood. The focus of this study will turn in later Chapters to the very matter that needs to be clear before any such appraisal work proceeds. This study addresses the significant question: 'What is the economic nature of the outputs of mental health care?' When more clarity exists about the outputs, then useful evaluations of the outputs are possible.

The Economics of Mental Health Care: Scope and Definition

With this overview of several key issues in economic method, attention is now directed to two issues of definition.

The first issue is general and refers to the scope of health economics and mental health care. The issue arises because, in economics, 'utility' is useful as a conceptual tool, and some discussion of the distinction between 'utility' and 'mental health' is therefore important in a study of the economics of mental health care. The second issue relates to the definition of output in the health sector generally, and in mental health care, in particular.

In his didactic discussion of the definition of the economics of health care, Evans (1984) concludes that health economics 'restricts attention to a particular set of goods and services which have somehow been identified as having a special relationship to health status...' (p. 3). He continues with a caution that '...unless this special relationship and health status itself are defined narrowly, the economics of health care can easily become the economics of everything.' His basic argument is that although health is an essential part of well-being or welfare, it is obviously not the same as well-being.

Evans' caution about health economics is not a trivial matter when economic studies are undertaken in the mental health care sector. It is argued that if health is equated with utility, then all economics is health economics, a nonsensical state of affairs. The focus of the economics of health care needs to be narrow rather than wide, not just for the reason of avoiding demarcation disputes between the disciplines. The value in clarifying a set of commodities uniquely related to health, according to Evans, is that it provides a clear distinction between health care and other commodities. For example, unlike most commodities that are purchased because they directly increase our utility, health care is not purchased for that reason. Indeed, health care can temporarily lower a person's utility. Rather, when people seek health care, it is in **anticipation** that it will improve their health and, in turn, individuals' levels of utility are improved or at least restored to some previous level.

Evans' argument is that the ability to delineate such distinguishing characteristics of health care makes it possible, then, to clarify the characteristics of health care that make it 'different' as a commodity. In economics, the only differences in the nature of the commodity that matter are those that carry implications for economic welfare.

Definitional problems are more intense with mental health care. While the definition provided by Evans has relevance for the economics of mental health care, the definition is not without qualification. Some psychiatric conditions can be improved greatly with health services, and income maintenance eases the financial burden of the illness. However, there are instances where medical and hospital services, narrowly defined, serve only a minor role in alleviating the suffering of an individual with a mental disorder, and in these cases, Evans' definition is too narrow for the economics of mental health care. Mental health care, more broadly defined, is this: Services that alleviate (or attempt to alleviate) the symptoms and reduce (or attempt to reduce) the disabilities causing the suffering of having a mental disorder. Where psychiatric treatment alone cures a mental illness, then clearly a narrow definition of mental health care applies. Where the illness is incurable, then a broader definition of mental health care is needed. The precise nature of the services that help will vary with the type of symptoms and disabilities suffered by the individual. However, the principle is the same: the alleviation of symptoms and the reduction of disabilities from mental disorders is a multi-dimensional phenomenon. Economics has an important conceptual contribution to make in regard to multi-dimensional phenomena and individual welfare.

The second issue is the problem of specifying or defining output in the health sector. This is an all-pervasive problem and arises in many contexts, e.g. in the literature on the health production function and in the literature associated with health institutions, such as hospitals. See, for example, Connelly and Doessel (2000) for the former, and Butler (1995) for the latter.

In the context of health institutions, one can argue that the output of, say, a hospital is an improvement in the consumer's health status. But there are several problems associated with measures of such a concept, e.g. the absence of an all-embracing, holistic health status instrument. There is also the issue of causality: did the hospital services cause the change in health status? Clearly, there are other mechanisms (diet etc.) that contribute to the consumer's changed health status.

Another concept of hospital output is that of 'a treatment for an episode of illness', the measure of which is the case, admissions, or patients treated. This measure has often been invoked in empirical studies since the pioneering studies by Feldstein (1965), and is the basis for the much discussed disaggregated case-mix measure, Diagnosis Related Groups (DRGs). See below for further discussion.

A third concept of hospital output is that of accommodation, for which the measure is the occupied bed-day (OBD). OBDs are readily and easily calculable, as are comparable measures for hotels, motels, jails etc. The key attribute of this concept is that it has **a temporal dimension**, i.e. a day. This is an attribute that is not central to the other two concepts of output, improved health status and the case (whether the latter be a simple count of all admissions, or some disaggregated case-mix measure such as DRGs).

Paradoxically, although all health services, whether diagnosis, treatment or care, have this temporal attribute to them, the temporal dimension is not acknowledged in all health output measures: it is absent in two concepts of output, *viz.* 'improved health status' and 'a treatment for an episode of illness'. Note that the latter can be measured by a simple count of all admissions or it can be measured by a derived case-mix measure (e.g. DRGs). In contrast, and in spite of its temporal dimension, note that the OBD tells as little about the health status output of a hospital as it does about the health output of hotels and motels.

It is clear that the accommodation concept of health output may, in the context of an institution like a nursing home, be used as a 'gross' measure of output. Given the nature of the physical or emotional conditions of nursing home residents, a measure such as the OBD may be relevant.[3] It may also be relevant to psychiatric institutions that provide only care services to those residents who are not responsive to any therapy.

But the following question is relevant: given that many mental health services are not provided in an institution, why place an emphasis on the output of an institution as a definition of mental health output? The complexities associated with mental health care will be considered further below with an approach which applies across services, whether in institutional or in non-institutional contexts.

The Complicated Nature of Mental Illness and its Treatment

It might be useful to consider in some schematic way the complexities of the phenomena with which we are dealing. In this context heterogeneity of location of service provision, whether the attending medical practitioner does, or does not, have specialist qualifications in psychiatry, and whether the hospital does, or does not, have a dedicated psychiatric unit, are not considered. Wallen's (1987) econometric analysis indicates that such variables are statistically significant in explaining resource use by psychiatric patients. The emphasis is placed on a number of other attributes of the all-encompassing term, 'mental health care'. The purpose of this Section is to 'unpack' this term.

First, consider how mental illness consists of various illnesses/conditions such as depression, bipolar disorder etc. For each illness/condition, severity is widely variable. Health status instruments can provide empirical scores about severity. Some health status instruments are general, e.g. SF36 (Ware *et al.*, 1993) and some are more specific. For example, consider the Panic and Agoraphobia Scale recently devised by Bandelow (1995). This instrument has been developed specifically for use in randomised clinical trials (RCTs) of new therapies, including drugs, for the treatment of agoraphobia. The factors that the instrument separately addresses are as follows: panic attacks, phobic avoidance, anticipatory anxiety, impairment of social and work relationships, and the assumption of somatic disease.

---

3 The term, 'gross', in the discussion of nursing homes has been used quite deliberately. In a recent analysis of the output of nursing homes in the United States, Cohen and Spector (1996) used a measure of the span of time from date of admission to date of mortality, and numbers of bedsores as the measure of output, rather than (simply) the equivalent of OBDs. Such a study is, essentially, concerned with moving 'behind the veil' of the temporal dimension of care services or, put otherwise, the output of the nursing home is time-related, whereas the output of an acute hospital is not (now) time-related. Similarly, the output of a hospice is time-related.

Measures of severity, whether general or specific, are often expressed in ranges (of scores obtained from administration of such instruments), such as 10.1-15.0, 15.1-20.0 etc., and are then collapsed down to, say, a threefold classification, e.g. 'mild', 'moderate' and 'severe'.[4]

Consider next a commonly-invoked **functional classification** of outputs in the health care sector, *viz.*, diagnosis, treatment and care.[5] Regarding diagnosis, the use of diagnostic tests essentially provides information about the presence or absence of an illness/condition (Doessel, 1986). Having determined a person's illness/condition, there is then a separate issue, which is that of applying appropriate treatment technology, such as that found in the available therapies, in an attempt to reverse, or else stabilise, the natural history of the illness. This process can be appropriately described as the 'treatment' function. It may be provided in an institution, usually a hospital. The other aspect of a functional classification of the outputs of health care is that of 'care'. Where no efficacious therapies exist for some illnesses/conditions, then 'care' is undertaken. This function is often performed in separate institutions such as nursing homes, hospices etc.

These dimensions of complexity, or heterogeneity, are brought together in Table 2.1 which recognises multiple mental illnesses (1,2,3, ..., n), as well as a threefold classification of severity (mild, moderate, severe) and a threefold classification of output in the health sector, i.e. diagnosis, treatment, care. Table 2.1 is, in a sense, a depiction of our knowledge, or ignorance, about mental illness at a point in time. For example, for Mental Illness/Condition 1, Table 2.1 indicates that there is no reliable diagnostic test that indicates the presence of this illness/condition in 'mild' or 'moderate' cases. The only reliable test diagnoses 'severe' cases. Similarly, in terms of the three measures of severity with respect to treatment or therapy, the entries in the cells for Mental Illness/Condition 1 indicate that a therapy exists for 'mild' cases only. 'Care' services for Mental Illness/Condition 1 are thought to be 'appropriate' (A) for 'moderate' and 'severe' cases, whereas they are thought to be 'not appropriate' (NA) for mild cases. And so on, for other mental illnesses/conditions.

---

4 It is instructive to observe that not only was Wallen (1987) able to classify psychiatric patients using a four-fold severity classification scheme (based on a concept of disease or illness staging), but that severity was shown to be a statistically significant determinent of resource use for those patients.

5 There are, of course, more detailed classifications of outputs in the health sector. See, for example, Cooper and Bennett (1984), for an early application. Such classifications arise from the reform of the **form** of government budgets initiated in the US Department of Defense in the 1960s (Hitch and McKean, 1960; Hitch, 1965). See Burkhead and Miner (1971) for an account of these early developments. See Commons *et al.* (1997) for an account of performance contracting for treating substance abuse patients. Culyer (1980) provides a neat overview of the characteristics of 'performance budgeting', 'program budgeting' or 'output budgeting', as it has been variously called.

Some qualifications are relevant in regard to Table 2.1. First, Table 2.1 presents 'what exists' at a particular point in time, given existing technologies and current preferences and conceptions. For example, the development of a new drug for an illness for which there was no previous therapy would involve a change in one, two or three cells of Table 2.1, from the 'NE_{TR}' notation to the 'E_{TR}' notation. Second, Table 2.1 does not take into account multiple diagnostic tests or therapies for a particular illness/condition, nor does it recognise the relative efficacy of such tests and therapies. In addition, Table 2.1 regards some phenomena, e.g. severity, as being discrete in nature whereas, in reality, the measurements of such phenomena are continuous. Also, the varying degrees of efficacy of mental health therapies have not been recognised. Finally, Table 2.1 does not take account of the fact that discretion, or medical 'fashion', i.e. the ability to 'shift the goalposts', is possible. For example, the deinstitutionalisation movement involved a shift of what was considered 'appropriate' and 'not appropriate' in some dimensions of Table 2.1.

It is also relevant to note that the distinctions indicated in Table 2.1 do not imply any one-to-one, or unique, relationship with respect to institutional or non-institutional forms in the provision of some mental health services, irrespective of whether reference is being made to diagnostic, therapeutic or care services.

Table 2.1 The existence and/or appropriateness of diagnostic tests, treatment and care for various mental illnesses/ conditions

Mental Illness / Condition	Diagnosis			Treatment			Care		
	Mild	Moderate	Severe	Mild	Moderate	Severe	Mild	Moderate	Severe
1	NE_D	NE_D	E_D	E_{TR}	NE_{TR}	NE_{TR}	NA	A	A
2	NE_D	E_D	E_D	NE_{TR}	E_{TR}	E_{TR}	NA	NA	NA
.									
.									
.									
n	E_D	E_D	E_D	NE_{TR}	NE_{TR}	NE_{TR}	A	A	A

Notes:

'E_D' indicates that a diagnostic test for an illness/condition 'exists', and 'NE_D' indicates that a diagnostic test does 'not exist'.

'E_{TR}' indicates that a treatment for an illness/condition 'exists', and 'NE_{TR}' indicates that a treatment does 'not exist'.

'A' indicates that care services are thought to be 'appropriate' for a particular illness/condition, and 'NA' indicates that care services are thought to be 'not appropriate' for a particular illness/ condition.

It is important to note that this approach is applicable either in an institutional context or a non-institutional context. Put otherwise, the approach is not tied to a specific setting.

Such heterogeneity, as indicated in Table 2.1, highlights the importance of recognising patient case-mix in any particular institution or approach to service provision for the mentally ill. Since Feldstein (1965), case-mix has been acknowledged as a fundamentally important variable in several studies, for example, in the analysis of hospital costs. For a detailed account, see Butler (1995). As a very important case-mix classification, DRGs have now become a major analytical tool in some countries for various aspects of hospital management (Fetter, Thompson and Mills, 1976; Fetter, Shin, Freeman *et al.*, 1980; Fetter, 1991; Fetter, 1999). It is important to note in this context that while case-mix issues are **not** confined to general hospitals, they **may well turn out to have been 'easy' in general hospitals**, compared to the difficulties of case-mix in psychiatric institutions or for services in community settings for people with mental illness (Taube *et al.*, 1984; Horgan and Jencks, 1987; Wallen, 1987). For an account of a specifically-designed system of case-mix for mental illness, see Whiteford, Thompson and Casey (2000, pp. 407-8).

Conclusion

In this Chapter some issues in economic method have been examined. These included the use of the rationality assumption in economics for studies of mental health care; the distinction between positive and normative method in economics; the relevance of the individualistic framework of conventional economics; the economic meaning of the presence of 'consumer ignorance' in mental health care; and, finally, the role of social investment appraisal in mental health care.

Attention then turned to definitional matters, first, regarding the scope of economics of mental health care, and second, concerning the problem, in health economics generally, of specifying the output. The final Section of the Chapter suggested an approach to dealing with the heterogeneous nature of the treatment of mental illness, in view of the existence of degrees of severity of the illness.

In the next Chapter attention will turn to the Welfare Economics of mental health care. Since this study is fundamentally concerned with economic welfare, a framework is needed for examining mental health care problems where an economic dimension is involved, and it is appropriate to employ a framework that sheds light upon economic welfare. A useful framework of study is conventional Welfare Economics, which is the topic of the next Chapter.

3 The Welfare Economics of Mental Health Care

Introduction

In this Chapter, the conventional Theorems of Welfare Economics are presented. This is with a view to examining the degree to which these conventional Theorems are useful when *Homo Economicus* has a mental disorder. To the extent that the premises are not applicable to mental health care, then the economist's efficiency criteria for attaining net social benefit require modification. Suitable modifications provide economists, and policymakers, with a standard for knowing what constitutes a positive change in welfare.

The Welfare Economics of (general) medical services was first addressed in the economics literature in the early 1960s in Arrow's (1963a) paper entitled 'The Welfare Economics of Medical Care'. That paper is regarded as seminal. It serves also as a foundation for explaining the institutions that replace markets in the provision of medical services. For Arrow, particular characteristics of health and/or health care explain the historical existence of non-market institutions, including eleemosynary ones, in the health sector. Arrow's work assists in providing an understanding also of mental health care.

Initially in this Chapter, general issues in the Welfare Economics of mental health care are explored. A discussion follows of the Welfare Economics of (general) medical services, after Arrow (1963a), and attention turns lastly to the characteristics of mental illness and mental health care that explain *a priori* the institutional and market arrangements in mental health care.

The Welfare Economics of Mental Health Care

In order to investigate the Welfare Economics of mental health care, let the economic well-being of buyers and sellers in mental health consist of two components: quantities of services bought and sold; and the individual's budget constraint. In other words, a simple definition of standard of living is employed. The purpose here is to consider how deficiencies in resource allocation affect the level of economic well-being. Note that the definition of living standard is just one aspect of Sen's more comprehensive definition of the standard of living, discussed in Chapter 1.

Next, assume initially the conventional definition of the norm for the common good (i.e. well-being). The norm is that the common good is determined by an arrangement of buyers and sellers such that the flows of services for sale and for purchase are (taking the position of both buyer and seller) available at prices for which buyers and sellers are unable to influence market quantities traded, or prices. In such an arrangement, consumer surplus and producer surplus are maximised.

Additionally, assume that the going prices are such that they make equal the total amounts of services offered for exchange and the total amounts which buyers altogether are willing to purchase, with no restrictions imposed upon supply and demand. Put simply, 'market success' occurs when the allocations achieved with markets are efficient; and when the allocations are not efficient, then there is market failure of some kind. Market failure implies a choice: whether to accept the allocative inefficiency due to the market failure as the best approach to society's well-being; or whether political intervention in the marketplace will improve well-being; or whether another non-market alternative will improve well-being.

The purpose of the model of the so-called 'competitive equilibrium' is not to idealise a personal preference for free markets. The competitive model defines a conceptual economic arrangement for specifying the way in which the economic well-being of society is served, given our present understanding. It also defines a basis from which to judge the presence of increases or decreases in general welfare.

Specifying a norm begs the question, of course, as to what purpose the norm serves. Since the early decades of the twentieth century, the economic needs of society have no longer been considered to be best served when national output is maximised. Rather, the common good is understood in terms of the outcome of Pareto optimality. This occurs when no other allocation of resources could result in anyone in the society being better off without someone being made worse off. Pareto optimality suggests a very exact interpretation of society's economic welfare.

Now, two theorems about the economic welfare of society assist in the identification of a Pareto optimal state.[1] The First Theorem of Welfare Economics stated most simply (Ledyard, 1987, p. 326) is as follows: if there are enough markets,[2] if all producers and consumers behave competitively

1 Comprehensive statements are found in intermediate textbooks such as Varian (1984). For a survey of two formative decades, see Mishan (1960).

2 The conventional explanation, stated simply is that '[a]lthough there are no definitive guidelines as to what constitutes "enough", the general principle is that if any actor in the economy cares about something that also involves an interaction with at least one other actor, then there should be a market for that something: it should have a price. ... This is

and if an equilibrium exists at all, then the allocation of resources in that equilibrium will be Pareto optimal, and such an allocation is attained with the competitive equilibrium, provided that all costs are in fact priced in the market, and all interdependencies between firms and producers are internalised.

The Second Theorem is as follows: provided special conditions applying to production sets and utility sets are satisfied, then almost every Pareto optimal state is attainable if competitive equilibria are modified, that is, markets can be 'completed', either by a system of lump-sum taxes and transfers that re-distributes purchasing power more fairly, or if property rights are re-specified.

The Third Theorem, not stated here, is concerned with the preconditions required in order to aggregate reliably the heterogeneous preferences arising in society. Distributional paradoxes arising with the Third Theorem are irreconcilable. For an account of the theoretical nature of these issues, see Arrow (1963b) or Feldman (1987).

The implication of the Theorems above is summarised as follows in respect of mental health care, in a manner after Arrow (1963a). Given that the conditions of the Theorems are satisfied, then a mental health services market (or, as is the case in Arrow's paper, the medical services market) could be 'trusted' with the resource allocation function, and government would execute policies to distribute income equitably.

Perhaps of great importance here is that, because the 'real world' of mental health services differs from the conditions of the competitive model, then the separation of allocative and distributional processes for the mental health care sector of the economy is virtually impossible (Arrow, 1963a, pp.15-16). In any case, the competitive model could only ever serve as a universal, prescriptive standard for economic efficiency subject to strict conditions.

The Competitive Model and Medical Services

The deficiencies in the competitive model are well-established, and the literature on these deficiencies is vast. Four of the standard objections are given here (Bator, 1958; Feldman, 1987). First, the preferences of consumers are far from being exogenous and are subject to many influences from the market, such as advertising and other more subtle forms of persuasion. See also Bowles (1998). Second, instead of competitive practices abounding, the real world is replete

---

true whether that something is consumption of bread, consumption of smoke from a factory, or the amount of national defence' (Ledyard, 1987, pp. 326-27). Ledyard then outlines pervasive informational asymmetries inducing market failure. Of course, having too few markets is not simply solved by creating more markets. Creating another market is pointless if in that market, an equilibrium does not exist, such as in the well-known case of increasing returns to scale. For the existence of an equilibrium, see the conditions of the First Theorem, above.

with monopolistic behaviours. Third, externalities and public goods are assumed away for the sake of the model and yet in reality they are all pervasive. Fourth, distributional issues remain unsettled.

Arrow's paper next examines the 'real world' medical market. His aim is to find where the actual market differs from the competitive model. He addresses this by considering the institutional organisation of the industry and the 'observable mores' of the medical profession. He also explores the presence or absence in medical services of the major preconditions for the model. Arrow's primary focus is the absence of marketability of medical services. By this, he means the tendency for a free market to fail to provide a mechanism for medical services to be offered and demanded.

To be able to shift the risks of illness to others 'is worth a price which many are willing to pay', but the markets for this are not well-formed (Arrow, 1963b, p. 17). With illness being unpredictable by nature, the provision of insurance against risk is an important adjunct to medical care. The seminal contribution of Arrow was thus to the theory of health and hospital insurance. Arrow discusses the likelihood, in the face of uncertainty, of medical information also being a commodity. This is especially apparent with the sellers of medical services tending to have more market power over information than the buyers of these services. Another way of stating this phenomenon is that medical services are characterised by information asymmetry between producers and consumers. Essentially, then, it is the prevalence of both risk and uncertainty that, according to Arrow, explains the special features of the medical market. The market fails to achieve Pareto optimality, and both government and other social institutions 'step into the optimality gap' (Arrow, 1963b, p. 20).

In all, Arrow addresses three characteristics of health care which have economic significance: the uncertainty with which illness strikes; the dominant presence of interpersonal effects of consumption (that is, externalities are present to the extent that people's consumption of health care affects not just their own well-being but others') relative to other commodities; and the fact that the provider of health care usually has a far greater knowledge of health care than the consumer, relative to the providers of many other commodities.

Arrow drew attention to the notable absence of markets in medical services. To the extent that markets do not function, then government-subsidised or -provided services in medical care are common. His explanation of the development of this phenomenon is that when illness strikes, it brings with it not just the temporary impact of the illness itself but also the risk of delayed or incomplete recovery. One missing market is that for the complete bearing of risks. To the extent that insurance covers an individual's risk, incremental gains in welfare occur. Apart from the possibility of lost income-earning capacity, the two main losses arising with illness which are risked by individuals are loss due to treatment costs and the loss due to discomfort brought on by the illness.

Another missing market is the market for information. According to Arrow, the individual suffering an illness cannot, when needing to decide how much of his or her budget is best consumed on treatment, judge the worth of a treatment as ideally as he or she would want. The medical practitioner knows more about the efficacy of the treatment, but the medical practitioner does not know the individual's preference set well enough to advise the patient on the ideal amount of his or her budget to spend on treatment, relative to other utility-producing activities.

The medical market is characterised, therefore, by payment systems that do not incorporate a component insuring for the probability of treatment failure. Where this component is absent, various social institutions come into play. The institutions that Arrow mentions include: a degree of trust characterising the provision of medical services; other non-market institutions that have eleemosynary motives; the tendency for decisions to be delegated to medical practitioners or others; and the presence of licensing and educational standards for providers of medical services.

Arrow also refers to a range of other characteristics of medical care: product uncertainty; restricted entry; increasing returns; price discrimination. To give no further reference to those matters here is not to imply at all that they are irrelevant to mental health care. Many, if not all, are relevant to the analysis of mental disorders. While some of the economic characteristics of the treatment of physical ailments are relevant to the treatment of mental disorders, and these will be indicated below, others are not. Some dimensions are unique to mental health care.

The Competitive Model and Mental Health Care

Though sharing many features in common with other medical services, the market for mental health has some unique characteristics. There are some other characteristics that have more in common with markets for disability services than for medical services. The important differences will be described in this Section. It is argued that these features have implications for the attainment of an optimal level of well-being from economic transactions in mental health care. In a contrasting approach to the technical matters herein, the Appendix to this Chapter illustrates the suitability of goods and services available for people with a particular physical illness, compared with those for people with a mental illness.

The background for this Section is the contribution of Arrow (1963a). This was discussed in the previous Section where it was explained that Arrow depicts the presence of uncertainty as a definitive feature of the demand for medical services. Arrow's seminal contribution to the economics of medical care arose out of his theory of (ideal) medical insurance. While Arrow's paper is largely concerned with physical ailments, it is apparent that uncertainty is also prevalent in the consumption of services for mental illnesses. It can be argued, in fact, that uncertainty looms larger for mental health services than for physical health services. Hence, to the extent that mental health services have the characteristic of uncertainty in common with medical services, then Arrow's paper also serves as a foundation for the economics of mental health services. Indeed, it has already spawned a burgeoning literature on insurance for in-patient and out-patient mental health care, of which McGuire's *Financing Psychotherapy* (1981) is a forerunner. Chapter 4 surveys the literature.

Further studies of market failure in mental health care reveal other features. For example, Frank (1990) notes that few transactions in mental health care are simple and bilateral but, rather, are characterised by agency, familial and (generally more complex) 'other' relationships. Other features include the presence of regulations and of government departments, as well as payment occurring via third parties (which means people other than the buyers of the service).

Other instances of market failure noted by Frank include the lack of information in mental health care on prices, quality, outcome and appropriate levels of consumption. Also, externalities are pervasive where the benefits of treatment and care extend to people other than those undergoing the care and treatment.

The following Sub-sections address these and some of the other aspects of mental health services which have significance for economic well-being.

Uncertainty and Consumer Preferences

The existence of, and expression of, an individual's preference set is fundamental to the processes that achieve economic well-being for the individual. However, mental illness causes disorder in the existence, and/or the expression, of a person's preferences over treatment, over other mental health services, and indeed over the consumption of any good or service at all. In other words, the nature of the condition can affect choice. It particularly affects the person's ability to express those preferences in the market for mental health care. Note, though, that individuals with a mental illness know, to varying and elusive degrees of reliability, **some and even many things** about their own preferences over treatment and support services, and indeed, over all goods and services consumed in their budget, as well as goods and services not yet available. There is a clinical tension here that has important economic implications. Put otherwise, the nature of the person's preferences is a matter of degree not kind. The issue at stake here (for people with mental disorders, as for all people) is of a continuous, not a discrete, nature.

One achievement of successful mental health care surely is to restore the individual's ability to form and express 'healthy' preferences in order that the person might live in society as painlessly as possible. However, there are other important economic implications of this issue of uncertainty over consumer preferences, as follows.

In the presence of treatment, influences upon patients' preferences present complex issues. With mental health care in particular, it is difficult for **any** person to know fully the preference set of another individual, and yet, for a service provider, knowing where the disorder starts and the individual's personality stops is vital in the treatment and care of the individual with mental illness. Put otherwise, given a person has a preference set, then some part of this is due to personality, some part is due to illness and, to some elusive extent, the two overlap. The service provider has the difficult task of working out what is personality, and of devising appropriate treatment, without influencing a patient's preferences according to the provider's own interests. Arrow's point is that the individual suffering an illness cannot, when needing to decide how much of his or her budget is best consumed on treatment, judge the worth of a treatment as ideally as he or she would want. As has been stated already, Arrow's key contribution to health care was to direct attention to a crucial market missing in health care: the problem of the imperfect marketability of information. One aspect of the so-called information problem in markets is that, regarding mental health care, the supplier of treatment becomes involved in varying ways in the **formation** of the consumer's preferences, that is, in imposing provider preferences on patients. The supplier, perhaps a medical practitioner, usually knows more about the efficacy of the treatment or services that the patient consumes than do the patients themselves know. Medical practitioners, as well as bureaucrats and other service providers, have historically had a large influence on the shape of the preference set of persons with mental illness.

Instances where providers influence patient preferences are diverse. A general economic framework has been provided by Doessel and Marshall (1985), conceptualising the different instances where provider preferences are imposed on patients. They use characteristics space to examine choice of alternative health treatments, and then apply this framework to illustrate two contrasting examples. In the first example, the case is examined of the supplier failing to provide information to the consumer about the consumption technology. That is, information about the quantities of characteristics in the treatment (its efficacy), as well as information about the price, is concealed. The efficiency frontier is not what the consumer thinks it is. Next, Doessel and Marshall conceptualise the possibility of the supplier advising the consumer to substitute the supplier's preferences concerning the characteristics of a health treatment for the consumer's own preferences. In this instance, consumer preferences are juxtaposed with provider preferences in the same characteristics space (p. 1325).

Two other aspects of uncertainty and consumer preferences are worthy of a brief remark. First, the neglect by society in general of people with mental illnesses has resulted in a highly constrained preference set for those people who need useful treatment and services merely to live their lives. The economic perspective is that the various institutions and institutional processes in mental health care that have historical origins, and still are evolving, operate as blunt instruments in addressing missing markets in the supply and demand for support to people with a disorder of individual preferences.[3] This matter will be considered again in a later Sub-section.

Second, sometimes of course, the preferences of some individuals are socially unacceptable. Where this is the case, it should be treated as a special case of market failure in mental health care that arises from the unacceptability of consumer preferences. That is, it is not an issue of uncertainty about consumer preferences. The two issues are quite separate. Socially unacceptable preferences will be considered next. Following that, market failures in attaining exchange efficiency in the presence of chronic/incurable conditions are re-addressed.

Socially Unacceptable Preferences

Some individuals with mental disorders exhibit socially unacceptable preferences. Societies express disapproval of individuals' preferences and behaviour both with benevolent and malevolent motivations. Disapproval is expressed by varying degrees of restriction upon the individual. At worst, political dissidents can be incarcerated in psychiatric institutions, as illustrated in Solzhenitsyn's (1978) *The Gulag Archipelago*. In contrast, in the eighteenth and nineteenth centuries in England the social neglect of demented individuals caused outrage among some Quakers who initiated benevolent efforts to provide individualised care for such people. The efforts came to be known as the 'moral treatment' movement (Rosenblatt, 1984; Lewis, 1988; English and McGarrick, 1989).

In democratic societies, the variance in standards of acceptance implies important and extremely difficult questions. For example, there is the question of which individuals are to be committed to involuntary psychiatric care in institutions, for whatever reasons and for whatever care. See Kafka (1925); also Human Rights and Equal Opportunity Commission (1993), Eisen and Wolfenden (1988, pp. 369-75), and Kirby (1985) for Australia; and, for the US, Morrissey and Goldman (1984).

Chronic Illness and the Nature of Demand and Supply

Some mental disorders are not curable. Where no cure is available, many of the consequences of chronic mental illnesses are similar to those of chronic physical illnesses and conditions, because having a psychiatric illness interferes with the functioning and independence needed for living and for enjoying life. A key difference, however, is that both under-production and over-production of services for chronic mental illness are severe, and are more likely to occur than for chronic physical illnesses.

---

3 Here is another case where such a comment as this should not be taken as, to repeat words from Chapter 1, a personal indictment of highly dedicated people who work in various services, or who give care in their home, and who face critical, 'coal-face' decisions affecting disadvantaged and vulnerable people.

The temporal pattern of the problems of the chronically ill person is highly variable from one condition to the next, and from one person to the next. The demand for mental health care is, thus, not standardised.

Agency relationships in mental health care are pervasive. Until recently, institutional decisions in mental health care often defined the boundaries of service delivery. Institutional definitions of mental health care are not equivalent to the economic notion of demand for mental health care. Nor are the services delivered by bureaucracies equivalent to the economic notion of supply of mental health care. See also Chapter 6.

Income and the Nature of Demand

The symptoms and disabilities that arise with a **physical** condition interfere with the individual's ability to do what is necessary to live one's daily life, as well as to enjoy what one likes. In most cases, pain and limitation adversely affect the ability to have the sensations of enjoyment and living, and the desire to reverse this state is the simplest reason that sick people seek the services of healers and helpers. Higher income may lead to an increased likelihood of improvement.

The symptoms and disabilities that arise with **psychiatric** conditions, as with physical ailments, interfere with activity, decision-making, enjoyment (except with temporary manias or euphoric states, such as in bipolar disorder) and motivation. However, having considerable income rarely enables an individual to escape mental disorder. High incomes seem seldom to help people escape the consequences of mental illnesses and disorders, except where stays in a private hospital ease symptoms or where suitable private nursing support can be purchased to ameliorate symptoms.

The Under-Consumption and Under-Production of Consumer Aids and Aides

Appropriate consumer aids and aides are likely to assist people with mental illnesses to live their lives. Why is it that these are both under-consumed and under-produced? Without attempting a comprehensive explanation here, some interesting issues are considered.

With physical ailments, a patient is likely to notice any malfunctioning of a part of the body, but the disorder is not always apparent in the case of a mental illness. Individuals may believe, at least to some degree, that nothing is wrong. However, apart from the few people with mental illnesses who are proven to be dangerous, many of the mentally ill are 'gravely disabled people who are too disorganised to avail themselves of vitally needed care' (Lamb, 1984, p. 529). Alternatively, the stigma experienced by an individual diagnosed with a mental illness means a person may prefer not to seek treatment.

People with mental illness may not seek help for more than one reason. Let us consider briefly here the issues surrounding failure to seek help. People may not be aware of the need or they may not expect their needs to be met, having had little success from help in the past. Weakness of will and failing to 'pull up your socks' is another reason, but this is exceptional; what may appear to be apathy or weakness of will may actually reflect the fact that help is neither adequate nor forthcoming. Because mental disorders affect a person's ability to take the necessary steps to improve his/her own well-being, people with mental disorders may appear to be weak-willed and, if they are neglecting themselves, this is to be taken as their own choice, even fault. No grounds exist for supposing that the presence of weakness of will is any more prevalent in these people than in the general population. Indeed, it could well be that individuals with mental disorders develop a stronger will than the average person, just in order to survive. Individuals with mental disorders may be struggling ineffectually to maintain their well-being, and this is due partly to the disabilities and symptoms present with the illness, and partly to the absence of useful treatment and support. It is, therefore, too simplistic to cast aside the under-consumption of consumer aids and aides with an assertion that people with mental illness prefer to live the way they are now; that they could get better if they wanted to and if they would only help themselves.

The assumptions of conventional Welfare Economics imply that, with enough information, income and technology available, individuals have the ability to maintain and improve their well-being, should they wish to do so. This statement both represents and misrepresents the attempts by individuals with a mental disorder to maintain and improve their well-being, in an extraordinary mixture of personal strengths and serious limitations with which a person with a mental disorder presents. For people with mental illnesses, services that enable the development and expression of consumer preferences of the individual with the mental illness, particularly those with a chronic condition, are being severely under-consumed. Blind people have 'Seeing Eye' dogs; deaf people have hearing aids; but markets for aids and aides for people with mental illnesses are missing, or consumers are severely under-consuming. Note that the presence of under-consumption of services implies that the under-production of services is, in aggregate, occurring also.

Multilateral Transactions

According to Frank (1990), various parties, beyond the individuals receiving care and treatment and their families, are interested in the outcomes of mental health care. Government represents voter interests in altruism, in prudent expenditure and in tax minimisation. Service providers represent both their own interests (financial, professional, ideological) and act as agents for the consumers of their services.

Frank continues with the following claim:

> [I]t is very difficult to rely on 'shopping' behaviour to discipline the market. Even those parties that represent consumer interests (third party payors [*sic*] and government) face a difficult and costly task of monitoring quality, outcome and quantity of care. This set of circumstances underlies one of the most fundamental (and unique) sets of tensions found in the health and mental health sectors of the economy. That is, providers view regulations, payment methods, and external quality control as costly incursions into their enterprises. Payors [*sic*] and government are interested in assuring that dollars for which they are responsible are appropriately spent. These opposing perspectives inevitably result in conflict (Frank, 1990, p. 190).

Externalities

When private benefits do not equate with social benefits and private costs do not equate with social costs, then the consequence of 'spillover effects' (also referred to as externalities and cause the disparity between private and social costs and benefits) is that the market solution is not Pareto optimal. The result is under- or over-production of commodities subject to beneficial external effects, or of commodities subject to adverse external effects, respectively. Some externalities arising in the presence of mental illness are given below.

One externality is a 'caring externality'. Given that individuals care about each other, then individuals whose well-being is reduced, because others are not receiving enough treatment or care in their state of ill-health, are experiencing a negative externality (Culyer, 1980). Another dimension of this is that the quality of care which individuals expect to be available for themselves, should the need for treatment or care arise, is likely to differ from the quality of care that individuals demand due to the so-called caring externality (Pauly, 1981).

Second, externalities exist in regard to care-givers. Individuals in society are believed also to care that care-givers, say in the home, are exhausted or that family life is breaking down, due to the demanding circumstances of looking after a family member with a serious mental disorder. Both these effects result in a divergence between private marginal benefit and the social marginal benefit.

Before discussing another externality, a point of clarification is needed. Mishan (1981; 1982) points out that some reactions would not be categorised as externalities, since society, in its ethical capacity, does not count reactions arising from envy, spite or cruelty as any part of the concept of the externality. Mishan notes, for example, that a person who indulges his spite by throwing a brick through another person's window undoubtedly inflicts a loss of welfare, but economists would not count such an event as an externality (Mishan, 1981, pp. 392-93). Likewise is the case of the person who is affronted by the beggar asking for money, where again, the ethical society would not regard an externality as having arisen. Essentially, then, '...normative economics, if it is to be an acceptable guide to allocation or economic policy generally, has to be rooted in the ethics of the community' (Mishan, 1981, p. 393).

Two other types of externality, which have arisen due to deinstitutionalisation, are 'legitimate instances' of people being affronted by particularly odd or difficult behaviours of some individuals. Consider one instance, a person suffering with dementia who shouts so constantly that the level of well-being of neighbours is reduced. In the former era when people with mental illness were routinely institutionalised, the 'shouting' externality was internalised in several ways, by labour being employed to care for such a person and premises being constructed that would give a person with such unpleasant behaviour a place to live. In the present era of deinstitutionalisation, the 'shouting' externality is no longer internalised.

In another instance, consider again how unusual or unpleasant behaviour distresses other people. That reaction causes people with mental illness to feel outcast, feeling the stigma of their illness. Before deinstitutionalisation, some people with mental illness felt they had a community where they were accepted, albeit a hospital. With deinstitutionalisation, many people with mental illness are hidden away still, neglected, living in inner-city hovels, in the 'communities of acceptance' shared by other outcasts. Or these people are living lonely lives hiding away from people generally. Due to the lack of internalisation of this stigma externality, the living standard of people with mental illnesses has declined and their housing standard is thought to be very low.

In this era of deinstitutionalisation, it would appear that the benefits of community acceptance and the costs of reducing community rejection of the mentally ill are seldom being counted by policy makers (Cousens and Crawford, 1988).

Jointness in Production

Jointness in production occurs when a change in the rate of output of one product brings about a similar change in the other product(s). Joint production is not of itself a market failure. However, with the complicated nature of any multi-product firm or service provider, the achievement of appropriate regulation of the sector is fraught with problems.

One problem has arisen with the changes through time to the provision of mental health care. Historically, psychiatric hospitals were responsible for the joint production, institutionally, of the entirety of services consumed by someone with a serious mental disorder. Presently, the regular health, social and disability services designed for the needs of the general community are available for people with mental disorders living in the community. A person with a chronic disorder can often be in need of the entire range of these services. People with chronic mental disorders find the task of generating the range of support they require from the existing highly fragmented array of services impossibly difficult, largely due to the very nature of the condition they suffer.

It is increasingly the practice at present to have case management. Case management is a bureaucratically-developed product for co-ordinating care, and providing, from the myriad of services available, access to appropriate services. Continuity of care is a desired goal of case management but this goal is not always achieved. One problem that inhibits continuity of care is the absence of funding mechanisms suited to community care. See, for example, McGuire and Riordan (1993).

Statistical Significance and Elasticity of Inputs in the Mental Health Production Function

The relationship between mental health inputs and mental health status can be expressed by a production function for mental health status. When an input is a statistically significant variable in the mental health production function, then it is statistically significant that the input contributes to mental health output. Where the application of an input results in no change at all in mental health status, other things being equal, then the input will not be in the production function.

Once statistical significance is established, the degree of responsiveness of the output to a particular statistically significant input can be expressed by its elasticity. An inelastic mental health production function with respect to one input implies that mental health status is not very responsive to a change in that variable. Also, substitutability of one input for another can be measured by the elasticity of input substitution. For an early empirical application (not in a mental health context), see Reinhardt (1972) and more recently Gerdtham, Löthgren, Tambour and Rehnberg (1999) and the literature cited therein. This type of analysis does not commonly occur in the context of mental illnesses. In fact, there are only several studies of which we are aware, that have formally estimated a mental health production function. Healey, Mirandola, Amaddeo *et al.* (2000), using both fixed- and random-effects estimation techniques, have analysed changes in mental health status (measured by the Global Assessment of Functioning, GAF, scale) for a group of 662 first-ever patients, referred over a four-year period, to a community-based mental health service in Verona, Italy.

It is difficult to summarise all of their conclusions briefly, but some of their results are very interesting. First, the effect on mental health status (of service consultations) was, generally, not large. Second, there were differential impacts from different service providers (psychologists, psychiatrists etc.). Third, the efficacy of service provision varied by diagnosis, using a four-fold classification, *viz.* affective disorders, schizophrenia, neurosis and other diagnoses. Fourth, the effect of in-patient care varied by diagnosis, being statistically significant only for persons diagnosed with schizophrenia.

A second study, Lu (1999), analysed the experience of 3,221 individuals who were interviewed in a community setting in Puerto Rico in the period

October 1992 to May 1994. Outcome was measured as a change in need for mental health services. An important characteristic of this study is the use of instrumental variables (IVs). Conventional regression analysis produced the conclusion that, for two measures of mental health treatment, mental health services had a negative (but statistically insignificant) effect on mental heath status. Other explanatory variables were case-mix (measured by using the Psychological Symptom and Dysfunction Scales), age, gender, education, income, etc. However, data such as were available from this non-experimental setting may be subject to the selection bias problem. To address this problem, a number of IVs were applied and the results were quite different: thus treatment is productive. The results are supportive of the concerns on the credibility of evaluation results using observation data sets when the endogeneity of the treatment variables is not experimentally controlled (p. 68).

Consider now some illustrations. Psychiatrists employ the so-called 'rule of three' when giving a prognosis for schizophrenia. One-third of cases are treatable and a cure can be effected; another one-third of cases have little benefit, if any, from treatment but the person's mental health status is reasonably stable; lastly, one-third of cases have an extremely poor prognosis with the person's condition deteriorating seriously and treatment mostly quite ineffective.

In regard to the first one-third of cases, a period of hospitalisation (with its complex mix of inputs) precedes recovery and is known to play a vital role in alleviating the symptoms of the case and eventually effecting a cure. The hospitalisation input in the production function will therefore be statistically significant, other factors held constant, and the mental health production function may be highly elastic with respect to the range of inputs jointly provided by a hospital. For the other two-thirds of cases of schizophrenia, however, quite a different outcome results. The second third of the cases suffer recurring episodes of schizophrenia, in spite of treatment. The last third of the cases are virtually untreatable. In spite of the untreatability, repeated applications of inputs may occur with these cases: continuous medication; and/or regular medical or clinic visits year after year; and/or prolonged hospitalisation. While the application of these inputs may sometimes alleviate the severity of the condition, in most instances relatively little change at all occurs, the outcome being, rather, that some satisfaction is gained in having the condition supervised. In the second one-third of cases, hospitalisation may be a statistically significant variable, but the mental health production function with respect to hospitalisation is relatively inelastic. In the last one-third of cases, mental health care inputs in the production function (bundled into 'hospitalisation') would be expected to be statistically insignificant, although the definition of efficacious treatment may, in the process of failed outcomes, become subtly reduced to 'supervision'.

In an era of deinstitutionalisation, it is an empirical matter to establish whether the substitution of out-patient inputs for in-patient inputs (which *a priori* reduces costs) produces the same, higher or lower mental health status. Results of some empirical studies of deinstitutionalisation are discussed again in the literature review in the next chapter. However, these studies have not applied the economic theory of production.

Finally, in some conditions or instances of mental illness, an explanatory variable can be negative and significant, for example, where mental health status deteriorates once an individual is institutionalised. For example, some institutions are iatrogenic in providing care for individuals with dementia.

Regarding severe cases of people with a mental illness, where individuals are a threat to themselves or to others, then an externality is present. Lengthy institutionalisation may be the only input thought relevant for dealing with the problem. Where it has been legally deemed best to remove the individual's freedom and to support that person's life inside an institution, then the input is likely to be statistically significant. Note, though, that mental health care is the output of the joint production of at least two 'bundled' inputs, namely, 'loss of freedom' and 'treatment'. For further discussion of jointness in production in mental health care, see Chapter 9.

Many instances are thought to exist of individuals who are imprisoned for a minor crime, but a mental disorder goes undiagnosed. The prevalence is difficult to quantify (Human Rights and Equal Opportunity Commission, 1993, Ch. 25). Once in prison, treatment needs are seldom addressed properly and in such cases, year after year of prison life or repeated imprisonment is to little avail, certainly doing nothing to improve mental health status. With even the most basic treatment, prolonged deprivation of freedom may not be needed at all, but many such individuals are too disabled by their condition to advocate mental health care for themselves whilst in prison.

This brief discussion of the application of the economic theory of production in the context of mental illnesses and disorders is hypothetical, in the sense that such studies, with two notable exceptions (above), have not been undertaken. Health production functions have been estimated not only for the general population (Auster, Leveson and Saracheck, 1969; Newhouse and Friedlander, 1980; and Ettner, 1996) but also for specific groups, e.g. children (Corman, Joyce and Grossman, 1987; Bishai, 1996) and the elderly (Hadley, 1982; Hadley, 1988). For a recent review of the health production function literature, see Connelly and Doessel (2000). It needs to be said, however, that the sub-group of the population suffering mental illnesses and disorders has not been extensively examined using this technique, which is but one of the tools in the economist's tool-kit. The problems of defining the health status output measure, and the relevant inputs, and of having the relevant data, are formidable obstacles that contribute to this lacuna. The conceptual and practical problems of undertaking such studies are not easily overcome.

Conclusion

Economists know well that, in all industries in the economy, the assumptions that make Pareto optimality achievable are not conditions that can be attained. For various reasons, markets are not perfect, externalities abound, some goods are public in nature, information is limited and asymmetric, and prices are not set to marginal costs.

The model of perfect competition depicted briefly in this Chapter is a theoretical construct, and the discussions that have ensued out of that model represent only one aspect of health care. In this Chapter, consideration has been given to the standard conditions known to result in Pareto efficiency; to some of the main factors thought to be inhibiting the attainment of that state in mental health care; and to some more general economic issues that arise in the economic analysis of mental health care. Conceptual and practical problems are likely to be more intractable in the analysis of mental health than in health care generally.

Appendix 3.1

Differences between Mental and Physical Illnesses

The purpose of this Appendix is to illustrate in a stark fashion the differences in services confronting people with mental illnesses compared with those with a physical illness.

Consider a fictitious character, person M. In the illustration that follows, a contrast is made between the services for individuals who have an illness that is well-served by health care and those for an illness that is not well-served by health care. To achieve this contrast, let person M's affliction first be heart disease. Having considered the nature of consumer preferences with heart disease, then let person M's affliction be mental illness, not heart disease.

In the normal course of dealing with heart disease, the availability of suitable goods and services would enable person M to:

a. admit and accept that he/she has heart disease;

b. identify, with professional guidance, the limitations that heart disease places on his/her life, for example, through realising the importance of the need to change diet, not to smoke, to have regular exercise such as daily walks, and to avoid stress;

c. take responsibility for making some necessary changes such as

  i. employing the help he/she needs;
  ii. having regular check-ups with a physician (probably subsidised by government);
  iii. undergoing bypass surgery, for example (probably subsidised by public or private health funds);
  iv. making other necessary changes like eating foods recommended by nutritionists and dieticians, and walking or exercising regularly;
  v. making the best of life, even though Person M has heart disease, by bringing pleasure to his/her own life and to others.

Now let Person M instead have schizophrenia. If similarly suitable goods and services were provided, Person M would:

a. admit, accept and live openly with schizophrenia, assisted by professional guidance;

b. identify the limitations that it places on his/her life in order to live within these;

c. take responsibility, with help and guidance, for making the necessary changes such as

  i. employing the necessary help (subject to the availability of public or private funds). For example, it may be necessary for there to be a formal arrangement where Person M can employ the services of people to give him/her domestic support when his/her thinking patterns do not enable him/her to cope with daily living;

ii. making his/her own changes where possible;

iii. adopting an appropriate attitude to his/her own life, and to others;

iv. making the best of life, even though person M has schizophrenia, by bringing pleasure to his/her own life, and to others.

Are goods and services for chronic mental illness and disorder enabling such facility for living? Some successes are documented. However, living with constant inability to access what is needed to cope with life with a mental disorder must be, for all who are involved, like a paraplegic living in an economy where a wheelchair cannot be acquired.

This list above of supports for living, when compared with what is actually the situation with mental illness, highlights the contrast with physical illness. When the lack of availability of support is recognised, the contrast is obvious. Clinicians and service providers would mostly be aware of this problem but let others (including economists) also be aware.

4 A Survey of the Economics of Mental Health Care

Introduction

The economic nature of the outputs of mental health care is fundamentally important. Often it is implied, though seldom actually acknowledged, in the literature that little is known about the outputs. The issue has been present throughout the upsurge of economic research into mental health care for three decades, but, as yet, much is unresolved about the economics of the outputs.

A significant proportion of the literature on mental health care and economics originated in the United States (US), with research largely focussing on public policy concerns. There is virtually no Australian literature on the economics of mental health and mental health care. Most policy decisions over the use of mental health care resources in Australia are, therefore, made in ignorance of information on consumer behaviour and producer behaviour, and on the relative efficiency of alternative types of therapies and treatment settings.

The work undertaken in this Chapter suggests a place for this study within the literature. This Chapter is concerned also with identifying some 'pegs' upon which to 'hang', or classify conceptually, the insights derived from the progress of knowledge. The sub-specialty of economics and mental health care is now very broad and yet, in terms of the purpose of the present work, the prior literature available for this study is limited.

It is relevant to observe that, in spite of this Chapter being called a survey, that term has a somewhat limited meaning in the present context. At various points in this book, i.e. not only in the survey chapter, there are discussions of more recently-raised issues of an economic nature which now form part of the literature. As an illustration, recently, economists working at the coal-face of mental health care have addressed several tasks: they have considered the definition of the output of mental health services; they have analysed the prices of those outputs through time; and, hence, they have raised issues in regard to the productivity of mental health care. In this book, these three inter-related issues (outputs, prices and productivity) are, for example, considered also in Chapters 5 and 11, and in somewhat greater detail than they are in this survey Chapter. While the contents of this Chapter may have appropriately been described some years ago as a survey, such a description has rapidly become rather limited. That this is the case is a comment on the extent to which the issues addressed in the economics of mental health now are multitudinous.

Historical Forces

The account of the expansion in the US of studies concerned with economics and mental health care, as recounted by McGuire (1990, 1992), is briefly retold here as background, since much of the available literature is not Australian.

The impetus for the economic analysis of mental health care in the US came in the late 1970s when President Jimmy Carter formed the President's Commission on Mental Health. The terms of reference of the Commission were 'to review the mental health needs of the Nation and to make recommendations to the President as to how the Nation might best suit those needs.' Of the thirty-five task groups created, only one relied on economic analysis, and this panel was formed to consider 'the cost and financing of mental health'. Of the fourteen people on this panel, McGuire notes that only two were economists. While both panellists were 'senior public policy/health economists', neither was actively involved in research in the economics of mental health.

McGuire acknowledges the limitations in the scope of the report of the above-mentioned panel, since practically no research literature was available. The small number of publications to that date had examined one small component of economic concerns, namely, the financial loss due to the illness (e.g. Fein, 1958; Rice, 1966, cited in Conley *et al.*, 1967).

In the late 1970s, the National Institute of Mental Health (NIMH) in the US began fostering a sub-specialty (now) called economics and mental health. By the early 1980s, the NIMH sponsored biennial conferences on economics and mental health care. During the 1980s its Research Program had three components: demand and supply issues; prospective payment studies; and assessments of the impacts of managed care and alternative delivery systems in providing cost-effective care. In 1985, the NIMH announced its invitation for research on reimbursement issues, an initiation which continues (Rupp, 1996, cited in Moscarelli, Rupp and Sartorius, 1996). Indeed, because of its strategic importance, many of the economic issues under study are thought to be due to the NIMH (McGuire, 1990).

The 1997 special issue of *Administration and Policy in Mental Health* was devoted entirely to mental health economics. The Guest Editors' Introduction makes several remarks that summarise the emphases in present topics under study (Frank and McGuire, 1997). Observing (in regard to the US) the 'expanded reliance on market mechanisms to allocate mental health resources, privatization of formerly government functions and the application of incentive schemes to influence behavior of providers and managers of mental health services', Frank and McGuire note that 'concern for cost remains a driving force' and that '[while] all the evidence is not yet in, in principle, and partially in fact, managed care with its attendant privatization and new forms of contracting gives new options to policymakers' (p. 275).

Internationally, endeavours are occurring within the mental health division of the World Health Organization (WHO). Its task is to develop multinational initiatives on mental health policy and care that take into account the use of economic information (Gulbinat *et al.*, 1996). The WHO is directing attention to policy development in mental health care in both developed and developing countries. For a comprehensive handbook of the breadth of international studies that come under an umbrella called 'mental health economics', see Moscarelli, Rupp and Sartorius (1996).

In Australia the purpose of the National Mental Health Strategy, adopted in 1992, is to address the need for reform of the mental health care system. Twelve 'priority areas for reform under the National Mental Health Strategy' are defined, as follows: consumer rights; the relationship between mental health services and general health services; linking mental health services with other sectors; service mix; promotion and prevention; primary care services; carers and non-government organizations; mental health workforce; legislation; research and evaluation; standards; monitoring and accountability (Mental Health Branch, Commonwealth Department of Health and Aged Care, 1998, p. 2 and Appendix 13).

Although funding issues and economic behaviour in mental health care have implications for several, if not most, of those priority areas, the design of funding itself is not counted as a direct concern. Put otherwise, the National Mental Health Strategy does not identify issues of funding and economic behaviour as a separate area of priority. Moreover, no studies into any aspect of economic behaviour that arises with mental health care are funded by the Mental Health Grants of the National Mental Health Strategy (Mental Health Branch, Commonwealth Department of Health and Family Services, 1997, Appendix 11).

Economic Studies of Mental Health Care and of the Outputs

Several surveys (Taube and Burns, 1988; McGuire, 1990; McGuire, 1992; Frank and McGuire, 1999) indicate some of the existing economic dimensions of mental health care.

Cost of Illness Studies

The earliest work of an economic nature undertaken with respect to mental illness was the estimation of the cost of illness (Fein, 1958). Cost of illness studies measure direct illness costs (involving payments being made) due to medical and hospital care services, as well as indirect costs (involving resources being lost) due to reduced productivity, estimated by earnings foregone. However, the term burden of illness is also currently in use because present estimates try to consider all social and economic costs of illness.

Broadly speaking, the emphasis in the literature concerning burden of illness studies is on the measurement problems that arise in achieving reliable estimates of the costs, or financial losses, of mental illness for each diagnostic category (and, subsequently, for mental illness in total). The problems addressed in that literature include: counting the full range of costs correctly; taking account of overlapping costs that arise with co-morbidity; estimating offset effects; and estimating losses due to the difficult measurement problems arising with the so-called family burden of mental illness.

It is instructive to note that, in this literature, subsequent to the common beginnings in Fein's study, two subsequent origins are recognised, and the presence of this produces some variation in illness cost estimates. There is a group of studies in the *genre* of Dorothy Rice and colleagues at the National Center for Health Statistics, that originated with Rice (1966, cited in Conley *et al.*, 1967), the latest study being Hodgson and Cohen (1998, cited in Triplett, 1999). Another group of studies originated from Levine and Levine (1975) and the (now) Research Triangle Institute. In this *genre* are the studies of Frank and Kamlet (1985), Parsons *et al.* (1980) and Mark *et al.* (1998) (condensed as McKusick *et al.*, 1998) (all cited in Triplett, 1999) and others. The latter group provides higher estimates of expenditures for treatment of mental illness than the former (although, Triplett notes, that the variation may not be due entirely to different methodology).

Let us focus now on the key measurement issues addressed in the cost of illness literature. Recent studies (e.g. those cited in Triplett, 1999, some of which are listed above; also Rice, Kelman *et al.*, 1990, cited in Frank and McGuire, 1999; and Rice and Miller, 1993) take a wider range of costs into account than was the case with the earlier cost of illness studies of mental illness. Recent studies incorporate indirect cost estimates of reduced or lost productivity, and also mortality cost estimation, i.e. the value of lost productivity due to premature deaths, as well as estimation of the value of time spent on care by family members. Other direct costs include public and private expenditures related to the co-incidence of crime as well as the administrative costs of social welfare programs.

Estimating the resources used in treating mental illnesses is complicated. The estimation of at least two of the indirect costs is difficult. First, co-morbidity of mental illnesses with other conditions increases the cost of treatment (Rice and Kelman, 1989). One of the most common co-morbidities with mental illnesses is substance abuse, including alcoholism. This is estimated by Goodman, Nishiura and Hankin (1995, cited in Folland, Goodman and Stano, 1997, p. 585). In the presence of co-morbidity, offset effects occur. Offset effects arise when the use of psychiatric services correlates, mostly positively, with a reduced use of medical services (Kessler *et al.*, 1982; Goodman, 1989). The present estimation work of the offset effect faces some measurement difficulties. These are considered by Wells and Sturm (1995). Note that some of the limitations are associated with definitional problems with the output of treatment episodes. Frank and McGuire (1995) also argue that the issue with offset effects is that if, for example, coverage for psychotherapy is increased, the question, then, is how much more offset will there be. The evidence for offset effects is weak but the estimation of offset effects has been in regard to initial treatment, not marginal treatment. According to Frank and McGuire, '[t]he estimates of health reform costs disregarded marginal offsets, which was probably the right thing to do' (Frank and McGuire, 1995, p. 112).

One other co-morbidity effect about which little is known occurs where individuals with mental illness are unable to organise themselves enough to seek medical help for their physical illnesses, let alone seek help with their psychiatric condition. To the extent that this occurs, studies of the financial losses due to mental illness underestimate treatment costs.

During the 1990s, an important advance occurred in studying a second indirect cost effect of financial loss due to illness: estimation of family costs. Estimation of the family burden of mental illnesses, i.e. the pain and suffering endured by patients, their families and friends (Rice and Miller, 1996), adds a further difficulty to estimating the burden of mental illness. The most comprehensive empirical study at present is Franks (1990).[1]

With the improved accuracy of illness burden estimation, some segments of the population perceive a political use of these monetary measurements of financial loss from illnesses/conditions. Protagonists of the cause of mental health see such estimates as assisting the political process of allocating the appropriate expenditure levels across the spectrum of all illnesses and conditions. Estimating financial loss due to illness is said to be 'a vital link between clinical care and political decisions', e.g. to place in order of priority expenditures on disease categories (Muller and Caton, 1983, pp. 93, 94). At one level, such a statement about the political process is true. On the other hand, though, the issues faced by government range widely; and cost of illness estimates of the impact of complex conditions like mental illness are not enough in themselves to inform the political process. In the absence of better knowledge about the wider issues, decision-making by government, therefore, suffers a 'disability'. The Sub-sections following discuss some of these other issues.

---

1 There is another aspect of family burden. This involves studies of the factors that determine the supply of informal care (i.e. including care by family and friends). See, for example, Knapp, Beecham *et al.*, (1994), Tessler and Gamache (1994) and Holmes and Deb (1998). For one discussion about services for families of people with schizophrenia, see Dixon (1999).

Financing Mental Health Care

From the 1960s and 1970s, a new approach was being taken in research, involving new topics and different types of empirical approaches and studies. The impetus was found in the study of **economic behaviour** associated with mental illnesses and the delivery of services. This new approach is the hallmark of the 'new' economics of mental health care.

The single theoretical issue redirecting the work initially was the effect of insurance coverage upon demand for mental health care and upon mental health expenditures. This arose largely from the seminal work of Arrow (1963a), outlined in the previous Chapter.

Information asymmetries pervade financing and reimbursement in mental health care. Indeed, two information asymmetries, in particular, 'hit mental health markets with special force' (Frank and McGuire, 1999). The **level of probability of loss** due to a particular individual's condition is often unknown to the insurer; as well, there are situations where **the actual loss in real income or well-being experienced by the sick person is unknown** (Pauly, 1986). The former, namely, adverse selection, is the much-studied phenomenon whereby purchasers of insurance know better than insurers *ex ante* the probability of their falling ill. The latter is moral hazard. According to Arrow (1985), the essential problem with moral hazard is that particular economic actions, 'hidden actions', cannot be observed accurately, but information on these is needed in order to develop (first-best) efficient contracts. In practice, this means that providing better coverage, i.e. lowering the price for the patient, increases the quantity demanded of the service. Adverse selection or 'hidden knowledge' arises when a party to a contract hides information with guile, or else when access to information is limited. In practice in health insurance, this means that, given utility-maximising individuals, those policy-holders who are more likely to use benefits will choose better coverage and those less likely to use benefits will pay lower rates, while profit-maximising insurers would prefer to have a relatively large proportion of policy-holders being less likely to use benefits.

The problems of correcting the inefficiencies due to moral hazard and adverse selection in health care generally (and it seems more so in mental health care) are immense, and will be discussed briefly again in the next Sub-section. The economic approach to these problems is that, while moral hazard and adverse selection are not necessarily 'correctable inefficiencies', inefficiency from 'excessive' moral hazard and adverse selection (excessive in reference to the opportunity cost of alternative policy responses) is not a trivial matter (Pauly, 1983, 1986).

Pauly (1968) and Zeckhauser (1970) showed that relatively more cost-sharing, i.e. a higher patient co-payment, is necessary in services where the own-price elasticity of demand of that service is higher than for services generally. They showed that cost-sharing should offset the gains from risk protection against the losses from moral hazard. Until the early 1980s in the US, the degree of cost-sharing in mental health care via insurance coverage which was needed to attain economic efficiency was still of an unknown magnitude.

Evidence became available early in the 1980s of the reluctance of private insurers to cover mental illnesses adequately, due to adverse selection and moral hazard (Sharfstein and Taube, 1982). Shortly after, an important empirical matter was established. It was shown that the own-price elasticity of demand for mental health care is greater, particularly for out-patient services for which adequate data are available, than for other health services (Manning and Newhouse *et al.*, 1987; Keeler, Manning and Wells, 1988; McGuire, 1989b). What became very clear from this research is that broadening insurance cover to include mental health care results in immense problems of economic efficiency. This is demonstrated by simultaneously occurring over-insurance and under-insurance, as happens with moral hazard and adverse selection (McGuire, 1989b; Ma and McGuire, 1997; Frank and McGuire, 1998).

Numerous empirical studies have been undertaken concerning these fundamental efficiency problems in the insurance arrangements for mental health care. Some of these are broadly reported below. First, some findings about the economics of financing and reimbursement arrangements are reviewed. Empirical findings about other specific demand and supply issues are then addressed.

Financing and reimbursement issues The above-mentioned studies and policy responses that arose from the recognition of missing markets and market failures are reviewed briefly here. Before turning to these matters, a comment by Mark Pauly (1986), following, provides a context for the thrust of what is to be discussed in this Section. Pauly noted the following observations, just prior to the explosion in the 1990s of schemes in the US for financing and reimbursement in mental health care, which seek to reduce 'excessive' moral hazard and adverse selection:

> It is, however, remarkable that the major thrust of Arrow's article (1963) did not stimulate much subsequent work. His major point was that many of the peculiar aspects of the medical care sector – not only the existence of insurance but its form, not only the licensure of providers but their proposed deviations from profit-maximising behaviour – can be explained as public and private institutional substitutes for the absence of a competitive market insuring against all uncertainties. There has been little attempt to elaborate on this proposition, and little empirical testing. The empirical question of whether *new* or *additional* steps could be taken to repair the failure of markets to provide for risk has also been largely dormant although ... some recent work on ... the behaviour of physicians as agent may be interpreted this way (Pauly, 1986, p. 631).

This comment accentuates the changes occurring under an umbrella called 'managed care', an approach which has been rising in relative importance within schemes for financing and reimbursement of mental health care since Pauly's comment. Some of these changes are reviewed below. The comment also anticipates a recent study by Ma and McGuire (1997) which points to the need for theory that is adequate to address the complex contractual arrangements presently flourishing in the US insurance industry. Note that although Australia's system of financing and reimbursement of mental health care differs markedly from that in the US, a broad understanding of the issues of financing and reimbursement of mental health care is extremely useful.

Arrow's 1963 paper produced a stream of empirical studies. These were mainly concerned with schemes where mental health care was being reimbursed through a fee-for-service system. Recall here some basic principles of economic behaviour. The conventional model underlying insurance coverage for fee-for-service medicine is that the interaction of demand and supply for mental health services determines the level of service use. An estimated consumer demand curve therefore is useful because it provides predictions about levels of service use, in the presence of given variations in out-of-pocket expenses that are levied by insurers and are incurred by consumers.

The earliest econometric studies of this model (McGuire, 1981; Horgan, 1986; Taube, Kessler and Burns, 1986; Watts, Scheffler and Jewell, 1986, in regard to out-patient care; and Scheffler and Watts, 1986, in regard to in-patient care) investigated demand responses to various co-payment (or 'cost-sharing') arrangements. The studies showed that the own-price elasticity of demand for these mental health services is relatively price inelastic, but the own-price elasticities are higher in absolute value than the estimates for general health care services.

In the earlier studies such as those mentioned in the previous paragraph, a simplifying assumption was that consumers face a single insurance price. More recent studies incorporate greater complexity. Present econometric models incorporate, for example, more realistic assumptions about pricing, acknowledging that consumers face 'pricing blocks' such as a deductible, a region of co-insurance and a region of higher uncovered pricing (e.g. Manning and Frank, 1992). Another important assumption relates to incorporating demand responses where expectations about price exist. These are addressed in Ellis and McGuire (1986), for example, where the model bases consumers' spending decisions on their 'expected' end-of-year price. Keeler, Manning and Wells (1988) also incorporate a price expectation. Improved data collection, such as that enabled by the Rand Health Insurance Experiment, is discussed in several studies (e.g. Keeler, Manning and Wells, 1988; Newhouse *et al.*, 1994).

The available evidence in all the studies, both the earlier ones and the more recent ones, indicates the presence of relatively higher price elasticities of demand for out-patient mental health care, i.e. relative to general medical services. The results also indicate that the demand for mental health visits is relatively responsive to price changes in all but the highest income groups (Frank and McGuire, 1986; Watts, Scheffler and Jewell, 1986).

The magnitudes of the own-price elasticity of demand vary across the studies. A partial summary is given in Table 4.1 below. For a discussion of these magnitudes, see Frank and McGuire (1999).

Table 4.1 Variations in the magnitude of the price elasticity of the demand for mental health care/substance abuse (MH/SA) and for (general) health care reported in five studies

Study	Type of Elasticity	MH/SA Estimates	Health Care Estimates
McGuire (1981)	Point	-1.00	
Taube *et al.* (1986)	Point (level of use)	-0.54	-0.13
Horgan (1986)	Point (level of use)	-0.44	-0.16
Ellis and McGuire (1986)	Point (level of use)	-0.37	
Manning *et al.* (1989)	Arc	-0.80	-0.30

Source: Frank and McGuire, 1999, Table 3, p. 86.

According to Pauly (1968), discussed above, and Zeckhauser (1970), a relatively high elasticity implies that insurance for mental health care requires higher levels of cost sharing, particularly for out-patient services, than that for medical services generally. This is an important policy implication. The main conclusion is that, in the presence of insurance schemes where reimbursement is through fee-for-service, the occurrence of moral hazard and adverse selection causes expenditures upon mental health care to be very high while, simultaneously, people with mental illnesses mostly remain relatively under-insured.

In contrast to this policy implication is another highly influential notion about financing policy. Mental health care is approached from another perspective by advocates of fairness for sufferers of mental illness. Such advocates exert pressure to have an issue addressed that, they argue, is a higher need than the economic fundamental of cost-sharing, just noted above. For nearly two decades now, 'parity' in insurance coverage for mental health care has been advocated by some. For recent comments, see Hanson (1998), Mechanic (1998) and Szasz (1998), for example. Parity refers to a contention that the insurance benefit paid for mental health care should be equal to that paid for general health services. Parity gives rise to important efficiency consequences. These differ with different types of financing arrangements for mental health care such as managed care, discussed below, as opposed to insurance coverage for fee-for-service medicine (Frank and McGuire, 1998).

In the light of all the policy issues just mentioned, various problems with demand-side cost-sharing were discussed again throughout the 1990s. Rice (1992) argued that there are at least two qualifications to the conventional model: the possibility that providers also determine service use, to a degree; and the possibility that consumers may be less rational than the model assumes them to be.

Consider also that for over a decade now, it has been established empirically that the demand for mental health care is not uniform. Variations in mental health services occur for different sub-groups of the population, other than income groups (Horgan, 1986; Taube *et al.*, 1986; Wallen, Roddy and Meyers, 1986).

Frank and McGuire (1999) approach non-uniform demand from another angle, explaining various difficulties with interpreting the conventional notion in economics of 'demand' with respect to mental health care:

> The normative interpretation of mental health care demand ... has long been problematic. Long standing issues of asymmetric information and imperfect agency relationships that were noted in the early study of health care markets (Arrow, 1963) temper the normative interpretation of all health care demand schedules as marginal benefit schedules. The demand for mental health care has a special set of constraints upon consumer information. Demand for mental health services may be influenced by fear of stigma, Veblen's 'bandwagon' effects (McGuire, 1981) and unclear information about efficacy of specific treatments. In addition, many mental disorders affect the capacity of individuals to make decisions in their own best interests (Rubin, 1978). For these illnesses, placing a strong normative interpretation on observed demand behavior is unlikely to be justified (Frank and McGuire, 1999, p. 33).

'Managed care' was brought to the forefront of attention in the 1980s and 1990s (Frank, McGuire and Newhouse, 1995). Managed care is an alternative set of social institutions for addressing the rationing problems associated with coverage for privately provided mental health services. 'Health plans' involve more than an insurance policy; providers are paid upon meeting particular terms of treatment. With managed care, the essential notion is to minimise moral hazard by rationing care in ways **other** than 'demand-side cost sharing' which, in practice in the past, has meant making adjustments to the price faced by the consumer.

Various administrative arrangements that address moral hazard are implemented by managed care organisations. Mostly, they involve: selecting a network of mental health care providers; defining a population of enrolees; developing clinical criteria that define the levels of care to which enrolees are directed; determining contractual financial incentives for providers in order to limit care, as well as giving feedback to providers about their own treatment patterns, their peers' and the pattern for the 'clinical norm'; and determining 'medical necessity' for defining the need for, and the benefits of, treatment for each level of care (Frank and McGuire, 1999).

There are, of course, many 'other ways' of rationing within managed care. However, economically speaking, they all ultimately reduce to administrative arrangements, developed by a managed care organisation, which involve variations on either price rationing, or quantity rationing, or quality rationing, or trade-offs among these.[2] The types of managed care, from an economic viewpoint, are summarised elsewhere. See Enthoven (1988) and, in the context of mental health, Frank and McGuire (1999).

---

2 Quality variations are conceptualised here as variations in the quantities of characteristics in a product.

Harrow and Ellis (1992) address the existence of variations in provider behaviour in the presence of different reimbursement systems. The results estimate the effect of reimbursement policies on in-patient length-of-stay, as well as the magnitude of that effect, and the effect of reimbursement policies on frequency of out-patient visits. See also Frank and Lave (1986). As with insurance coverage for fee-for-service medicine, one implication of the rationing devices used in managed care is that distortions are likely from adverse selection (Cutler and Zeckhauser, 1998). Profit-maximising managed care organisations are likely to provide services that encourage 'good risks' and dissuade 'bad risks' within the insurance pool. Since mental health care often involves long-term treatment, thereby incurring high costs, it is likely that profit-maximising managed care organisations will under-provide mental health services.

In the 1990s, a special feature of mental health care benefits is that the benefits are being 'carved out'. This means that health insurers subcontract benefits for mental health care where it is possible to disaggregate diagnoses into categories of services consumed. Separate contracting, or carving out, is therefore possible at least in principle, for the management of the risk of the expenses incurred by psychiatric treatment, although the transaction costs of the sub-contracting process are unlikely to be negligible (Frank, Goldman and McGuire, 1992; Frank, McGuire and Newhouse, 1995; Frank, Huskampf, McGuire and Newhouse, 1997).

The welfare implications of managed care and of insurance for fee-for-service medicine are immense, and these cannot be addressed here. For an overview, see Frank and McGuire (1999).

Note briefly some final points. First, mention has been made already that the efficiency consequences of parity under managed care are different from those encountered by insuring for fee-for-service payment in mental health care (Frank and McGuire, 1998).

Second, an estimation is yet to be undertaken of the welfare loss associated with moral hazard, as a per cent of Gross Domestic Product, under both types of institutional funding arrangements.

Third, the range of services, other than treatment, that are needed to support people with mental disorders is another dimension of financing. How broadly should the benefit range in order to cover the risk of the full extent of expenses being incurred due to a mental illness? The needs of individuals with serious mental illness include housing, social services and so on. To the extent that services associated with mental illness incur costs that are insurable risks, then financing and reimbursement together need to be designed to provide better coverage for mental illnesses (Arons and Frank, 1993).

Fourth, note that because a group of people suffering mental illnesses and disorders goes untreated, then most health care systems address 'access to care' as one of the goals for improvement in the system. In the light of the above discussions, though, it is important to note that lack of treatment is assumed to be an 'access' problem. There is a misconception here, namely, that increasing the supply of practitioners or reducing the price will improve access to care. The preceding discussions have shown that increasing the supply of medical practitioners in order to solve the co-existing problems of under-treatment for some and over-treatment for others is likely to have limited success.

Fifth, in spite of the greater level of understanding of the efficiency problems arising in each of the various approaches to reimbursement, a range of complex contractual arrangements has evolved in the US. It would appear that the conventional theoretical view, based on the idea of a trade-off between moral hazard and risk, has become far from adequate (Ma and McGuire, 1997). Ma and McGuire argue, moreover, that other markets are also missing in mental health care financing. One such market is medical practitioners' input of effort which is, at the margin, non-contractible. Effort, as an economic phenomenon, can behave in a manner after the 'hidden action', previously discussed in this Section, which has efficiency implications. Ma and McGuire also note that insurance payments for treatment are based on reports of, or claims about, treatment, not on the actual treatment itself (its quantity and quality). Because the actual quantity of treatment is difficult to verify, a degree of under-reporting of the diagnosis/treatment will occur, whether there is co-payment or a capitation contract. Contractual arrangements to ensure truthful reporting are modelled. Of course, the social institutions embedded within such modelling in the US are quite a different approach from Mishan's (1981) notion of the 'virtual constitution' to addressing the ethical outcome.

Lastly, given the need for improving the ways that mental health care is financed, incentives should be structured in order to encourage socially desirable outcomes/outputs. See Dickey and Cohen (1993). McGuire and Riordan (1993) present one study of the crucial issues behind engaging the (community) provider to serve the public interest in contracting for community-based, public mental health services. The incentives of the financing system partly determine outcomes. Adequate services for the seriously mentally ill are a major responsibility of government, and such matters are conceptualised in later Chapters.

Other economic behaviour issues Present studies involving either supply issues or demand issues make assumptions, either implicitly or explicitly, about the nature of the outputs, assumptions which often have had to be made because of urgently needed empirical results for policy-making. Another issue arising from Arrow's seminal work is that insurance schemes attain first-best efficiency when based on health outcomes. While the notion of an 'episode of care' has subsequently become important, this notion also is far from adequate, given the heterogeneity of mental health care, examined in Chapter 2.

For example, with particular purposes such as prospective payment (Goldman *et al.*, 1987; Keeler, Manning and Wells, 1988) for cure, the treatment episode is the appropriate unit of treatment output. However, attaching predictions of resource costs to diagnosis/treatment/care of psychiatric illness is fraught with difficulty. Diagnosis-Related Groups (DRGs) are known now to be an unreliable predictor of treatment costs (e.g. Taube, Lee and Forthofer, 1984). For an overview of the problems of prospective payments for in-patient treatment and care based on DRGs for psychiatry in the US, see Wallen (1987) and White and Dada (1993). Other methods are being devised to predict resource consumption (e.g. Windle, 1991; Whiteford, Thompson and Casey, 2000, pp. 407-8). In regard to out-patient treatment, Dorwart, Rodriguez and Causino (1993) address methods of determining fees for the services of medical practitioners who treat mental illness. A resource-based relative value scale for psychiatry is provided but the authors point out the pitfalls in the measurement of psychiatric work. One common problem across all approaches is that the relationship between payment systems and the outcomes of mental health care is elusive. This is partly because observation is impossible when the market is missing, and partly also because the heterogeneity of the output is not acknowledged adequately.

Another issue is whether or not public spending on psychiatric hospitals replaces charitable giving towards care for the indigent. Frank and Salkever (1992) find that public psychiatric hospitals tend to increase the total amount of care to indigent people with mental illnesses rather than replace charitable giving.

The substitutability of inputs in the production of mental health services is another important economic issue. The relevant concept for determining the presence, and degree, of substitutability is 'cross-price elasticity' and its measurement. Note that while 'input substitutability' is a specific issue (relevant at several places throughout this study, such as in Chapters 3 and 10), three studies are mentioned here in this Chapter to introduce the approaches to the issue. Deb and Holmes (1998) applied a two-stage demand analysis. First, a consumer makes a decision to seek, or not seek, mental health care. Second, assuming 'yes' to the first question, the consumer then makes a decision whether to see a medically-qualified provider or a non medically-qualified provider. *Inter alia*, their cross-price elasticity estimates indicate that consumers regard the services of these two groups as substitutes. Frank (1985a) estimates the cross-price elasticity of demand for the services of social workers and psychologists compared with psychiatrists. The study indicates that major portions of the services provided by each profession are close substitutes in demand. In an earlier (and contrasting) study, Knesper, Belcher and Cross (1989) compare the practices of psychiatrists and psychologists. They use multiple regression models to explain variations in services by these provider groups.

One other issue in demand studies under insurance is that of the possible differences in the nature of the outputs of treatment under public insurance systems and private insurance systems. Implications from such studies are likely for Australia's mental health care system, and elsewhere, as shown by the next study to be considered. During the period of comprehensive national health insurance in Canada studied by D'Arcy *et al.* (1981), the rate of health care utilisation for psychiatric conditions increased by 49 per cent. Most persons had conditions diagnosed and treated by General Practitioners (GPs) rather than by private psychiatrists or the public outpatient sector. Sixty-five per cent of persons whose conditions were diagnosed by GPs had neuroses, compared with 31 per cent of those whose conditions were diagnosed by private psychiatrists. Personality and behaviour disorders were the largest diagnostic category among public sector outpatients. More than 60 per cent of patients hospitalised during the six-year study period were diagnosed with one of the psychoses, compared with 37 per cent of patients hospitalised in the private sector. The public sector accounted for 66 per cent of all psychiatric care costs in 1974, although it treated only 14 per cent of all psychiatric patients. The private sector accounted for 34 per cent of all psychiatric health care costs but treated 93 per cent of patients.[3]

A study of some of the difficulties presented by Canada's universal health insurance system (el-Guebaly *et al.*, 1985) raises other relevant issues for Australia's system of comprehensive health insurance, such as the selectivity of psychotherapists about whom they treat; the length of waiting lists in the public system; and the matter of the 'double allegiance' of therapists to the government and to the patient.

The need to understand the economic, and not just the medical, nature of mental health care outputs has remained an ongoing challenge in the emerging field of mental health care economics. Irrespective of whether research on mental health care relates to the financial burden of the illness, or whether studies are concerned with economic behaviour in mental health care, or, as is addressed below, whether economic evaluation work is to be done, a pervasive concern is how to conceptualise economically the nature of the outputs.

Social Investment Appraisal in Mental Health Care

Alongside the upsurge of interest in the US in the economics of financing mental health care, there has been increasing attention directed to issues surrounding social investment appraisal. Commonly referred to as 'evaluation studies', such work is undertaken across a range of issues that include institutional *versus* community care, in-patient care *versus* out-patient care; treatment in various types of hospitals; various types of treatment for people with schizophrenia or other conditions; nurse therapist treatment *versus* medical or psychiatric treatment of neurosis, to name a few.

Frank (1993) reviews the research in recent decades indicating the particular mental health treatments that are cost-effective. He next considers the issues surrounding how, and whether, such information is applicable to

---

3 The percentages of patients treated in public and in private in-patient facilities do not sum to 100 per cent in the original text.

developing policy about funding that is economically efficient. Frank points out where complexities arise over the nature of the objective functions of agencies that deliver services. This complexity creates difficult funding problems. He also discusses possible explanations, particularly distributional issues overlooked in social investment appraisal studies, for why desirable technologies fail to be adopted by agencies that deliver mental health care.

A review of 91 'economic evaluation' studies in mental health care (Evers, van Wijk and Ament, 1997) concludes with a discussion of the requirements of successful economic evaluation, and a comment that very few economic evaluations are adequately comprehensive or attain sufficient quality. The authors re-emphasise that studies must apply the principles of social investment appraisal, and they also draw attention to additional problems in social investment appraisal of mental health care. First, in the absence of appropriate criteria for defining the illnesses, cost measurement is imprecise. For example, definitions vary over time as to socially acceptable behaviour, and thus as to whether people are diagnosed with, or without, a mental illness. This affects the breadth of costs that are included. Second, data are generally inadequate, not being recorded in a form useful for social investment appraisal. Third, medical difficulties arise in diagnosing a condition reliably. Fourth, in some instances, patients' lack of rationality makes them an inadequate source of personal or clinical data. Fifth, treatment is not always 'proved' effective. Sixth, for an individual the success of treatment can vary over time. Seventh, the use of 'foregone wages' as a measure of productivity loss is not useful when people with psychiatric conditions are often unemployable. Indeed, people often have lost their jobs even before initial diagnosis. Lastly, the estimation of the effects of stigma, criminality, homelessness and any sort of externality is difficult. For a discussion of social investment appraisals within the context of its historical development, see Knapp (1999).

Goodman *et al.* (1994, cited in Folland, Goodman and Stano, 1997) examined substitutability between in-patient and out-patient alcoholism treatments. Insurance claim data from a large American employer-based insurance company were used. Price indices were computed for various treatments and these indices were used to calculate substitution elasticities across differing types and locations of treatment. The best substitute for in-patient alcoholism treatment was found not to be out-patient alcoholism treatment, which is a relatively less costly treatment, but rather in-patient psychiatric treatment. When they compared alcoholism treatment and psychiatric treatment, out-patient psychiatric treatment was found to be a closer substitute for in-patient psychiatric treatment than out-patient treatment for alcoholism as a substitute for in-patient treatment. A caution with these results is that they are specific to this insurance plan. However, the general implication is that potential savings in substituting out-patient care for in-patient care are limited, even though the cost of out-patient care is less, because the two inputs are not close substitutes.

The issue of the substitutability of psychiatric care and general practitioner (GP) care was investigated in regard to the treatment of depression (Wells and Sturm, 1995, also cited in Folland, Goodman and Stano, 1997). The finding emerged that, although substituting GP care for specialist care reduces treatment costs, the health outcomes are worse. The interpretation of such a result is not at all clear, however. While it is likely that the health outcomes are poorer with GP treatment because patients do not receive enough appropriate care during a visit to a GP, the authors caution, on the other hand, against a conclusion that psychiatric care is more efficient. This is because the higher rates of appropriate care from specialist practitioners are accompanied by greater use of ineffective minor tranquillisers and high cost visits.

Three other reviews of evaluation studies (Hu, 1981, cited in Wolff and Helminiak, 1993; Berk, 1982; O'Donnell *et al.*, 1988) draw attention to the absence across the literature of clear and comparable definitions of costs and of complete coverage of the range of costs. The cost-benefit analysis undertaken by Weisbrod, Test and Stein (1980) is a noteworthy example of a study that covers the costs of hospitalisation relatively completely.[4] While the study also valued loss of earnings due to hospitalisation for mental illness, its coverage of family burden and the costs to the community is limited.

A problem in many studies is that the costing of informal care in the community is inadequate. See the problems addressed in comparisons made by Wolff and Helminiak (1993), of four community-based US programs for the seriously mentally ill. Another common problem arises in the economic nature of the outputs that are being costed. For example, a readmission to a hospital may represent something of the nature of the illness itself; it may represent good treatment; or it may indicate that previous treatment produced no output. The implication is that even the use of an appropriate notion such as the episode of care, the notion employed in the important US study estimating the own-price elasticity of demand for out-patient mental health care (Keeler, Manning and Wells, 1988), requires careful qualification. Knowledge is very limited about effective treatment of many psychiatric illnesses.

While studies that evaluate loss of earnings incurred by patients' families, friends or neighbours due to the patients' illness are worthwhile (Berk, 1982), often the definition of the family burden and costs to the community are narrowly estimated (O'Donnell *et al.*, 1988; Goldman, 1983). Such costs as non-market (household) production and travel costs are often overlooked.

The estimation of the cost of care-givers' time in dollar terms usually requires valuing the time lost to household production due to the illness, and applying the expense of hiring a housekeeper to perform the caring tasks in the home (Posnett, 1996). Although such estimation is an important inclusion, current methods are

---

4 However, the difficulties associated with measuring the opportunity cost of capital in this study and the importance of including patient information that is disaggregated by case mix are discussed in Dickey, McGuire *et al.*, (1986).

not entirely satisfactory (Franks, 1990; McGuire, 1992). Time is valuable to people in ways other than earning a living. As well, while voluntary care-givers often are motivated by altruistic reasons, government-provided community care programs that are poorly funded often wear thin the altruism of care-givers. See Chapters 8, 9 and 10 of the present study. O'Donnell *et al.* (1988) conclude that '[u]nless informal care is costed comprehensively there will remain a possibility that community care only appears a more efficient alternative because it transfers part of the burden of care from statutory providers to informal carers ... and so a change in the distribution of costs may be falsely interpreted as a reduction in total costs' (O'Donnell *et al.*, 1988, p. 7).

Before concluding this Sub-section, it should be noted that a survey of the literature evaluating the cost-effectiveness of alternative medications is not undertaken in this study. An example of a recent cost-effectiveness study (as part of a large randomised control trial for the treatment of refractory schizophrenia) in mental health is that of Rosenheck, Cramer, Xu, Grabowski *et al.* (1998). This study, comparing the efficacy of clozapine and haloperidol (in terms of symptoms and side effects) and costs, found that the clozapine treatment, although more expensive was the most cost-effective.

In the health systems of some countries, ways of incorporating both clinical and economic guidelines that promote effective and efficient mental health care are being considered (Mason, Eccles *et al.,* 1999). However, a final comment about the evaluation of mental health care programs is suggested by the conclusion of Rubin (1982) from a study of the problems of method and measurement in comparisons across settings. Rubin places the controversies over evaluation studies in a wider context, noting that 'even as more is learned about the effectiveness and costs of alternative systems of care, there will remain the question of how much noninstitutional and institutional care the taxpaying public desires .... The structure of tomorrow's mental health system will depend on how that question is answered' (Rubin, 1982, p. 754).

Issues of Expenditure Trends, Output, Input Prices and Productivity

There is now a literature addressing issues surrounding the measurement and interpretation of spending trends in mental health care, and the output of mental health care. Other issues are extremely important and relate to input prices and productivity. This literature involves individuals and research groups at several institutions, including the Brookings Institution and the National Bureau of Economic Research.

The focus of the literature is upon medical care generally, i.e. not only mental health care; and there are several strands, addressing some highly inter-related issues. For example, many topics that are presently under study can be observed in the American Economic Association 1998 *American Economic Review: Papers and Proceedings*. In Triplett's (1999c) *Measuring the Prices of Medical Treatment*, there are topics like: the calculation of price indexes, specific to an illness, disease or condition, incorporating also technological, and other quality, improvements in treatment (Frank, Berndt and Busch, 1999); real expenditure trends in health care (Triplett, 1999a); and measuring the output of health care by estimating the willingness to pay for additional insurance when additional coverage for an (expensive) medical innovation is available (Pauly, 1999). See also the papers in Cutler and Berndt (forthcoming).

While the specific findings in this literature are very recent, its conceptual underpinnings (which include publications from the 1960s) involve broadly ranging inputs. For example, the present literature has developed from studies by Griliches (1971) on outputs in the services sector; Reder (1969) on using medical insurance prices to measure quality; Scitovsky's (1964) work on the definition of health output; and Rice's (1966, cited in Conley *et al.*, 1967) work on estimating the economic cost of illness. If one common thread linking this diversity could be discovered, it is likely to be the problem of conceptualising the output in health care. For an overview of the conceptual origins, see Triplett (1999a and 1999b).

Attention will now focus on the main concepts in, and some of the results of, this literature, but note also that in this literature there are several more studies that are relevant to this book, and these are considered in greater detail in the appropriate place in Chapter 5. Given that the two fundamental concerns of this recent literature, *viz.* health expenditure trends and price indexes, are not new, then what is new about this literature? Triplett (1999a, 1999b) and Triplett and Berndt (1999) explain that, in the past, expenditure trends in (mental) health care were, *inter alia*, calculated by determining the prices of particular inputs, such as those involved in medical or hospital provision. Such reporting about organisational units is useful, but this approach does not relate the inputs to the output (which, of course, is the entity that the individual consumes and which has direct effect upon an individual's well-being). It also does not indicate the trend in expenditures upon care and treatment for the illness. Hence, apart from the accounting meaning in these data (with its emphasis on institutional providers, on funding agencies and on the recipients of funding), there is little economic meaning. Data about the outcomes of the health sector are not reported.

By way of contrast, consider the economic approach. This involves finding the incremental change in an outcome, e.g. health status, that is due to a marginal or incremental change in a particular input or inputs, holding constant all other influences on health. When such an amount is established (in real terms), then it is also possible to determine through time the incremental effect upon the output of technological and other quality improvements in an input.

Let us now consider some of the different approaches to this issue which are adopted by various researchers. There are several stages in Triplett (1999b). First, he uses existing estimates of the direct costs of treating illness (i.e. he uses cost of mental illness studies, such as some of those cited in a previous Sub-section, which disaggregate medical expenditure according to the ICD-9 classification). This step provided Triplett with the relevant cost data.

Those cost estimates are the raw data of expenditure trends and it is necessary to separate (spending due to) price movements from (spending on) the output (cost is the unit price of treatments multiplied by quantity of treatment output). In other words, the problem in economic accounting regarding medical care is to be sure that an improvement in medical care is counted as an increase in medical output and is not counted as medical inflation (Triplett, 1999a, p. 238). The solution is to apply relevant illness price indexes to illness costs.[5]

Price indexes for the health sector have undergone enormous transformations during the 1990s. In Triplett (1999b) the applicability of the newly developed Producer Price Indexes (PPI) of the US Bureau of Labor Statistics (BLS) to tracking health expenditure trends is considered.[6] Triplett notes that, in spite of the superiority of the PPI compared with the Consumer Price Index (CPI), the PPI has a major limitation. In illnesses such as depression, where new, efficacious pharmacotherapies enable medication to be substituted for hospital care, then cost of treatment is falling, but the PPI does not reflect this. Two studies by Frank, Berndt and Busch (1998, 1999) about the cost of treating depression provided Triplett with illness-based price indexes. These first price indexes for treating depression are based on prices for the inputs associated with the American Psychiatric Association (APA) guidelines for the treatment of depression.[7] The significance of these price indexes is that they are developed for an illness that has undergone major technological improvements in its pharmacological treatment. Frank, Berndt and Busch's results are important: they report a falling price index for treating depression in the 1991-95 period.[8]

Of course, the Frank, Berndt and Busch price indexes are only for depression and Triplett is concerned with expenditure trends for mental illness generally. With other price indexes not yet developed, Triplett uses what he has available, and so provides two sets of real expenditure growth trends, one with an adjustment based on the ratio of the PPI to the CPI and another with Frank, Berndt and Busch (1998, 1999) indexes. These trends are for four time periods, 1972-80, 1980-85, 1985-90 and 1990-95. See Triplett (1999b, Table 12). In that Table,

5 Note that Triplett (1999a) also provides an analytic framework showing how two previously independent sources of information about health care, *viz*. price indexes for illnesses and cost-effectiveness studies, can be fitted together. Jointly, this framework furthers the data that are available for separating price movements from changes in medical outcomes.

6 Berndt, Cockburn and Griliches (1996) provide strong evidence that the Consumer Price Index has been biased upward in reporting mental health care inflation. The PPI in the US now provides a superior indicator of (and a much lower rate in regard to) mental health care inflation. For further discussion of this point, see Chapter 5.

7 Rather than developing a price index for one treatment, say, psychotherapy, Frank, Berndt and Busch regarded as equivalent all APA guideline treatments that resulted in equal clinical outcomes, and developed a price index accordingly.

8 This result is discussed further in Chapter 5.

Triplett shows that inflation in mental health care has been lower, not higher as has generally been thought, than the CPI since the mid 1980s, and it may even have been negative through the whole period (Triplett, 1999b, p. 49).

Consider the following implications noted by Triplett in regard to his research:

> A great deal of effort has been put into medical care cost containment in the US. The data in table 12 suggest that medical care inflation is not the driving force behind the run-up in medical care costs, at least in mental health care. In the case of mental health care, the aggregate level of services has improved, judging from the best picture that can be assembled from the US aggregate statistics, but the rate of growth of the real quantity of mental health care services has slowed in the post-1990 period of cost containment. If these numbers are anywhere near correct, they suggest that health care cost containment may have social costs – curtailment of health care that has real impacts on health – that are more severe than are generally recognized.
>
> And if the numbers are not correct, or if they need refinement before they can be used to inform public debate (the need for refinement in these estimates is hardly debatable), it is also the case that decisions on health policy are being based on statistical trend estimates that are at least as defective, and probably far more misleading, than the ones developed here (Triplett, 1999b, p. 52).

Note that further refinements to price indexes for depression can be found in Berndt, Bir, Busch *et al.* (2000). In this study, the problem of off-frontier production is addressed (which was not addressed in the earlier studies that considered only APA guideline treatment). What is meant by off-frontier is that, unlike prior analysis, the authors include in this study all consumers, i.e. those who partly, and those who completely, follow the suggested medication. In addition, they obtained expert clinical opinion, using a two-stage Delphi process, to assess outcomes. Ultimately, they obtain Laspeyres, Paasche and Fisher-ideal price indices. Their conclusion is summarised as follows: 'The results ... suggest that incorporating off-frontier treatment variations over time does not materially change findings from previous research on treatment of depression: the cost of treating an episode of depression has fallen from 1991 to 1996' (p. 14). To take account of the possibility that changing patient-mix has caused this result, various hedonic equations are estimated and it is concluded that 'the source of the spending increases [on depression] is volume (quantity) increases, and not price increases' (p. 14).

It should not be thought that these issues are confined to the health sector: similar concerns exist in the analysis of other industries, e.g. retail trade, life insurance, property insurance, electricity generation, etc. Some of these issues have arisen also in the context of the literature on computers and the productivity paradox. For an overview of this voluminous literature, see Diewert, Nakamura and Sharpe (1999), which is an introductory essay to an issue of the *Canadian Journal of Economics* devoted to the theme 'Service Sector Productivity and the Productivity Paradox'. It may be noted in passing that the approach taken in the health sector involves concentrating on the third type of measurement error (mismeasurement of outputs and inputs) highlighted by Diewert and Fox (1999).

Some Unresolved Matters

From time to time, there emerges in the literature explicit identification of the problems of conceptualising the economic nature of the outputs in mental health care. More often, the problems are in the literature as an undercurrent. The case being made in this study is that the economic nature of the outputs is not well understood.

One dimension of measurement difficulties is in valuing and costing the outputs. A matter outlined below may be thought to be 'old hat' by an economist. However, the subsequent debate that occurred in the early 1970s exposed issues that are still heard in the literature.

In 1972 Halpern and Binner of the Fort Logan Mental Health Center, Denver, Colorado, published a paper (Halpern and Binner, 1972) on a technique they developed, Output Value Analysis, for measuring program performance at the Fort Logan Center. The technique took only some of the concepts from cost-benefit analysis but, needless to say, had many difficulties.

In a critique of the study, Robert Arden, Supervisor of Long-Term Economic Forecasting of the American Telephone and Telegraph Company, points out several underlying problems in using the technique as an output measure (Arden, 1979). Arden also re-analysed the data using cost-effectiveness analysis.

In a subsequent debate between Arden and Binner in the 1979 issue of *Administration in Mental Health*, much of the disagreement was over the issues of measurement in regard to the computation of economic productivity, the computation of subjectively valued benefits and comparisons in the use of cost-effectiveness/cost-benefit analysis. However, Arden (1979) takes up a substantive issue with Halpern and Binner. Arden (1979) points out that 'cost-benefit analysis helps to assess the economic efficiency of alternative projects. Measurement of project outputs should include only those items that represent a change in society's output. ... In output value analysis it is not clear that the value of the estimated response is an addition to society's output or a redistribution of that output to patients by way of program treatment so that they may obtain greater pleasure from their lives' (p. 263).

Another unresolved issue is the development of indices that represent treatment outcomes. This area has grown considerably in recent decades. The Rosser index, the Nottingham Health Profile, the Sickness Impact Profile, SF-36 are concerned with health status measurement, and differ according to their purpose. See Maynard (1993). Both the Nottingham Health Profile and SF-36 attempt to grasp the multi-dimensional nature of health outcomes. Other indices such as the Psychiatry Severity of Illness Index (cited in Windle, 1991) predict resource consumption. Neither health status indexes nor resource use indexes are useful if the requirement is to value the outputs. For an overview of the data and techniques required in valuing health outcomes, see Shiell (1997, pp. 9-10).

Yet another dimension of the outputs problem, namely, the complex nature of the production function, was identified early in the 1970s. Romans (1973, cited in Frank, 1981) acknowledged the presence of multi-dimensional outputs and jointness in the production of mental health care, as follows:

> If the alternative methods of achieving the output are perfect substitutes for each other (i.e., one method is not subject to diminishing returns relative to another method), the decision problem comes down to simply choosing the method with least costs per unit of output. However, most production processes are not of this type. Typically, there are numerous methods of production, each subject to diminishing returns, so that least-cost production is a combination of many methods. For example, in the production of mental health services there are many treatment options – individual and group psychiatric counselling of many types, drugs, electro-shock treatment, rest, milieu, etc. The chances are that cost-effective treatment is going to be a *unique* combination of several of these (Romans, 1973, cited in Frank, 1981, p. 167) (emphasis added).[9]

Romans (1973) also correctly emphasises that little is known about the substitutability of inputs in the production of mental health care.

A fourth dimension of the problem of defining the outputs appeared in the mid 1980s, when Frank (1985b) suggested that the design of a mental health rationing system, e.g. an insurance scheme, was affecting the choice of technology. He contrasted two similar populations having different insurance schemes. One scheme encouraged few ambulatory cases and few visits per case; and the other scheme, with different co-payments and deductibles, encouraged many. Frank noted that 'if the outcomes of treatment technologies are unclear, it is impossible to decide which technologies are providing maximum benefits per unit of expenditure' (p. 26).

It has already been noted in this Chapter that Fein (1958), and others subsequently, have quantified a portion of the cost of mental illness by estimating medical and hospital expenditures and productivity losses. The results of studies that estimate the financial loss due to illness are difficult to interpret. What is being produced that causes the very treatment costs which are being aggregated?

---

9 What is interesting is that, without doubt, the combination of several of these inputs is a unique combination for an individual in a particular situation. That is, the appropriate combination is different for different people, and probably not fixed even for the individual because it varies across time and context.

Finally, in regard to evaluation studies, care givers' time is not yet well understood in an economic sense.

From time to time, problems of an essential nature emerge in the mental health care economics literature. Unfortunately, work that attempts to address one of these problems, that is, conceptualising the nature of the outputs, is largely missing. The issue deserves attention at this very time when the entire field of economics and mental health care is burgeoning.

The Outcomes Movement

Having considered from many angles the importance of an economic understanding of the outputs of mental health care, it is useful here in the literature survey to ask whether the so-called 'Outcomes Movement' could shed light on the issue. Such a clarification is necessary because an economic study about outputs may seem at odds, even anachronistic, with some other strands of research. For example, both Health Services Research and epidemiological research use the term, outcomes, and in the 1990s out of the field of Health Services Research arose a new flurry of activity called Outcomes Research.[10] It is from this that The Outcomes Movement has evolved. This Section addresses two questions: 'In which field does a study of outputs belong, and why is little reference made to Health Services Research?'

Initially, the following comment by Phillips and Rosenblatt (1992) is enlightening:

> Some of the major work currently underway in health services research involves the measurement and evaluation of health outcomes. 'Outcomes research' is the new byword, with millions of dollars in research money flowing into this area. Outcomes management, defined by Ellwood (1988, p. 1551) as a 'technology of patient experience designed to help patients, payers, and providers make rational medical care-related choices based on better insight into the effect of these choices on the patient's life', is viewed by many as an important approach to solving our health care system's ills. The traditional measures of outcomes have been mortality and morbidity and, more recently, the resultant benefits/costs (Epstein, 1990). However, increasingly more attention is being placed on the patient satisfaction and quality of life measures... (Phillips and Rosenblatt, 1992, pp. 195-96).

In a recent overview of the achievements and shortcomings of the Outcomes Movement, Shiell (1997) concludes that the Movement 'challenges decision makers to demonstrate the effectiveness of the services they provide (although) the economic perspective on health outcomes, described here, poses a yet bigger challenge. Decision makers must demonstrate not only what they

---

[10] For a review of three books from within the Outcomes Movement, see Salzer (1999) which appeared in the first issue of the journal, *Mental Health Services Research.*

have achieved but must also show that what has been achieved is what is valued most highly by those who benefit and those who must pay' (p. 13).

Out of the Movement, particularly over the last decades, has grown interest in the development of indexes that represent treatment outcomes. However, as explained previously in this Chapter, neither a health status index nor a resource use index is applicable if the requirement is to value the outputs.

Let us now consider outcomes and outputs, and recast some of Shiell's work in the following manner. In the economics discipline, outputs are the end product of transforming inputs into goods, although that rather simple notion is cast in a framework of rich conceptual interrelationships. Consider the entry under the term, output, in *The Macmillan Dictionary of Economics* (Pearce, 1986):

> ... This transformation process is formalised by saying that output is a function of the various quantities and qualities of inputs used, which is a verbal expression of the PRODUCTION FUNCTION. Output need not coincide with goods that create UTILITY. Such outputs would command zero or negative prices in markets ... (and) consumers would either pay to be rid of the good or require to be paid to accept it. Nor need output be a 'tangible' good... (p. 315).

The above dictionary entry reminds us that economic theory has a conceptual 'coat peg' for something that is likely to happen in reality: the output 'need not coincide with goods that create utility'. In markets, of course, prices exist and consumers' economic behaviour is defined as that sort of human behaviour which weighs up (or economically evaluates) how well a good or service serves one's own preference set. The consumer decision involves three variables: the quantity of the good to purchase, its price, and the income of the individual.

Economists are well aware that not all outputs have market prices. The technique of cost-benefit analysis is suitable in those instances where social investment appraisal is required. (See also Chapter 2.) The fundamental notion behind this technique is the decision about the worth of a public policy or program. How well do government outputs serve the preference set of society, given that 'society' involves the users (the direct beneficiaries of the outputs), payers and providers?

In Chapter 2, the issue was raised about the techniques of social investment appraisal being predicated on a value judgement that individual preferences should count in deciding what society prefers. It was noted that even democratic societies do not allow individual preferences to count in all instances. Dasgupta and Pearce (1972), in their text on cost-benefit analysis, mention a number of instances wherein government argues that so-called 'informed opinion' knows best what is good for people. They mention '*some* categories of mental health patients' (p. 20, emphasis added). The present study lays a conceptual framework for that very case which Dasgupta and Pearce, along with many social investment appraisal researchers, simply 'gloss over': mental health patients.

Chapter 3 pointed to the importance of clarifying what the outputs of mental health care would be like if they created utility. (This is largely the work of Chapters 5 and 6.) If resource costs are attached to outputs without such an understanding, the results mean very little. It is also necessary for such a clarification to be quite precise as to when and how individual preferences might, or might not, count with respect to mental health care. Hence, it is necessary to pay attention to the extent to which economic irrationality may, to varying degrees of severity, afflict people who suffer with mental illnesses and disorders.

Chapters 5, 6 and 7 consider a way of thinking about how government[11] is economically rational, or perhaps not, in its provision of services for people with mental disorders and illnesses. There, a framework is given for what it means, in an economic sense, when government budgets (bureaucratically determined) constrain the provision of these services. These Chapters also juxtapose this framework with how the mental health production function would relate, in a theoretical sense, to the indifference map, doing so within an economic conception that defines the role of economic rationality in mental health services.

Thus, a framework is begun here which ultimately suggests an approach to the hoary problems that afflict economic evaluations: how to value individual preferences; how to aggregate these individual preferences in society; and how to attach resource costs to the outputs.

In summary, this study does not fit easily into Outcomes Research. Its home is found within the discipline of Economics.

The Research Process and Apparent Precision

Economic research that provides information for policymakers' decisions can improve the policymaking process. The precision of decision-making can be improved. In a young field of research where little is yet understood, research outcomes often leave as many questions unanswered as answered, both for policymakers and researchers alike.

With the pressure to provide research outcomes that improve the precision of pressing policy decisions, equally important but more fundamental issues usually are left pending. In the US for example, precise economic research that informs policymaking in mental health services already has a vital role (Windle, 1991; McGuire, 1992). Now, if the present study had pursued the trends in the extant literature, mostly from the US, it might have delivered some comparative cost studies of different treatment settings, or it might have calculated the direct and indirect costs of schizophrenia, or it may have attempted some demand analyses, or it might have investigated the welfare

---

11 Government may be the producer of mental health services but it can also act as financier of mental health services provided by the private sector or the voluntary sector.

implications of a funding issue. These are worthy types of studies figuring importantly in the US field.

However, the questions addressed in this study offer a different precision from the types of studies already in the literature. The questions are original in two senses. First, the conceptual frameworks presented in the Chapters that follow are new in the literature on mental disorders. Second, this study is somewhat different because it addresses 'first questions', or original questions, that one should ask concerning economic behaviour relating to individuals whose well-being is impaired by a mental disorder. Those questions arose out of an awareness of our personal discomfort that the economic literature had not conceptually clarified some issues. It was thus discomfort about the precision of what really is known already.

A study by Doessel and Marshall (1983) on a similar issue, the nature of care of disabled people, comments in a similar way on three aspects of the economic literature that are 'unsettling', regarding care for aged and for disabled people:

> First, there is no mechanism in these analyses whereby preferences can be incorporated. ...Second, the output(s) of the services being produced by the care industry are not identified, defined or discussed. Third, the existence of joint production of the services needed by the handicapped is little recognised (p. 108).

Now with the pressures of policymaking, an apparently more precise research study might have involved, say, conducting controlled case studies of expenditures on a small sample of in-patients with schizophrenia at a psychiatric institution and in some other setting, e.g. out-patient care. While information of an empirical kind is precise in one sense, levels of spending do not, however, mean very much to an economist until the meaning of the outputs of such institutions is clear. Available hospital or government health department data on Admissions, on Average Length of Stay (ALS) and on Occupied Bed Days (OBD) do not answer a question as to the meaningful measurement of the treatment outputs for mental illness. It is a theoretical issue, then, to know what concept is to be measured regarding the treatment of mental illness.

While in the previous Chapter the complicated nature of mental illness and its treatment was considered, the following paragraphs will elaborate some of the problems of empirical research in the economics of mental health care. For example, when an individual enters a psychiatric hospital/unit, he or she is expecting to commence an episode of treatment. There are admissions data available for various treatment institutions. Whether this is a person's first admission, or one of many re-admissions, or whether the individual has been visiting outpatient clinics or private consulting rooms in the interim, can be known, at best, from individual medical records.

Furthermore, considerable clinical debate revolves around whether a re-admission reflects something of the nature of the illness itself or whether it represents good treatment (since the individual in between treatment episodes is assumed to be coping quite well with daily life) (Schanding *et al.*, 1984, p. 171). Yet another view is that re-admission indicates that previous treatment produced no output (in the sense that health status essentially did not improve).

Change in health status is not a readily measurable phenomenon (Schwartz and Griffin, 1986; McGuire, Henderson and Mooney, 1988, pp. 21-30) but it is essential to the question of outputs and, thus, to questions about what 'society' can look to purchase from its institutions, or from any other treatment/support services for people with mental disorders.

Consider yet another 'black box' problem. During the length of hospital stays, in-patients sleep in a bed. OBD data are commonly available from hospital data-sets. But it is not clear whether, with respect to chronic cases, this is a measure of treatment, and thus medical output, or how much of it represents accommodation, or whether the two are interconnected. And if the latter is the case, it is still not clear what the outputs of the institution are.

Again, from such data sets, ALS can be calculated. During a length of stay, an individual undergoes medical treatment, including specific therapy sessions; he or she may also undergo a social rehabilitation program, an organised recreational program, or other products of the 'active treatment' type (English and McGarrick, 1989, pp. 2082-83). Also, he or she will do other things, sleep, for instance. Sleeping can in itself represent the consumption of a therapy or treatment. In other cases, however, sleeping can be interpreted as the consumption of a joint product (Lloyd, 1983, for example) which comes with any in-patient treatment (Goldman and Regier, 1983). During a length of stay, the individual may be consuming such 'products' as sleep and recreation.

It may also be that individuals simply may need **time,** as mentioned earlier in this Chapter. Some individuals need time: time in order to consume time and time in which inner processes can work to restore health. Our society expects many things to happen fast and wants people back at work as soon as possible.[12] But of its nature, psychiatric rehabilitation cannot produce the rabbit from the hat.

Furthermore, the products mentioned in the previous paragraphs may not need to be consumed in the joint treatment-plus-accommodation product of a hospital setting. Sometimes, as examined later in this study, it is clinically preferable that some of the product is consumed in the setting of the community. Deinstitutionalisation started in the US as an outcome of several factors: the discovery of powerful psychotropic medications; concern for human rights; and rapid acceleration of the costs of in-patient care. For a discussion of the deinstitutionalisation movement in the US, its purposes, motivations and results, see Morrissey and Goldman (1984) and Pepper and Ryglewicz (1985); and in respect of these issues in Italy, see Scheper-Hughes and Lovell (1986).

---

12 A definition of welfare in terms of lost work time, or maximisation of Gross Domestic Product, is a narrow definition. There are other definitions which economists use, all of which are noted briefly by Cullis and Jones (1985, pp. 128-29), in reference to another health care issue.

For the present study, a more nagging concern replaced the lure of empirical research by way of case studies, cost studies, demand studies. The emphasis here has come to be one of seeking approaches to thinking economically about issues of funding and resource allocation in a climate of stigma, of consumer ignorance and of little opportunity, beyond the 'clear-cut' cases where society 'ought' to be imposing its norms on the individual, for the exercising of consumer preferences.

Conclusion

Four decades is a brief span of time, relatively speaking, in the aeons of growth in disciplined knowledge. Four decades of work is a briefer span of time if very little research activity occurs during the initial two, of those four, decades. Four decades of work is an even briefer span of time when the issue under study is a field within economics, itself a relatively young discipline. Such is the field of economics and mental health care.

Economists generally agree that 'access' to mental health treatment increases in the presence of insurance schemes that carefully address problems of under- and over-insurance. Much work yet remains to be done to address the social, housing, employment and other needs of the chronically mentally ill. The results of many evaluation studies, which are essentially cost studies, cannot yet be interpreted meaningfully because of a methodological vagueness over the measure of output that is (implicitly or explicitly) being employed. Additionally with evaluation studies, care-givers' time has not yet been given adequate economic meaning, and has been made more complicated in its measurement with the privatisation of formerly public services in mental health care into the realm of households and the general community.

It is also relevant to observe that there is very little published research in Australia on economic aspects of mental health care.

In view of the nature of the demand for economic research by US policymakers on matters in mental health care, and in view of the literature itself being recent, a cohesive body of understanding cannot yet be expected. The demand studies are successfully piecing together valuable empirical insights into consumer and provider behaviour regarding various (private) reimbursement arrangements in the US. Even so, some fundamental issues are not addressed in order to give these results meaning. For example, 'What is it that we buy with mental health care?' 'What does it mean, in an economic sense, to provide or finance particular mental health services privately, or publicly?'

It is appropriate at this point of the literature survey to reflect on the progress of this field. Reaching a view about the progress of the field can be difficult, since all sorts of myths surround progress in knowledge generally. Some of those myths are exposed by Koestler (1968) whose history of man's changing vision of the universe, though told in regard to quite a different field from economics and mental health care, suggests some lessons that are worth remembering.

One of the myths considered by Koestler is that the progression of scientific thought and understanding is, by nature, orderly and sensible. Put otherwise, Koestler is concerned with exposing an often-held misconception, namely, that human knowledge about the physical and social worlds advances in a linear fashion, and that it is subject to a relatively constant rate of increase through time. Although some may make a distinction between 'cumulative' and 'non-cumulative' knowledge (Brinton, 1950), a distinction that is more or less synonymous with the positive/normative distinction often invoked in economic discourse, Koestler's argument is that cumulative/positive knowledge is not devoid of 'dead ends' and 'blind alleys'. Koestler starts with the understanding contributed by various Greeks, like Pythagoras, Aristarchus, Plato and Ptolemy, but focusses largely upon the lives and contributions of Copernicus, Kepler, Galileo and Newton. Koestler's story of mankind's attempts, over several millennia, to understand the nature of the earth's place in the universe leads one to jettison a view of rational, efficient and orderly progression of knowledge, even if a restriction to cumulative knowledge were imposed. It is well known, of course, that the opposite occurred in regard to the understanding of the solar system.

The themes underlying Koestler's reflections offer universal application to an understanding of the myths in scientific progress. (Of course, this is not to imply that erratic events will always be the case in the advance of knowledge.) First, Koestler's history directs attention to the psychological processes underpinning discovery in science, in particular, to the struggle of the roles of inspiration and delusion within research. Put otherwise, a tendency that is so starkly evident even in those great minds of the past is a tendency present in us all, that 'while part of their spirit was asking for more light, another part had been crying out for more darkness' (1968, p. 14). Essentially, the scientific method has fixed the problem of delusion, but only to a degree. Second, Koestler offers in his Preface another point, drawn from his reflections about the history of the universe:

> The progress of Science is generally regarded as a kind of clean, rational advance along a straight ascending line; in fact it has followed a zig-zag course, at times almost more bewildering than the evolution of political thought. The history of cosmic theories, in particular, may without exaggeration be called a history of collective obsessions and controlled schizophrenias; and the manner in which some of the most important individual discoveries were arrived at reminds one more of a sleepwalker's performance than an electronic brain's (Koestler, 1968, p. 15).

In a century's time and more, will the progress of knowledge in economics and mental health care be seen as rational and orderly, not to mention humane? We hope for this.

5 The Outputs of Mental Health Care: I

Introduction

Let us conceptualise an individual's demand for mental health services.

To attempt this requires an explanation in four parts. First, attention will be directed to applying a development of (traditional) production theory, after Becker (1965) and Grossman (1972a)(1972b), to household behaviour. This application, called household production theory, will demarcate the role of individual rationality, and will conceptualise mental health as a vector within a utility function.[1] Initially, the conventional axioms of the theory of consumer choice are employed. Separability theory then enables the model to be based upon two vectors of commodities in the utility function. The conception of two-stage budgeting (Deaton and Muellbauer, 1980), rather than Hicks' composite commodity theorem, is employed. Lancaster's characteristics theory will then be applied in order to explain preference behaviour within sub-vectors of an individual's mental health vector.

Some of the assumptions of the theory of consumer choice are particularly unreasonable with respect to the commodity, mental health services; these assumptions will be introduced, and considered in the following Chapter.

Having laid this groundwork in Chapter 5, the next step is to employ the initial model to clarify the links in the mental health household production function between the demand for mental health and mental health inputs. This is the purpose of Chapter 6 where the relationship between mental health inputs and the output of the mental health care sector is examined.

---

1 When utility is most simply defined in economics, it is synonymous with economic welfare, happiness or satisfaction, as outlined in Chapter 1. Another of its meanings, also outlined in Chapter 1, is that an individual derives utility from a good or service, or event, if he or she prefers it to exist rather than not to exist. When an individual derives more utility from good X than from good Y, the economic connotation is that the person prefers good X to good Y. Utility, in its ordinal meaning, has explanatory power, given the present state of knowledge of economic phenomena. It is this interpretation that is employed in Chapters 5 and 6, with the qualification that only one aspect of Sen's (1987b) approach to the standard of living, briefly explained in Chapter 1, will be addressed in these Chapters 5 and 6.

It is stressed from the outset that, in spite of the clarifications aimed for here, this model carries with it the limitations of conventional choice theory. Additionally, the focus here, being just on economic behaviour, can throw light on only one small, but highly significant, aspect of economic welfare.

The Need for Care and the Demand for Care

Initially, let us consider the distinction between need and demand. Demand reflects a decision about which wants to satisfy. McTaggart, Findlay and Parkin (1999) in an elementary textbook in microeconomics, explain that 'if you demand something, then you want it, can afford it, and have a definite plan to buy it. Demands are different from wants. Wants are the unlimited desires or wishes that people have for goods and services' (p. 4.2).

The notion of 'need' can be considered from several aspects, but not all of these are relevant here. The issue of how 'need' and 'demand' can be distinguished is pertinent and has been examined by Fuchs (1983). He notes two non-economic approaches to health care, which have connotations of need. One is the '**romantic**' approach. Fuchs gives the example of the statement, 'Health is the most important goal.' Such a statement sounds convincingly plausible, and yet it shrouds one aspect of the reality of human behaviour. Smoking, over-eating and stressful living are a few of many instances of human behaviour which show that the choices we make affect our health; these choices reveal that, frequently, a higher value is placed on satisfying wants other than health. In other words, health is not always the most important goal. The romantic approach 'denies the *inevitability* of choice. [It tends to] categorize some desires as "unnecessary" or "inappropriate", thus protecting the illusion that no scarcity exists. ... The fact that we are constantly being confronted with the need to choose is attributed to capitalism, communism, advertising, the unions, war, unemployment or any other scapegoat' (p. 5). Denying the inevitability of choice is a romanticised view of life and, from an economist's perspective, confuses an important distinction between need and demand. Indeed, denying the inevitability of choice usually implies individual preferences being over-ridden when assertions are made that a particular goal is the most important one.

Fuchs refers to the second approach as '**monotechnic**'. This approach, Fuchs argues, is 'frequently found among physicians, engineers, and others trained in the application of a particular technology. ... Its principal limitation is that it fails to recognize the multiplicity of human wants and the diversity of individual preferences. Every problem involving scarce resources has its technological aspects, and the contributions of those skilled in that technology are essential to finding solutions. The solution that is optimal to the engineer or physician, however, may frequently not be optimal for society as a whole because it requires resources that society would rather use for other purposes'

(p. 5). There is a tendency for medical practitioners and others in the caring professions to adopt either the romantic or the monotechnic view.

When used as an instrument of social decision-making, both the romantic and the monotechnic approaches involve a normative notion implying that a third party makes a judgement as to what services are best for society, that is, a so-called 'need'. This may or may not be desirable. Clearly, there are instances when consumer preferences have to be adjusted or over-ruled as, for example, in mental health care when people are institutionalised in order to protect their own lives or others'. However, when statements are made that the 'objective' of particular health care services is to continue to meet 'the needs' of the recipients of the service, it is never clear, as Culyer and colleagues put it succinctly, whether the person making the statement 'means that *he* needs it, whether he means society ought to get it in *his* opinion, whether a *majority* of the members of society want it, or *all* of them want it. Nor is it clear whether it is "needed" *regardless* of the cost to society' (Culyer *et al.*, cited in Culyer, 1976, p. 13).

Demand for health care, on the other hand, refers to the claims of individuals upon health care resources. While seriously mentally ill individuals cannot make such claims for themselves and tend to be gravely neglected in society, there are many others, not incapacitated, who do have legitimate preferences. However, they are unable to exercise these preferences under present arrangements. This is because choosing among inputs is not perceived to be a role of consumers of mental health care.

The Rational Consumption of Mental Health

The Household Production Function

It is necessary to undertake an analysis of the demand for mental health, before analysing the demand for mental health care. Grossman (1972a, 1972b) employs a similar distinction with respect to health and health care. Grossman's insight was based upon the seminal paper by Becker (1965) placing consumer choice behaviour in the household production framework.[2]

In Becker's paper, it is argued that households obtain utility from the essential attributes for which goods are wanted, attributes to which he applied the term, 'commodities'. Commodities, as defined, cannot be bought in the market but, rather, are produced by the household through a combination of inputs of market goods, time and human capital. For example, meat, cereals,

[2] Becker's choice of the adjective, 'household', can be misleading in so far as 'household' connotes a place or a social arrangement. The intended meaning relates to the household being the basic consuming unit, whether the unit be the individual person or a grouping of individuals. The role of the household is studied again in Chapter 8.

vegetables can be purchased and, combined with time and preparation skill, can produce nutrition and flavour, i.e. a meal. Another example which Grossman suggests is that producing the commodity, recreation, requires the use of sporting equipment and time (Grossman, 1972b, p. 224); and there are many other recreational inputs that people employ, like listening to music, watching television, seeing a play.

Grossman points out that the demand for purchased goods and services is a derived demand. This is because these goods and services are inputs in the production of fundamental commodities. The point is simple, yet it is an illuminating and critical insight: 'Health' constitutes a fundamental commodity, and consumers are therefore seen as undertaking the production of health by combining inputs such as diet, exercise and housing[3] and, as one among many inputs, the health services provided by medical practitioners, hospitals, etc. Based on Becker's approach, consumers demand health because it directly yields them utility and, additionally, because health determines how much time an individual can spend earning income from factor market activities. Income spent on purchasable goods being consumed along with (leisure) time produces commodities that enter the utility function directly.[4]

The implication of this point is that consumers and producers may behave differently with respect to health and to health care.

The Household Production of Mental Health

Grossman's analysis of health is perhaps even more clearly applicable to mental health. While serious physical ailments can poorly dispose a person in every aspect of his or her life, a number of physical ailments tend, on the other hand, to be an affliction upon only some aspects of a person's utility function. For example, digestive ailments may inhibit both a person's enjoyment of food and the vital metabolic processes important to daily energy levels; a broken arm limits some physical activity but not all, and does not nullify enjoyment or the individual's efficacy; heart disease normally need not stop an individual's enjoyment, say, of a concert.

On the other hand, for people with mental disorders, the effects are often pervasive. Many mental disorders, from depressive disorders and anxiety states through to the schizophrenias and the dementias, afflict a person's approach to life, his or her judgement and decision-making, the purpose for living and, in essence, an individual's basic valuation of the utility of time. Physical movement also can become distressful.

---

[3] The historical importance of these as inputs has been shown by McKeown (1979).

[4] The critique of household production theory by Pollak and Wachter (1975) suggests that to deduce a notion of 'commodity prices' from the model is unsatisfactory in many applications with joint production, and they suggest ways to avoid this limitation. According to McGuire, Henderson and Mooney (1988, pp. 141-47), the Grossman model has remained highly influential in the study of health economics, in spite of its critics.

Healing for an individual with a mental disorder entails, first, knowing the mental health production function that is unique to the individual. *Inter alia*, this production function includes (purchased) goods and services[5] and time. Simultaneously, healing involves the minimisation of personally destructive stresses that arise from particular externalities bearing upon the individual.

When a complex mix of biological, social and emotional problems arises, it is unlikely that the individual can manage his or her mental health problems, and in many instances the individual, or the family, looks elsewhere for help. Sometimes help is sought through drugs such as sedatives sold virtually 'over the counter'. Mostly, the individual also calls on external sources of human capital. This may take the form of a particularly helpful friend or community group or a minister of religion offering useful advice or practical assistance; or it may be in the form of paid services, such as those of a medical practitioner (MP) or a psychologist. Alternative health advice also may be sought, such as through visits to a homeopath or to a yoga ashram.

Individuals often 'employ' structured professional assistance, but it may be also that professional assistance seeks them: in all cases, professionals need, subtly or openly, to convince an individual that his or her production function needs their services, before an individual will consume their treatment.[6] There are other instances: a homeless alcoholic may be bundled off to hospital; or teams from the Department of Health may make visits to mentally ill individuals living almost forgotten in the boarding houses of the inner city.

The foregoing discussion assumes no opinions, or indeed reliable knowledge, of the specific contribution of inputs to mental disorder, including iatrogenic inputs. Further attention to inputs is given in the next Sub-section.

Inputs in the Household Production Approach

Invoking the household production approach implies that the individual, or the individual's agent, faces choices (or makes choices by default). This does not imply that people with mental illnesses are the type of people who do not want good health and so choose illness. Rather, this approach entails the simple notion that, for all individuals, there are special combinations of inputs that contribute to mental health. A wide variety in the types of inputs is available: there are unsophisticated inputs, like taking more walks in the bush, or sitting in a chair listening to music more often, or taking up a new past-time, or playing sport regularly, or praying. There are also structured inputs such as counselling or therapy sessions or perhaps, where appropriate, 'cold-turkey' treatment for

---

5 They need not be personally purchased, as they may be government-provided. It is then the government that is the purchaser. In other words, this is a redistribution in kind. Nevertheless, the opportunity cost is inescapable.

6 This is not necessarily being pejorative of the professionalism of professionals.

drug addiction, each input occurring with, or under the supervision of, a professional. There are also inputs in the form of biologically invasive treatments such as medication or electro-convulsive therapy (ECT).

Together, these inputs combine to produce the commodities that enter directly into the utility function which is the essence of individual well-being. Because every individual has a unique utility function, the combination of inputs is a complex, delicate process. Individuals and their agents differ greatly in their ability to produce mental health, as indicated by the possibilities from the following examples. In suggesting these examples, the implication of the approach is definitely not to place blame on the individual for his or her mental disorder.

Occasionally, a few, 'simple' inputs can make all the difference. A few sessions of counselling may be all that is needed to ease a neurotic state; some assistance with household duties may ease the condition of a young, abandoned mother of three or an ageing widow, each suffering with a neurosis. Alternatively, for many suffering bipolar disorder, a vital input is the daily consumption of lithium, which can counteract the mood swings that afflict the individual.

For many, the treatment issues are more complex. Unfortunately, some individuals may try many types of treatments without a significant change in their mental health status. For other individuals, treatment can become their opportunity for manipulative or escapist behaviour, such that the treatment itself entrenches the disorder. The psychoses, where the aetiology of many of the afflictions is not yet well established by medical research, are deemed to be caused by a complex array of factors; and the more extreme the psychotic affliction, the more the individual creates an unreal, albeit perverse, world in order to maintain a semblance of a utility function. A manifestation of this is when a person, severely impaired with schizophrenia, actually enjoys talking back to the voices, or the benevolent ones at least. (At least in the sanctuary of institutional care, he or she is free to do so.)

All the examples presented in the previous paragraphs illustrate the possible complexity of the individual mental health production function. It is inescapable that individuals themselves embody the throughput of the production of this commodity, mental health (Williams, 1978).

Throughputs in the Household Production Approach

Many of the difficulties, discussed previously, of measuring the output of health care services for chronic illness can be minimised with the adoption of output budgeting. See, for example, Cooper and Bennett (1984). See also Footnote 5 in Chapter 2. Williams (1978) notes that part of the budgeting process requires the definition of the inputs and outputs for the task at hand. Outputs can be difficult to measure, and measures of throughputs are used instead. For example, from another area, the output of education is difficult to measure and instead, number of students attending school, or the throughput, is one measure commonly used. Williams' distinctions about outputs and throughputs are useful in isolating a precise difficulty in mental health care economics.

Consider an example. Recall, first, that many individuals diagnosed with one of the schizophrenias are unable to integrate thinking and feeling. These individuals are capable of operating in only one mode of the thinking-feeling spectrum within which normal people operate. They are unable to function as normal people do, somewhere between the extremes of this spectrum. Because thoughts and feelings are not integrated for people with schizophrenia, they can live in a world only of thinking or only of emotions. Normal persons may live by a dominant mode in operation with the other subordinate, or else may operate in a dominantly thinking or feeling mode for a particular task at hand. But individuals with schizophrenia are unable to mix the two modes at all, or even to learn to do so. The implication is that any counselling inputs that enter into a mental health production function for an individual with schizophrenia will enter with the fixed proportions of the bipartite modes to which the individual is limited. In such instances, the throughput would be a poor indicator of the output.

The preference ordering capacity of seriously mentally ill individuals is usually severely impaired, and a way of incorporating this problem into the theoretical framework being discussed here will be considered later in this Chapter and in Chapter 6. The Section following will investigate the case where individuals can order preferences.

Consumer Behaviour

The Axioms of Consumer Behaviour

Throughout this Section, it is assumed that the consumer can exercise the necessary faculties of having preferences. Rational behaviour by the consumer is also assumed. The strict meaning of rational consumer behaviour is behaviour that is in accordance with a systematic set of preferences.[7] In the theory of consumer demand (Hicks, 1946), individuals are assumed to behave as if they follow particular assumptions or axioms of rationality, as well as other axioms of general behaviour. These will be given below. The seven axioms together mean that the individual's preferences can order, and value, a set of goods. Also, the axioms make possible a testable theory of consumer behaviour possible. The reader ought to note that the purpose in this Sub-section on axioms is not to explore or debate technical or philosophical issues here in regard to the axioms. Rather, the focus should be more general, that is, upon recalling that some

---

7 For a discussion of the question, 'Are consumers rational?' in the context of the above axioms, see Green (1971, pp. 25-26).

important axioms underlie propositions about preferences. Further, the focus is on the wider importance of addressing preference sets in mental health care.

Consider a consumer faced with a choice from a set *S* of alternative consumption bundles of commodities (denoted by vectors $\mathbf{x}, \mathbf{y}, \ldots$).[8] Assume *S* is a closed and convex set in commodity space. In order to be able to develop a preference ordering, it is necessary to find a relationship between a pair of elements in *S*. Such a relationship is best illustrated with the statement: 'The consumer thinks that the bundle **x** is at least as good as the bundle **y**.' This statement can be represented symbolically as follows: $\mathbf{x} \succsim \mathbf{y}$. Note that rational behaviour is sometimes more easily understood if stated in its reverse, namely, that it would not be rational to choose **y** from a set of alternatives when **x**, another alternative in the set, is preferred to **y**.

The first four axioms, below, permit the definition of rational behaviour, just given:

Completeness: For all $\mathbf{x}, \mathbf{y}$ in *S*, either $\mathbf{x} \succsim \mathbf{y}$ or $\mathbf{y} \succsim \mathbf{x}$, or both (i.e. $\mathbf{x} \succsim \mathbf{y}$ and $\mathbf{y} \succsim \mathbf{x}$) (which means that any two bundles can be compared so that the consumer is able to order the available combinations of goods according to his/her preferences);

Reflexivity: For all **x** in *S*, $\mathbf{x} \succsim \mathbf{x}$ (which means each good is as good as itself, a trivial matter);

Transitivity: For all **x**, **y** and **z** in *S*, then if $\mathbf{x} \succsim \mathbf{y}$ and $\mathbf{y} \succsim \mathbf{z}$, then $\mathbf{x} \succsim \mathbf{z}$ (which means that if some combination of commodities **x** is preferred to another combination **y**, and **y** is preferred to **z**, then **x** will be preferred to **z**);

Selection: For all **x**, **y** and **z** in *S*, the consumer aims for his or her most preferred state.

All the axioms above refer to aspects of consumer rationality. Often, other assumptions about behaviour are made, as follows, in order for testable hypotheses to be developed:

Continuity: For all **y** in *S*, $\{\mathbf{x}: \mathbf{x} \succsim \mathbf{y}\}$ and $\{\mathbf{x}: \mathbf{x} \precsim \mathbf{y}\}$ are closed sets. It follows that $\{\mathbf{x}: \mathbf{x} > \mathbf{y}\}$ and $\{\mathbf{x}: \mathbf{x} < \mathbf{y}\}$ are open sets. [This is an assumption about separating the commodity bundles that are preferred from those that are non-preferred or, to put it another way, about the indifference curve being 'a curve or line rather than a "smudge" ' (Pearce, 1986, p. 25)];

Strong monotonicity: If $\mathbf{x} \geq \mathbf{y}$ and $\mathbf{x} \neq \mathbf{y}$, then $\mathbf{x} \succsim \mathbf{y}$ (which is an assumption that more is better or, put otherwise, that it is not possible

8 Reference is made here to 'commodity bundles'. Of course, it is possible instead to refer to 'decision alternatives', 'outcomes', 'goods', or whatever.

for the consumer to have so much of everything that he or she is completely saturated)(often this axiom is replaced with a weaker assumption, local non-satiation, which says that one can always do a little better, even if only small changes in the consumption bundle are possible);

Strict convexity (of preferences):
Given $\mathbf{x} \neq \mathbf{y}$ and $\mathbf{z}$ in S, if $\mathbf{x} \geq \mathbf{z}$ and $\mathbf{y} \geq \mathbf{z}$, then $t\mathbf{x} + (1\text{-}t)\mathbf{y} > \mathbf{z}$ for all $0 < t < 1$ (which is a rather strong assumption, enabling a diminishing marginal rate of substitution, a technical matter).

For a full exposition of the axioms of consumer behaviour, see, for example, Deaton and Muellbauer (1980).

The Maximisation of Preferences

The axioms above define a preference ordering which is depicted in the form of a continuous utility function U (**x**,**y**) which says that a person's utility is related to that person's consumption bundles. A preference ordering can also be depicted as a conventional indifference map.

The set of all groupings of consumption bundles that the consumer can afford, as manifested in the conventional budget constraint, is given by

$$\mathbf{p}_x \cdot \mathbf{x} + \mathbf{p}_y \cdot \mathbf{y} < \text{Income} \quad (5.1)$$

where $\mathbf{p}_x$ is the vector of prices of x_1 to x_n, and
$\mathbf{p}_y$ is the vector of prices of y_1 to y_n.

The maximisation of preferences is then:

$$\text{Max. } U(\mathbf{x},\mathbf{y}) \quad (5.2)$$

s.t. $\mathbf{p}_x \cdot \mathbf{x} + \mathbf{p}_y \cdot \mathbf{y} < \text{Income}$
where (**x**,**y**) are in X and Y.

Without elaborating on either the embellishments or the limitations of conventional theory (Deaton and Muellbauer, 1980), it is necessary to consider an assumption implicit in the conventional analysis just given and, in so doing, to clarify the place of mental health in the individual's choice set.

Separability

Separability assumptions are helpful in modelling consumer choices among various mental health care options, taking the consumption of all other goods as given. The assumption of separability enables the individual's consumption set to be defined into groupings of goods.

Hicks (1946) is the first to define a set of conditions for the existence of commodity and price aggregates or indices. Hicksian separability, i.e. the composite commodity theorem, asserts that if the relative prices of a grouping of goods remain constant, then the corresponding grouping of goods can be considered as a single good. For an exposition, see Varian (1984) or Deaton and Muellbauer (1980).

The strongest objection to Hicksian separability is that it relies on an external factor, the constancy of relative prices, to define groupings of goods (Deaton and Muellbauer, 1980, p. 122). Additionally, it requires the assumption that the elasticities of demand for all goods in the group, with respect to expenditures in the group, are unity. Put otherwise, the Hicksian approach would need the assumption of aggregating expenditures on the grouping of goods, mental health, into which mental health inputs with differing elasticities, namely luxuries, near-luxuries and necessities, would be aggregated. Such an assumption is unreasonable (Gorman, cited in Green, 1971, p. 152).

Another simple way of approaching the existence of groupings of goods is to **assert the separability** of preferences *per se*, because preferences naturally structure themselves into groups. In other words, 'if food is a group, the consumer can rank different food bundles in a well-defined ordering which is independent of his consumption of housing, fuel, entertainment, and everything else outside the group' (Deaton and Muellbauer, 1980, p. 122). It is possible to define the utility function in terms of separable groups, say, food, shelter, entertainment, within which there are sub-groups, comprising at least one good. One way of understanding this is in terms of a utility tree, as in Figure 5.1.

Figure 5.1 A possible utility tree of an individual

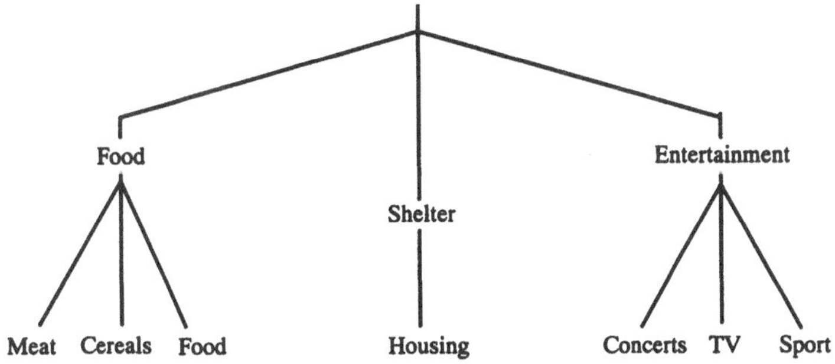

Source: Adapted from Deaton and Muellbauer (1980), Figure 4.1.

Can mental health be numbered within the 'natural ordering'? It can, considering that mental health, in Grossman's framework, is demanded for two reasons: first, mental health enters consumers' utility functions directly as a consumption commodity due to its direct influence on utility; second, it is an investment commodity because it determines the time available for work. These groupings are Becker-type commodities, and exist in Becker-type commodity space.

A simple, but important, notion of two-stage budgeting is suggested in Figure 5.1 (Deaton and Muellbauer, 1980). Broadly speaking, the consumer first allocates expenditure to the higher stage groups of commodities. For example, food, shelter, entertainment, mental health etc. are allocated first, followed then by the allocation of expenditure within commodity groupings among the relevant sub-vectors of goods and services. At each stage, only the information appropriate to decisions at that level is needed. Initially, an allocation is possible given knowledge of total expenditure as well as knowledge of commodity group prices. The notion here relates to a real price index, or else to a perceived one, for that commodity group. At the next stage of budgeting, each separate expenditure is a function only of prices within the commodity group and of group expenditure.

The relevant indifference map is shown in Figure 5.2 indicating preferences in commodity space. 'Mental health care' and 'the consumption of all other commodities' are the arguments of a person's utility function. The preferences shown here relate to a single individual. It is not assumed here that, across a population of individuals, every individual would have a set of preferences

Figure 5.2 Individual preferences for mental health care and other commodities

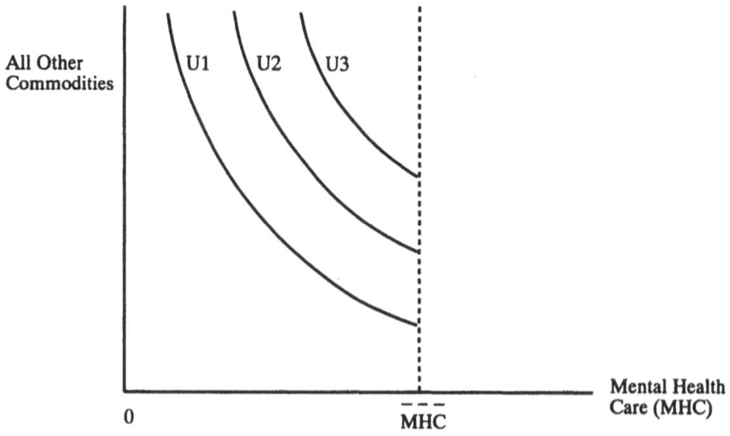

identical to this set. For example, a person who had no preferences for mental health care would have an indifference map such that each indifference curve would be a straight line parallel to the X-axis. The indifference curves in Figure 5.2 exhibit the usual characteristics: different points on the same indifference curve provide the same level of satisfaction or utility; and a higher level of satisfaction is associated with higher indifference curves.

It is important to note that Figure 5.2 has an important characteristic that is atypical of such a diagram in economics. The quantity of mental health care is bounded at a particular level, namely, $\overline{MHC}$. This bounded quantity of mental health care arises because it is unreasonable to invoke the usual assumption of non-satiation in this context. Once a person has reached a particular level of mental health status, it is conceivable that he or she will then cease to consume mental health services: satiation in mental health status will induce satiation in mental health care. (These two variables are formally linked through the relationship referred to as the mental health production function.)

Many modifications and extensions of this notion are possible, but are not within the limits of this study. See Deaton and Muellbauer (1980, pp. 122-36).

Choices within Characteristics Sets

It has been mentioned that the demand for mental health services is a derived demand, in that what the consumer really wants is improved mental health status. But health status is a multi-dimensional phenomenon (Doessel, 1987). Conventional economic theory associated with Hicks (1946) deals only with commodities that are uni-dimensional, but recent advances in the theory of consumer demand (Lancaster, 1966a; 1966b; 1971; Ironmonger, 1972) have shown how to incorporate multi-dimensional commodities into conventional economic theory. For an account of the Characteristics Theory of Consumer Demand, see Appendix 5.1 at the end of this Chapter.

Lancaster argues that the direct objects of utility for the consumer are the attributes or the characteristics of the commodity. What are the components of mental health status? Much of the literature suggests that people are looking for two gains to be made from mental health care: the alleviation of symptoms including the psychological pain they suffer; and the reduction of disabilities which represent the restriction caused by their condition. In economic terms, mental health status (MHS) is a function of two commodities, symptom alleviation (AS) and disability reduction (RD). Thus, we may write Equation 5.3:

$$\text{MHS} = f\,(\text{AS, RD}) \qquad (5.3)$$

Equation 5.3 can be considered in terms of Lancaster's (1966a, 1966b) and Ironmonger's (1972) characteristics framework. Accordingly, goods (including mental health care) are more appropriately perceived as 'consumption activities' (Lancaster, 1966a, p. 137) which produce joint outputs or characteristics which are 'embedded' in the goods. It can be conceived that various 'brands' of the inputs (which are the treatments/therapies/ 'unsophisticated' inputs available to the individual in the household mental health production function, as discussed in the previous Section) will service an individual with either symptom alleviation or disability reduction or, as is more likely, some combination of both. Combinations of AS and RD lead to improvements in the mental health status of the individual. This point will be reconsidered in detail shortly.

Figure 5.3 presents a geometric representation of the mental health utility function, stated in Equation (5.3). The arguments of that utility function, AS and RD, are indicated on the X- and Y-axes, respectively. Note that the characteristics space of Figure 5.3 is bounded in both dimensions, or components, of mental health status. See $\overline{AS}$ and $\overline{RD}$ in Figure 5.3. This produces a bounded space, namely, $0\overline{RD}M\overline{AS}$. This space is bounded as it is inappropriate to invoke the usual assumption of non-satiation. In this context, non-satiation means that an individual does not obtain more and more satisfaction, or utility, with ever-increasing 'reductions in disability' and ever-increasing 'alleviation of symptoms'. It is assumed that the individual requires these human characteristics up to a level that is 'normal', in the sense that the individual is virtually indistinguishable from other members of the community, abstracting from eccentricities that we all have. This implies that although

Figure 5.3 Individual preferences over the characteristics of mental health status

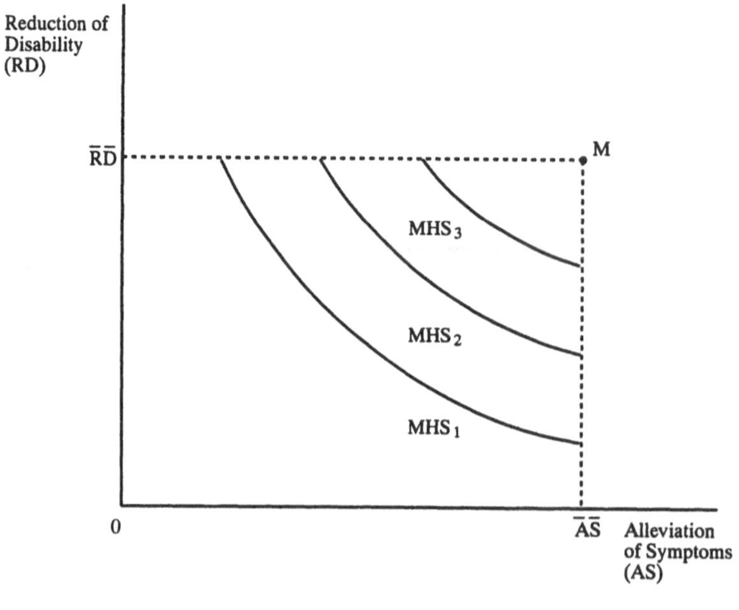

these distinctions are indicated in Figure 5.3 as points, namely, $\overline{AS}$ and $\overline{RD}$, these points are in fact simplifications of somewhat 'fuzzy' ranges of human behaviour.

It is relevant to comment on the indifference curves in the space of Figure 5.3. Given the way in which the characteristics have been defined, the individual's lowest level of mental health occurs at the origin and the highest level of mental health occurs at point M, where satiation in both characteristics of mental health occurs. In other words, indifference curves near the origin represent mental states of disorder that entail more distress and functional restriction. As the symptoms are increasingly alleviated and the disabilities increasingly reduced, individuals move outwards to higher indifference curves, each of which represents improved mental health status. That is, higher indifference curves represent mental health status increasing outwards towards the bounds of human potential.

As with the indifference curves in Figure 5.2, the preferences depicted in Figure 5.3 are those of a particular individual: it is not implied that all people will have the same preferences for RD and AS.

Lastly, it would be relevant to portray substitutes and complements in terms of indifference curves, as well as in terms of non-convex sets, but such qualifications will not be considered here.

The purpose of this analysis is to show when and how individuals can have preferences, even over side effects, and ultimately to define more clearly the outputs in terms of mental health status.[9] Since it is recognised that sometimes individuals will not know their preferences prior to treatment, this and other concerns will be considered in the next Chapter.

A Contrasting Approach to Conceptualising the Outputs: Price Index Issues

Before proceeding further, it is relevant to contrast the approach being considered here with a recent US literature. In that literature, a number of separate issues arise, associated with national accounting concepts and procedures to do with health accounts, as compiled by various national agencies (e.g. The Australian Institute of Health and Welfare and the US Health Care Financing Administration), and also published by the Organization for Economic Cooperation and Development (2000).

---

9 The clinical objections to the ICD system of diagnosis are not insignificant to the economist's concern with individual preferences. It is relevant also to the economist's interest in the specification of the output. Unlike ICD-10, DSM IV recognises the presence of symptoms and disabilities. Disease may impair a bodily system, function or organ, and manifest itself in the form of **distressing symptoms.** However, the **consequences** of disease arise in the form of limitations upon social functioning, so-called **disabilities and handicaps.**

Essentially, this recent literature revolves around various issues associated with the measurement of **price changes** in the health sector. The question of price change is important for a number of reasons, one being that if price changes are mis-measured through time, so too are real health expenditures. For a more detailed discussion, see Phelps (1999). It is helpful to understand that price change measurement within mental health care is only one part of the focus of that literature. Hence, attention turns to that issue within the broader scope of general health care, before focussing again on mental health care in particular.

Some of this recent literature just mentioned has focussed on 'nuts and bolts' matters: Griliches and Cockburn (1994) have shown that the specification of the regimen for off-patent pharmaceutical products, i.e. generic medications, as being 'new products' compared to their 'patent' equivalents, has resulted in overstated price increases for medications; Berndt, Griliches and Rosett (1993) have shown that by over-sampling 'older' medications and undersampling 'newer' medications, pharmaceutical price indices have overstated price rises;[10] and Ellison and Hellerstein (1999) have shown that ignoring institutional pricing factors (e.g. medications being covered by 'managed care' packages, legislation enabling and/or requiring pharmacists to dispense lower-priced generic pharmaceuticals, and public awareness of antibiotic resistance) has led to systematic overstatement of price rises for antibiotics, i.e. 'the price growth of antibiotics has been very modest over the last decade ... although it is contrary to what government statistics suggest' (Ellison and Hellerstein, 1999, p. 133). It must be emphasised that this conclusion is based on '... computations of traditional price indexes'. A similar exercise has been undertaken for antidepressive medications (Berndt, Cockburn and Griliches, 1997).[11]

Other 'nuts and bolts' issues (of a non-pharmaceutical kind) which have also been addressed, relate to the goods and services whose prices are measured. Historically, the (US) Bureau of Labor Statistics collected data on various inputs (X-rays, laboratory tests, hospital charges, medical practitioners' fees, etc.). Collecting data on inputs can create biases as the incorporation of technology improvements is extremely difficult, e.g. 'the average household stay for cataract surgery has fallen from seven days in 1952 to zero currently because the surgery has become an outpatient procedures' (Triplett and Berndt, 1999, pp. 3-4). An empirical analysis by Shapiro and Wilcox (1996) of cataract surgery has also demonstrated the importance of re-weighting in index

---

10 Berndt, Griliches and Rosett's results were confirmed in a subsequent study (Berndt and Greenberg, 1995) for a more recent period, 1987 to 1991, using a larger data set.

11 Some readers may note that some aspects of this recent discussion have a *déjà vu* dimension, as it retraces the general issue of 'list prices' *vs* 'transactions prices', a part of the Stigler and Kindahl (1970) critique of the procedures applied by the US Bureau of Labor Statistics for collecting price data in general. See Carlton and Perloff (1994, pp. 721-26) for a general discussion.

construction. For details of the revised Bureau of Labor Statistics procedures, see Kelly (1997) and Fixler (1999).

Although these new procedures are important, they are by no means the only work that is relevant in this context. By far the most important are those studies which are recognising, and attempting to take account of, quality changes in the provision of medical services. Quality change is a general issue that affects all parts of the regimens of price indices. See Moulton and Moses (1997) for a detailed account of the Bureau of Labor Statistics response to various critiques of the treatment of quality changes in the (US) PPI and CPI. The importance of changing composition of the regimen has been documented in detail for the treatment of heart attack: a 'fixed basket' Laspeyres index increased at an annual ratio of 2.8 per cent compared to an annual growth rate of 2.1 per cent for a five-year chain-weighted Laspeyres index, and at a 0.7 per cent growth rate for an annually re-weighted index (Cutler, McClellan, Newhouse and Remler, 1998, p. 1004). A similar conclusion holds for a more aggregated service index (medical management, cardiac catherisation, bypass surgery and angioplasty (Cutler, McClellan, Newhouse and Remler, 1998, pp. 1004-8). In this context there are several empirical studies of ischaemic heart disease (IHD) (Cutler, McClellan and Newhouse, 1999) and depression (Frank, Busch and Berndt, 1998; Frank, Berndt and Busch, 1999).

The analysis of IHD involves the construction of an index which 'measures a quality-adjusted cost of treating a health problem' (Cutler, McClellan, Newhouse and Remler, 1998, p. 991). The 'quality-adjustment' involves pricing improvements in health, which can involve both the length and quality of life, as well as mental and physical dimensions of personhood (p. 1008). In the empirical analysis, only extension of life is considered and valued. Given that mortality rates for persons (post heart attack) have consistently fallen (since 1984), one conclusion is that 'the real [cost-of-living] actually **fell** over the 1984-91 period' (p. 1016). Alternatively, '[t]he implication is that the cost-of-living index for heart attack care is actually falling over time, not rising' (Cutler, McClellan and Newhouse, 1999, p. 64). This conclusion is based on changes in treatment costs and changes in mortality.

The work on the treatment of depression (Frank, Busch and Berndt, 1998; Frank, Berndt and Busch, 1999; Berndt, Bir, Busch, *et al.*, 2000) is of more relevance in the present context. The 1999 paper begins with a DSM-IV-type discussion (definition, symptoms, persistence, prevalence etc.) and then moves on to consider alternative treatments, their efficacy, etc. In the spirit of Scitovsky (1964), who argued that the appropriate concept of output in the health sector was the treatment provided during an episode of illness, the next step is to consider 'treatment bundles', concentrating on outpatient claims and prescription drug use. After a consideration of available data, 'average supply (PPI) and demand (CPI) prices for five aggregated treatment bundles' (p. 88) were calculated for 1991 and 1995. From these raw data, five PPI price indices (Laspeyres, Paasche, etc.) have been calculated and all show price reductions in the period 1992 to 1995, the finding being that 'although all price indexes reveal a decline in the supply price of treating acute-phase depression..., the extent of the decline varies modestly with the choice of weights and substitution assumptions' (Frank, Berndt and Busch, 1999, p. 93). Furthermore, '[a]ll of these price reductions are rather dramatic and contrast sharply to changes in the [three] published medical ... indexes [which] estimate price increases for mental health-related services' (p. 95). Similarly, price falls characterise the demand prices for acute-phase treatment of depression: 'The price reductions have ranged from 22 per cent for the Cobb-Douglas and perfect substitution indexes to about 30 per cent for the fixed-weight Laspeyres' (p. 96). The suggested reasons for the calculated falls relate to the effect of managed care and to the technical changes in the treatment of depression, particularly in terms of pharmaceuticals and types of therapy. But one should also not lose sight of the fact that quantity has been specified in a way 'that attempts to incorporate outcome information in defining output' (p. 97). With respect to the effect of managed care, Berndt, Frank and McGuire (1997) have shown that the substitution of pharmaceutical treatment for (more expensive) counselling therapies has not been as great as anecdotal evidence has indicated.

In a sense, both of these studies (IHD and depression) have moved to a definition of output that is health-related, i.e. improved health status is regarded (or specified) as the output of the episode of care or treatment provided. In the IHD case, the output is increased life-years saved, and in the depression case, the following statement is crucial:

> Based on these observations from the literature, we view all the major treatment technologies as offering comparable expected outcomes for the average care of less severe acute-phase depression. For severe depression we view [tricyclic antidepressants] TCAs and [selective seretonin reuptake inhibitors] SSRIs alone as comparable to each other and to combinations of TCAs and SSRIs with psychotherapy (Frank, Berndt and Busch, 1999, p. 81).

It should be noted that the application of the Scitovsky output conception involves aggregating various types of treatment associated with an episode of illness. Scitovsky employed data from the Palo Alto Medical Clinic (in California) and, through time, calculated costs associated with treatments for such conditions as 'Otitis Media (children)', 'Appendicitis (simple)', 'Appendicitis (perforated)', 'Forearm fracture (children) – cast only', 'Forearm fracture (children) – closed reduction, general or regional anaesthetic,' etc. See Scitovsky (1967, 1979, 1985); and Scitovsky and McCall (1980). For a detailed discussion, in the context of the role of technology as an explanatory factor for rising health expenditures, see Doessel (1992, pp. 10-13).

The Scitovsky concept, when recently applied, takes account of changes in output. Consider the heart attack case: the analytic process involves the measurement of the output of care in physical terms, *viz.* improved mortality, and then the valuation of that change directly. But what of the improved quality of life that might accompany the increased years of life? It is not measured and, hence, the process leads to an underestimate: 'Because this figure does not consider changes in the quality of life [e.g. a gain in functioning], it probably understates the benefits of the change in treatment' (Cutler, McClellan and Newhouse, 1998, p. 135).

The point is that 'health' or 'health status' is a multi-dimensional concept and, hence, a 'change in health' will also be multi-dimensional. Multi-dimensionality is recognised in some contexts, e.g. the quality-adjusted life year (QALY) literature (Drummond, O'Brien, Stoddart and Torrance, 1997), where the multi-dimensionality is incorporated into a single measure. However, in view of our objective here, we do not wish to suppress the multi-dimensionality of changes in health status: our concern is to have an explicit recognition of the multi-dimensional nature of the outputs of the mental health care sector.

Summary and Conclusion

The purpose of the analysis in this and the following Chapters is to consider individual preferences over treatment inputs in mental health.

Initially, a distinction was made between the need for care and the demand for care, specifically important for matters relating to resource allocation. It was then suggested that it is helpful to think of mental health as entering the household production function as a commodity vector, following Becker (1965) and Grossman (1972a; 1972b).

Preferences for mental health and for all other commodities are shown to exist in commodity space upon the application of an appropriate separability function involving two-stage budgeting. This approach helps explain the relationship between mental health care inputs and the outputs of the mental health care sector. Also, it enables a clarification of implications arising from the rationality assumption, basic to the approach at hand, i.e. resource allocation in mental health care. In particular, an explanation is possible, within characteristics space, of preference behaviour relating to two mental health dimensions or characteristics: symptom alleviation and disability reduction.

While this approach could be useful for explaining individuals' preferences regarding voluntary in-patient care, or ambulatory care, it will be used in the next Chapter to indicate, in an economic sense, when society 'draws the line' and an individual is involuntarily committed to inpatient treatment/care.

The analysis provided in this Chapter will be extended in the next Chapter in order to provide an approach that defines more clearly the outputs of mental health care. In mental health care, special problems for economic analysis arise when dealing with preferences. These and other issues will now be considered.

Appendix 5.1

The Characteristics Theory of Consumer Demand

Introduction

From the start of Chapter 5, this study employs various concepts associated with the 'new' or 'characteristics' theory of consumer demand. As this conceptual framework may not be widely discussed outside a smallish 'club' of devotees of esoteric theory, this Appendix has the objective of providing a readable account of this development in the economic theory of consumer demand. The key concepts, *viz.* the arguments that enter the consumer's utility function, the efficiency frontier, the consumption technology etc., are described. It is shown how price changes for commodities and changes in the budget can be analysed. Discrete choice is also considered. It is relevant also that this conceptual framework has the implication that 'quality' is no longer a qualitative phenomenon: quality is, in principle, measurable in this framework.

In the 1960s there were a number of important advances in microeconomic theory. First, there was Becker's (1965) incorporation of time costs in economic theory. Second, Tullock's (1967) seminal paper entitled 'The Welfare Economics of Tariffs, Monopoly and Theft' was published. Third, Leibenstein (1966) introduced 'X-efficiency', and Niskanen (1967) published a paper that established a literature on 'the economics of bureaucracy'. A fifth contribution, the 'characteristics' theory of consumer demand, is the subject matter of this Appendix. This literature is, in part, concerned with how quality differences between commodities can be incorporated into economic analysis.

In the early to mid-1960s, three economists (who all happen to be Australians) were nibbling away at much the same bone. Ironmonger (1972) was concerned with how to incorporate new commodities into economic theory; Kolsen (1968) was concerned with asking questions such as 'does rail have an advantage over road transport for low value, bulky commodities over long distances (say, coal and iron ore) and high value commodities over short distances (say, computers)?' and Lancaster (1966a)(1966b) was concerned with more general theoretical issues. As it happens, not all of the approaches have turned out to be equally significant: the so-called 'new' characteristics (or attributes) theory of demand is now predominantly associated with Kelvin Lancaster. See also Lancaster (1971) (1972). However, one should not discount the contribution of Duncan Ironmonger (1972).

Some Important Concepts

The Utility Function

For Lancaster, 'Goods, as such, are not the immediate objects of preference, or utility or welfare, but have associated with them characteristics which are directly relevant to the consumer ... The consumer is assumed to have a preference ordering over the set of all possible characteristics vectors, and his (*sic*) aim is to attain his most desired bundle of characteristics subject to the constraints of the situation. The consumer's demand for goods arises from the fact that goods are required to obtain characteristics and is a derived demand' (Lancaster, 1966b, p.14).

Traditional demand theory, associated with Hicks (1946), assumes that consumers obtain utility from goods and services; put otherwise, it is goods and services that enter the person's utility function, i.e.

$$U = U(X_1, X_2, ..., X_n) \qquad (5A.1)$$

where U is the person's utility or satisfaction, and X_i is the quantity of the i th good or service.

Lancaster's argument, however, is that the characteristics possessed by goods and services are the arguments that enter the consumer's utility function, i.e.

$$U = U(c_1, c_2, ..., c_n) \qquad (5A.2)$$

where c_i is the quantity of the *i* th characteristic. This involves the assumption of what Lancaster calls an 'intrinsic commodity group', i.e. that complete separability characterises the consumption technology. (For a discussion of separability, see the sub-section on this topic in Chapter 5.)

Thus, the geometric representation of this situation can be depicted in 'characteristics space' with indifference curves having the usual properties. See Figure 5A.1.

The characteristics which consumers desire are produced jointly by goods and/or services. Lancaster says that demand theory requires 'two types of input-information about **things** as well as about **people**. As it stands in the generally accepted form, demand theory makes no use of information about things' (Lancaster, 1971) (emphasis added). The indifference curves in Figure 5A1 indicate something about people and the objects of their preference, i.e. characteristics. Figure 5A.1 indicates nothing about 'things'. Attention is now directed to 'things'.

The Consumption Technology

Lancaster's discussion of 'things' is under the term 'the consumption technology'. This notion is important as Lancaster argues that there is, in reality,

Figure 5A.1 Consumer preference for characteristics

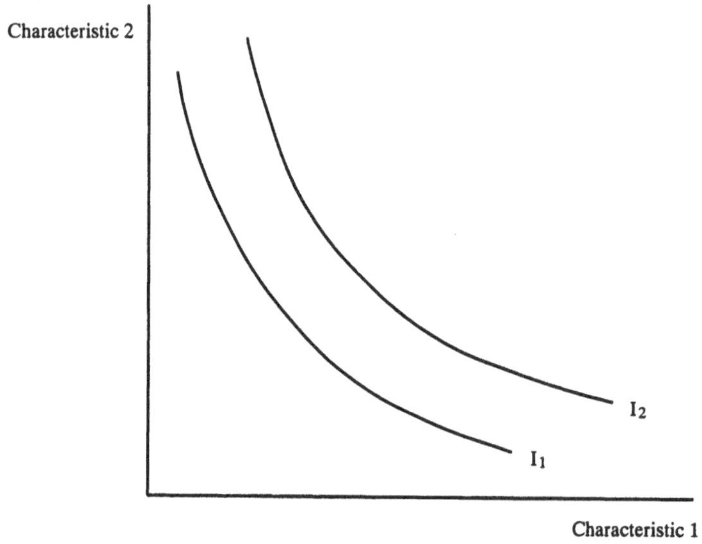

not a sharp distinction between 'consumption' and 'production': consumption activities have some features in common with production. This is brought out in the following statement:

> The jointness of the characteristics is really the core of the whole approach. If we eat an apple, we are enjoying a bundle of characteristics – flavor, texture, juiciness. Another apple may have the same flavor but associated with a different texture, or be more or less juicy. A single good may have more than one characteristic, and a single characteristic may be obtainable from more than one good. Goods which share a common characteristic may have their own characteristics qualitatively different, or they may give the same characteristics but in a quantitatively different combination. If the relationship between goods and characteristics was merely one-to-one in both directions, so that the only characteristic of an apple was appleness, then there would be no operational difference between the traditional approach to consumer theory and that being portrayed here (Lancaster, 1966b, p. 15).

Other dimensions of the consumption technology are as follows:

> It will be assumed that characteristics are, in principle, intrinsic and objective properties of consumption activities. Given arbitrary units, each consumption activity is defined by its inputs... and by the vector of characteristics which forms its output. It will be further assumed that the activities are linearly homogeneous, so that doubling the goods input gives double the characteristics.

> Essentially psychological effects, such as the consumer's relative interest in different characteristics ... are assumed to make their appearance in the preference ordering of the characteristics vectors, not in the relationship between goods and characteristics. The set of all possible consumption activities forms the consumption technology (Lancaster, 1966b, p. 15).

Having said all this, it is useful to illustrate these concepts geometrically. Different goods (beef, veal, fish) possess characteristics (protein, saturated fats, etc.) in different proportions. These characteristics are measured (cardinally) on the axes of Figure 5A.2, that depicts characteristics space. Note that the analysis can be applied to other phenomena, e.g. different types of cars that have comfort, safety, speed, etc. in different proportions. It is such differences that explain why a Mini is not the same as a Rolls Royce. For an ironic, but supportive, comment, see Scitovsky (1966).

The three rays from the origin (OB, OV and OF) indicate how the goods (beef, veal and fish) produce characteristics in different proportions. For example, if a consumer wants O P of protein, then he/she obtains this by jointly obtaining OS_1 of saturated fats from fish, or OS_2 of saturated fats from veal, and OS_3 of saturated fats from beef. The consumption technology then defines how goods are **imperfect** substitutes: perfect substitutes would have the same **ray** in the characteristics space of Figure 5A.2. However, some other assumptions must also be met for goods to be perfect substitutes.

Figure 5A.2 The consumption technology in characteristics space

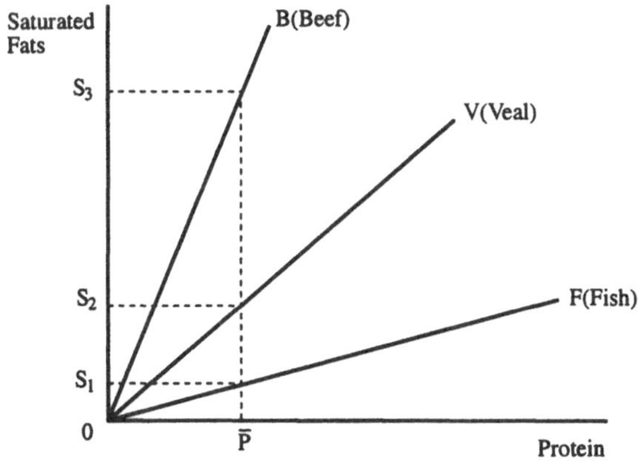

The Efficiency Frontier

Let us now impose a budget constraint, say \$x, on the consumer. If we know the prices of beef, veal and fish per kilogram, we can then specify the 'budget points' B, V and F in Figure 5A.3.

Changing the Budget If the consumer were to double the budget for food, i.e. the budget becomes \$2x, then the relevant budget points are B_1, V_1 and F_1 in Figure 5A.3. If the consumer wished to obtain a **combination** of veal and beef, then the budget point would be on the segment BV, i.e. a straight line joining the points, B and V. Similarly, if the consumer wished to obtain a **combination** of veal and fish, then the segment VF is relevant. The efficiency frontier is defined as BVF: 'an efficient consumer will choose combinations on ... the efficiency frontier for characteristics' (Lancaster, 1966b, p. 17).

Thus, doubling the budget gives a new efficiency frontier further out from the origin. In like manner, decreasing the budget shifts the efficiency frontier closer to the origin.

We have seen how a change in income can be incorporated in this framework. Attention is now directed to how price changes can be analysed.

Changing the prices for goods Let us assume that the price of veal falls. This means that, with the given budget, \$x, the consumer can obtain more veal. Thus, the budget point for veal will become V_1 in Figure 5A.4, and the efficiency frontier becomes BV_1.

Note that V_1F is a dashed line, a dimension that will be explained shortly. In like manner, if the price of veal were to rise, then the budget point for veal would become V_2. Note that in Figure 5A.4, BV_2F is also indicated by dashed lines. This has been done because BV_2F is **not** an efficiency frontier. The point V_2 lies **below** the line joining B and F and, in fact, in this case when the price of veal rises and the budget point for veal falls **below** the line BF, then BF **becomes** the efficiency frontier. The reason for this is as follows: when the price of veal is such that the budget point for veal lies on BF (as occurs at the point V_3), then the purchase of veal is essentially the same (in terms of the characteristics protein and saturated fats) as **a combination of beef and fish**. In fact, any budget point under a segment of an efficiency frontier can be described as an 'inefficient' point. Similarly, all points under BV_1 are inefficient points, and it is for this reason that V_1F is **not** part of the efficiency frontier. This may become clearer as the next step is taken by combining the indifference curves of Figure 5A.1 with the efficiency frontier of Figure 5A.3.

The Equilibrium Condition

Equilibrium is attained, and the consumer maximises his/her utility, at the point where the highest possible indifference curve in characteristics space is tangential to the efficiency frontier. See Figure 5A.5.

Figure 5A.3 The consumption technology with a budget constraint

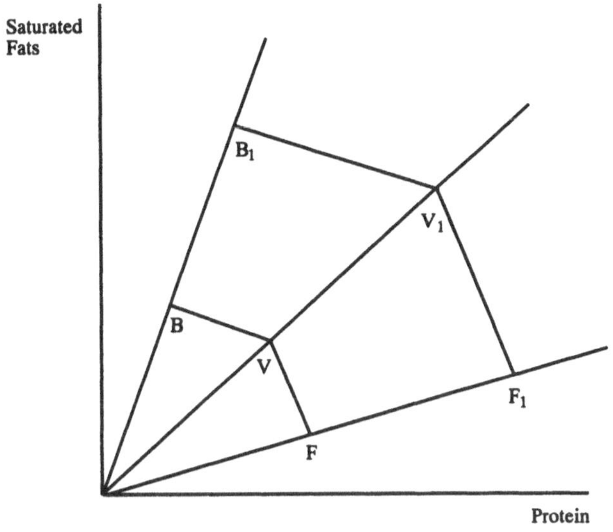

Figure 5A.4 Price changes and the consumption technology

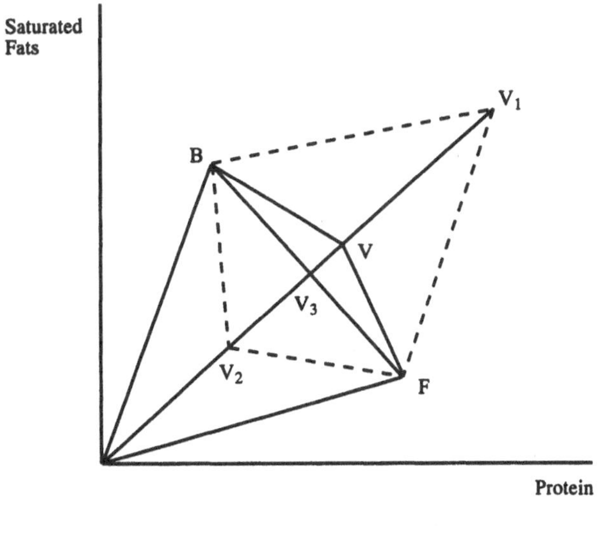

Figure 5A.5 Consumer equilibrium in characteristics space

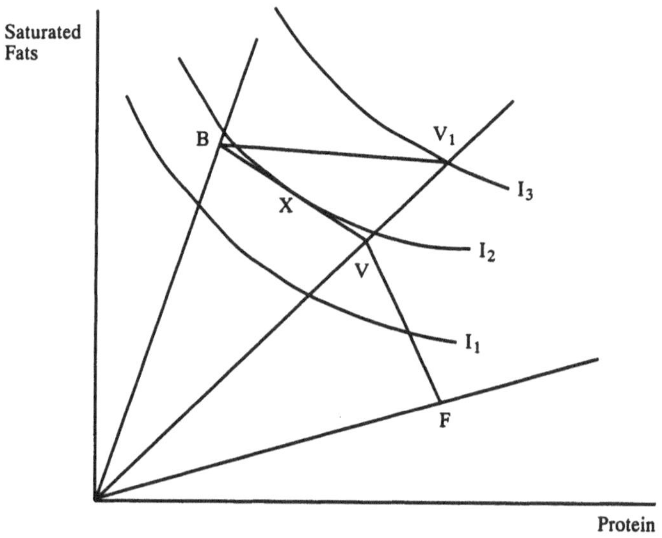

Figure 5A.6 An equilibrium corner solution in characteristics space

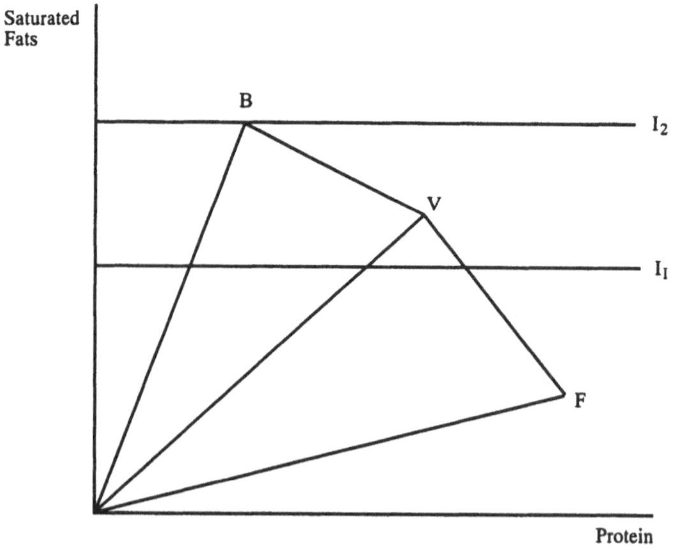

Figure 5A.5 brings together indifference curves in characteristics space ('information about people') and the efficiency frontier ('information about things'). Equilibrium is attained at the point X for the consumer whose indifference curves are shown in Figure 5A.5: he/she obtains maximum utility by a combination of beef and veal.

It is clear from Figure 5A.5 that if the price of veal falls (and the veal 'budget point' moves out further along the ray for veal to V_1), then the consumer will switch entirely to veal (represented by the point V_1). The consumer will make the change to veal because he/she can move to a higher indifference curve I_3. (This involves a corner solution, which will be considered below.[12]) In this case, the efficiency frontier becomes BV_1, as F becomes an inefficient point in that no 'rational' consumer would consume fish, given the relative prices of the commodities.

The reader should note that this is not the only conceivable situation. The indifference curves in Figure 5A.5 may **not** be representative of all consumers. Figure 5A.6 indicates the preference function of a consumer whose preferences may have been formed by the bumper sticker, 'Eat more beef.' Note that protein does not enter this consumer's utility function at all.

In Figure 5A.6, the consumer's indifference curves are horizontal to the x-axis, i.e. he/she obtains higher utility from saturated fats. The equilibrium position is at B, which is described as a 'corner solution'. It should not be thought that this preference map is an extreme case: Lancaster has analysed a number of cases of 'quite different' preference functions (Lancaster, 1972).

It is useful, at this point, to indicate that this conceptual framework makes it clear that there is a sharp distinction between **nutritional knowledge** and **nutritional advice**. The former term applies to knowledge or information about various foods, and the latter term relates to attempts to alter consumers' preferences for various characteristics associated with different foods. Dieticians often give not just information but advice as well, i.e. they tell people what they should do. Although related, knowledge about food and nutritional advice are two conceptually different phenomena. See Doessel (1988).

Some Other Cases

Attention is now directed to some other cases. It has been assumed that the characteristics are objectively observable and measurable, and that the relationships between characteristics and commodities are linear and additive.

---

12 A corner solution arises in optimisation problems when the optimum occurs where one (or more) of the variables has a zero value. Take, for example, the case of optimising between work and leisure. A corner solution is one where an individual's optimum is to work all the time, i.e. have zero leisure. An example of another corner solution is if an individual's optimum is to choose to have zero income (leisure all the time).

Also, it has been assumed that all characteristics are desirable. It has also been assumed that the commodities purchased are continuous in nature, rather than discrete. The characteristics approach is not invalidated by these assumptions, and some of these cases will now be considered.

Non-Proportional Relationships Between Characteristics and Commodities

The case of non-proportional relationships between characteristics and commodities can be illustrated by the case of people who face either various pharmacological treatments or various types of counselling/therapy available for a given illness/condition.

Assume that there are three available treatments: X_1, X_2 and X_3. With a given budget, a given consumption technology (the relationships between the characteristics and the three treatments), and the prices of the three treatments, the budget points A, B and C are obtained in Figure 5A.7. Given that combinations of treatments are possible, the consumer is not constrained to choose X_1, X_2 or X_3. All points on the efficiency frontier are possible points of consumption. The point of tangency is, as indicated in Figure 5A.7, at the point A which is a corner solution or, as Lancaster calls it, 'a vertex optimum'.

Figure 5A.7 Choice of alternative health treatments: Combinable treatments and non-proportional relationships between health status and treatments

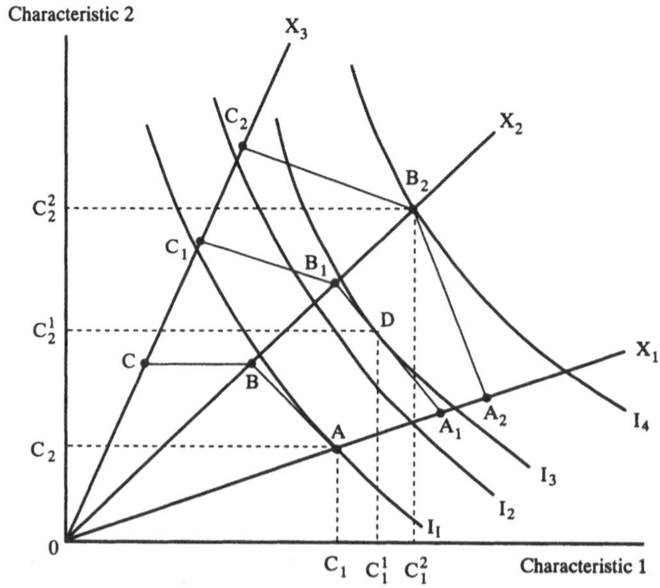

Assume now that the budget is doubled. The efficiency frontier is now A_1 B_1C_1. If the budget is increased, yet again, by the amount of the original budget, another efficiency frontier $A_2B_2C_2$ is obtained. In these cases, the prices of the alternative treatments are held constant. In Figure 5A.7 the equilibrium positions are A (a vertex optimum), D (a facet optimum involving a combination of commodities) and B_2 (another vertex optimum).

In other words, the way in which the frontier has shifted out is explained by the **technical relationships** between the characteristics and the three treatments. As indicated in Figure 5A.7, doubling the original budget has **not** produced a doubling of the quantities of the characteristics obtained from doubling the quantities of the treatments. Note that no facets of the efficiency frontiers, such as BC, B_1C_1 and B_2C_2 in Figure 5A.7, are parallel. This means that the technical relationships between characteristics and treatments are non-uniform between the alternative treatments.

It needs to be emphasised that the shapes and positions of various efficiency frontiers are **empirical** matters that must be determined in particular cases. The technical relationships between characteristics and commodities are factual matters that are to be established, not assumed.[13]

It is relevant to note that when a consumer purchases some of two commodities, such as at D, the shadow prices of the characteristics can be computed and this is possible by solving a system of simultaneous equations. However, this is not possible in the cases of corner solutions (Lancaster, 1971). Deaton and Muellbauer (1980) have made some suggestions for dealing with the problem of corner solutions. See also Green (1971).

Undesirable Characteristics

In the cases that have been considered so far, it has been assumed that all characteristics are positively desirable. There are, of course, many situations in the real world in which goods are jointly produced with 'bads', i.e. other commodities that are not desired. An example is the joint production of electricity and externalities such as heat and smoke. Such cases can also arise in the characteristics framework, an example being adverse side effects of a medical treatment.

In the characteristics framework, there are two ways in which undesirable characteristics can be analysed. One alternative is to treat the undesirable characteristic as a negative: this involves the insertion of a negative coefficient in the appropriate place in the technology matrix. In geometric terms this means that the analysis is no longer confined to the usual quadrant.

---

13 The reader should note that this point about relaxing the assumption of linear homogeneity, or proportional relationships, between characteristics and goods, may seem unnecessary if one has in mind beef, veal etc. and protein, but pharmacological and therapeutic contexts suggest that non-proportional relationships may be relevant in the health sector.

Figure 5A.8 Choice of alternative treatments: Combinable treatments with adverse side-effects

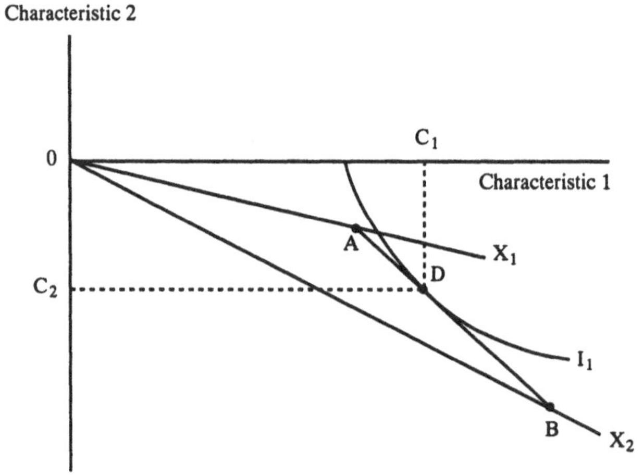

Figure 5A.9 The efficiency frontier in the case of discrete choice

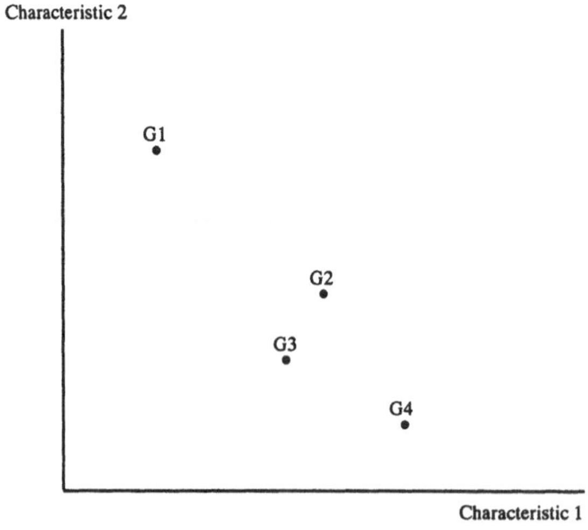

In Figure 5A.8, characteristic 1 is desirable and characteristic 2 is the undesirable side effect. With a given budget and the prices of the two (combinable) treatments, the relevant efficiency frontier is AB. Treatment X_2 provides more of the desirable characteristic than does treatment X_1 and it also possesses more of the side effect. D is the optimal point and involves a combination of the commodities. Note that both the shape and meaning of indifference curves are unchanged from the case of two positive characteristics.

The second method of analysis is to leave the coefficients in the technology matrix as positives and to alter the meaning of indifference curves. The indifference curves in the usual characteristics space would have a positive slope and, as one moves out in a south-east direction, the consumer would obtain a more preferred position (Auld, 1972).

Discrete Choice

Not all commodities are continuous in nature: some commodities involve discrete choice which implies a constraint on the consumer to buy only one of the commodities, as well as no choice with respect to the level of consumption of the commodity. Examples include consumer durable goods (like TV sets etc.) and diagnostic tests in medicine.

In Figure 5A.9, the points G_1, G_2, G_3 and G_4 represent the combinations of characteristics associated with four commodities and/or services. Since combinations of commodities are not possible, the efficiency frontier consists of only discrete points (G_1, G_2, G_3, and G_4) and **not** lines joining the points. Note that point G_3 is an inefficient point, as there is a point (G_2) that has more of both characteristics. In this case the efficiency 'frontier' is not a line but consists of the three points G_1, G_2 and G_4. Indifference curves can, of course, be indicated in Figure 5A.9.

This case involves some further complications in the treatment of prices and the budget. These matters, as well as some empirical results for diagnostic tests for the upper gastrointestinal tract, are discussed in Doessel (1986)(1992).

Conclusion

This Appendix has provided an overview of the characteristics (or attributes) theory of consumer demand. The important concepts of this approach have been considered, as well as some special cases. Not all issues have been addressed, e.g. the question of satiation. Furthermore, the difficult issues of measurement have not been addressed. However, the interested reader can consider such matters in the cited literature. See Auld (1972; 1974; 1975) for a consideration of this theory from the perspective of information and advertising.

6 The Outputs of Mental Health Care: II

Introduction

The purpose of the previous Chapter was to consider individual demand for mental health services. In Chapter 6, the limits on preferences of people with mental disorders are conceptualised. Once again in this Chapter, attention turns to the initial model of consumer demand in Chapter 5. It is employed again here in order to clarify the links between the demand for mental health and mental health inputs in the household production function for mental health. Doing so helps to explain the relationship between those inputs and the output of the mental health care sector.

Let it be stated once more that, in spite of the clarifications here, this model carries with it the limitations of conventional choice theory. Additionally, by focussing just on economic behaviour, light is shed upon one small part, albeit a highly significant part, of the subject matter of economic welfare.

The Limits on Preferences

Socially Unacceptable Preferences

Societies express disapproval of individuals' preferences and behaviour with benevolent as well as malevolent motivations, and can exercise this disapproval through varying degrees of restriction upon the individual. At worst, persons who are political dissidents can be incarcerated in psychiatric institutions. In contrast, institutionalised care in the form of the 'moral treatment' movement, which originated as a Quaker initiative, arose out of a sense of outrage over the social neglect suffered by demented individuals in the eighteenth and nineteenth centuries (Rosenblatt, 1984; Lewis, 1988; English and McGarrick, 1989). See also Chapter 7.

In democratic societies, questions over which individuals are to be committed to involuntary psychiatric care in institutions, for what reasons and for what care, are important, and extremely difficult, ones. At a general level, see Kafka (1925); also, Kirby (1983) for Australia; Morrissey and Goldman (1984) for the US; and also Eisen and Wolfenden (1988, pp. 369-75).

Apart from this political issue of unacceptable preferences, more common issues arise in the everyday world of personal interaction. Consider a person subject to some mental illness who is unaware of his or her condition and who also has a strong personal preference for listening to loud, 'heavy metal' rock music. This case is depicted in goods space in Figure 6.1.

In Figure 6.1, BC represents the individual's budget constraint. The individual's preferences are indicated by the indifference curves I_1, I_2, I_3. As indicated here, the optimal point of consumption involves a 'corner solution' at B, a position which involves the allocation of the person's entire budget to expenditure on stereo equipment and CDs; no part of the person's budget is allocated to mental health care. (Budget allocations to other goods, e.g. food, may also be zero.) Preferences such as those indicated here may have significant adverse effects, or external diseconomies, on the people living nearby. These neighbours may well describe these preferences as 'socially unacceptable'.

Figure 6.1 Consumer choice from 'unacceptable preferences'

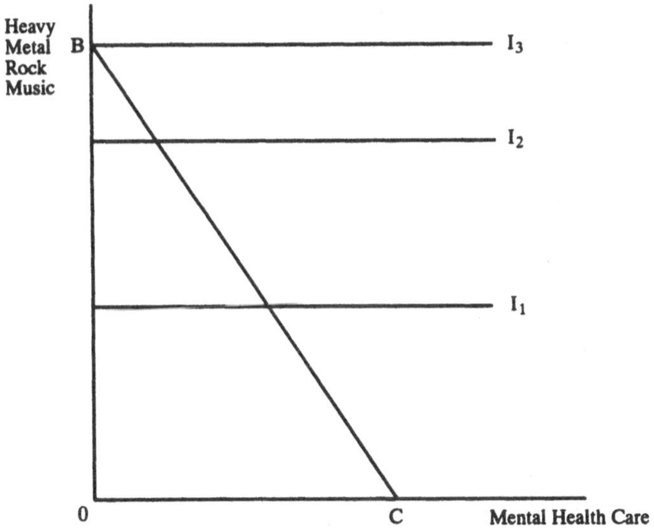

Impaired Preference Capacity

At least two of the basic axioms of the theory of consumer choice may be negated when individuals are severely ill, such as with the onset of an acute psychotic illness. Transitivity and monotonicity are, for example, likely to be negated. When a person who says he or she prefers A to B and prefers B to C but also says that he or she prefers C to A, then such a person is deemed to have an intransitive preference function. This would be regarded as 'irrational' behaviour. The choice mechanism is impaired. In Figure 6.2 indifference curves in Hicksian goods space for two goods, X and Y, show this case. Given the ratio of relative prices for the two goods, embedded in the slope of the budget constraint (not shown), the combination of goods indicated by the point C (OX_1 and OY_1) would be chosen. With an increased income, the combination at point B (OX_2 and OY_2) would then be preferred to the combination at C. Likewise, the combination at A (OX_3 and OY_3) would be preferred, in turn, to the combination at the point B. Such preferences are transitive. Intransitivity involves the preference of C over A, even though A is preferred to B, and B is preferred to C. In other words, the person does not order his or her preferences in the conventional way.

Irrational behaviour is also exemplified when an individual chooses A from a set of alternatives when there was another alternative A′ in the consumption set which the individual preferred. Such a violation of the monotonicity axiom also represents 'irrationality'. One example of the violation of the monotonicity assumption is when consumers of mental health care consume at a point less than their budget constraint. This is illustrated in Figure 6.3 in which the budget constraint is indicated by BC. Monotonicity implies that the combination of goods X and Y indicated by the point A′ is preferred to the combination at A, on the lower indifference curve I_2^{MI}. The violation of monotonicity, choosing the combination at A rather than A′, implies the reversal of ordering of indifference curves. In other words, I_2^{MI} is regarded as a 'higher' indifference curve (by a mentally ill person) than I_1^{MI}.

The purpose of this Sub-section is to shed light from an economic perspective on some instances where mentally ill individuals have an impaired ability to formulate preferences. It is important, though, to recall from the discussion of the rationality assumption in Chapter 2 that this Sub-section addresses just one aspect of the issue regarding the implications for economic behaviour of impaired preference ability.

Imperfect Information

Two features that characterise the demand for mental health services are consumer ignorance and consumer uncertainty.

It has been suggested by Sloan (1971) that there are three types of consumer ignorance which help to explain the tendency for mental health care services generally to be poorly matched to the users of those services. First, there may be an inability of the consumer to assess the services he or she receives; second, there may be an inability to choose among providers; and third, there may be a failure to use preventive services (Sloan, 1971, p. 4). Only the first two will be discussed here.

The inability of the consumer to assess mental health services is not unique or confined to such services: consumers of many services confront this same

Figure 6.2 Preference reversal

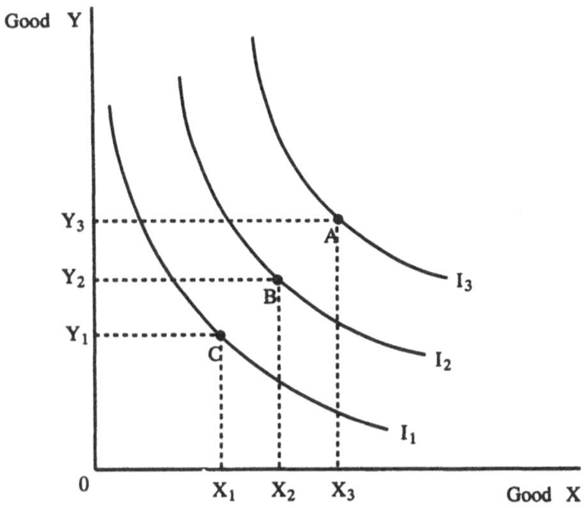

Figure 6.3 A case of violation of monotonicity

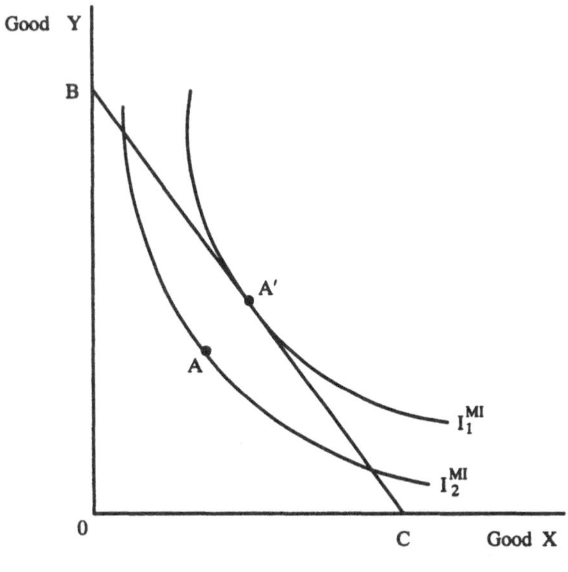

problem. The consequence is that arbitrary checks and balances may be introduced, instead of policy makers realising the root of the problem itself. Individuals cannot readily assess if they are being supplied a quantity of service that deviates from the equilibrium quantity (Enthoven, 1981).

Another form of consumer ignorance is the inability of consumers to make rational choices among providers. The individual may not know, or even think it useful to know, the various product types (the philosophical underpinnings of treatment models) among the various 'brands' of psychiatrists, psychologists, etc., nor their own preferences about treatment, before undergoing it. See Parloff (1976), cited in Rosenhan and Seligman (1984, p. 635 *ff*).

Additionally, information on prices charged for treatment or therapy is seldom known clearly. Mental health professionals are generally not alarmed by such an example of consumer ignorance. For example, it is seen as the job of the professional social worker to guide a patient, especially the poor, through the mental health delivery system. To have a social worker operate in this capacity is an illustration of the very high search costs for information regarding health care. It is a very expensive use of scarce social worker resources.

This discussion of imperfect information, although relevant to this Section on the limits to preferences, is central in the context of market failure. As such, it is of prime importance in a discussion of the normative role of government in mental health care, which is the subject matter of the next Chapter.

The separation of supply and demand is not always possible, in so far as the providers of care act both as agents for the consumer concerning the quantity demanded, and supplying the services. Further comment on the agency role will be left to the following Chapter.

The 'Imposed Indifference Curve'

With respect to the problems with preferences mentioned in the previous Sub-sections, the indifference map will be used now to show the stage at which society 'draws the line' with such individuals so that, with or without committal, these individuals will be institutionalised. In fact, it will become clear that one way of understanding the deinstitutionalisation movement is to conceive of it as a different 'drawing of the line', i.e. a shift to the south-east of what will be defined as the 'imposed indifference curve' (IC_I). It is useful to make the observation that although the term 'imposed indifference curve' will be employed, an alternative way of describing this concept is as a multi-dimensional or multi-attribute constraint. There is no formal difference in approach behind the alternative terminology.

Before proceeding further, it is helpful to consider the apparent 'contradiction-in-terms' in the words 'imposed indifference curve'. A reader may be perplexed by this, but there is an irony in the term, imposed indifference curve, that is intentional. It is (to economists) ironic that mental health care, having been delivered for years in a manner that is largely disengaged from the preferences of consumers, only acknowledges explicitly one set of preferences: a set of preferences of other people (judges, medical practitioners, etc.) representing 'society', and the preferences are imposed upon the individual for medical, legal or political reasons.

The 'Imposed Indifference Curve' in Characteristics Space (ChS)

In Figure 6.4, three indifference curves, MHS_1, MHS_2, MHS_3, show combinations of alleviation of symptoms (AS) and reduction of disabilities (RD) in characteristics space. These indifference curves exhibit the usual characteristics, i.e. that different points on the same indifference curve provide the same level of satisfaction or utility and, second, that a higher level of satisfaction is associated with higher indifference curves. Instances where society decides to 'draw the line', with respect to either behavioural or functional capability can be represented on this indifference map by adding a particular lexicographical ordering. In other words, individuals whose symptoms are such that they attempt to suicide or show other symptoms of serious depression, or who harm their well-being or the well-being of others to such a degree that they slip under the societal threshold, irrespective of how that is defined, are institutionalised in order that their symptoms can be treated.

Figure 6.4 The 'imposed indifference curve' (IC_I) in characteristics space (ChS)

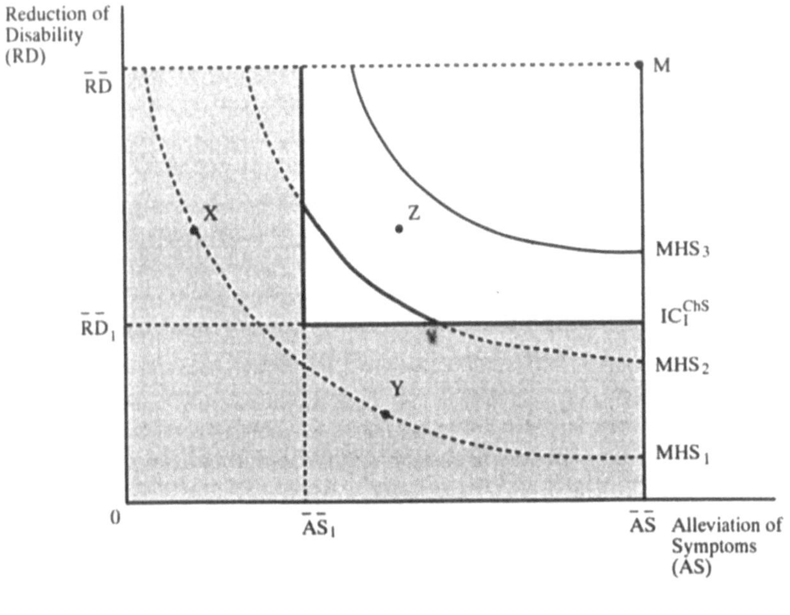

Additionally, when it is established that the degree of disability due to mental disorders, in such areas as nutrition, accommodation, communication or personal care, slips under the societal threshold, institutionalisation will occur. This is indicated by the shaded area for which the outer boundary is IC_I^{ChS}. The 'imposed indifference curve' IC_I^{ChS} thus depicts the preferences that society imposes on the individual.

Note that IC_I^{ChS} is not an individual's indifference curve. First, it is not part of an indifference map but is a single curve that has minimum, 'acceptable' values of both AS and RD (indicated by $\overline{AS}_1$ and $\overline{RD}_1$). This explains the right-angled shape of IC_I^{ChS}, which is a manifestation of lexicographical ordering.[1] Also, although the shape of IC_I^{ChS} appears to be that of an indifference curve representing perfect complements, the interpretation is not the same as that for an indifference curve. In the case of the 'imposed indifference curve', the interpretation is that society requires that individuals with mental illnesses will consume a minimum level both of symptom alleviation and of disability reduction. In other words, a serial or lexical ordering is present, since the implication of the lexical ordering is that minima must be achieved before any additions to the other characteristics are consumed or, as in this case, before any further preferences are satisfied.

In the presence of the 'imposed indifference curve', the individual's utility function is possibly non-existent or, more likely, is over-ridden by society in the shaded area of Figure 6.4. Society chooses for the individual the amount of AS and RD indicated by IC_I^{ChS}, as in Figure 6.4. The shaded area represents the area of enforced care, over which the medical profession, police, lawyers, families, neighbours and sick people themselves, tangle as to its boundaries.

The significance of the lexicographical ordering in Figure 6.4 is that 'society' regards $O\overline{RD}_1$ **and** $O\overline{AS}_1$ as the minima of RD and AS that are 'acceptable': if a person has a level of AS **or** RD below these minima, then institutionalisation will take place. For example, a person whose symptom alleviation and disability reduction can be depicted by point X will be institutionalised. Likewise, institutionalisation will occur if the person's combination of symptom alleviation and disability reduction is at the point Y. In both instances, the indifference curve MHS_1 is entirely inside IC_I^{ChS}. On the other hand, another instance can be considered where, for example, at point Z, the person has a level of disability reduction that is no better than it was at X but the level of symptom alleviation is higher. In this instance, the person is

1 Rawls (1971) defines a 'lexicographical' ordering (the less cumbersome word is 'lexical') as follows: 'This is an order which requires us to satisfy the first principle in the ordering before we can move on to the second, the second before we consider the third, and so on. A principle does not come into play until those previous to it are either fully met or do not apply. A serial ordering avoids, then, having to balance principles at all; those earlier in the ordering have absolute weight, so to speak, with respect to later ones, and hold without exception…' (pp. 42-43).

not institutionalised. MHS_3 is an example, on the other hand, of a higher mental health status that is considered to be beyond the bounds of institutionalisation. That is, MHS_3 is entirely to the north-east of IC_I^{ChS}. Such is not the case, however, with MHS_2 that has one segment that is not in the shaded area and two other segments that are in the shaded area. Those two segments of MHS_2 show a mental health status where one or the other of the characteristics of mental health has slipped below society's acceptable level, even though the other characteristic reaches society's minimum standard. That is, the mental health status is 'sufficient' in one dimension but is not 'sufficient' in the other. Mental health status is not high enough to ensure that, at some levels of AS, RD is high enough to reach society's acceptable level for reduction of disabilities, $\overline{RD}_1$, or else some levels of RD are associated with levels of AS that have slipped below $\overline{AS}_1$.

When individuals are institutionalised, they will remain 'in the shaded area', for the present, for three reasons: the first reason is that treatment cannot shift individuals out of this shaded area (explained in the next paragraph); the second is that the alternative of support and treatment in the community is not sufficient to support people outside of an institution; and the third is that, for financial motivations, as has been alleged in the United States, government adopts sweeping deinstitutionalisation (Pepper and Ryglewicz, 1985).

In-Patient Psychiatric Treatment of Mental Disorder in Characteristics Space

Assume, in a manner after Green's interpretation (1971, pp. 156-64) of Lancaster, that there are three types of treatment of mental disorder (T_1, T_2 and T_3) with differing proportions of symptom alleviation (AS) and disability reduction (RD). As before, IC_I^{ChS} represents the combinations of AS and RD which 'society' regards as 'minimal', in the sense that if a person exhibits less than these quantities, then societal intervention (compulsory in-patient treatment, and accommodation, meals etc.) will take place. The shaded area IC_I^{ChS} of Figure 6.5 represents a region of functioning that 'society' regards as unacceptable, and societal intervention takes place. These characteristics were indicated in Chapter 5 in Equation (5.3). The three treatments, which produce the characteristics in different proportions, are represented as rays OA, OB and OC from the origin in Figure 6.5. The points A, B and C indicate quantities of AS and RD, obtained by spending a given amount on mental health care. In this instance, the 'given' amount can be understood in terms of the mental health care budget, as discussed later. If homogeneous divisibility is assumed, then expenditure on mental health care can reach any point along AC, the efficiency frontier. Treatment OB is inefficacious because higher patient satisfaction is achieved by combinations of characteristics along the AC efficiency frontier. Because AC is below IC_I^{ChS}, the individual will remain institutionalised. It is fundamentally important to

Figure 6.5 Three alternative treatments for mental disorder in characteristics space (ChS)

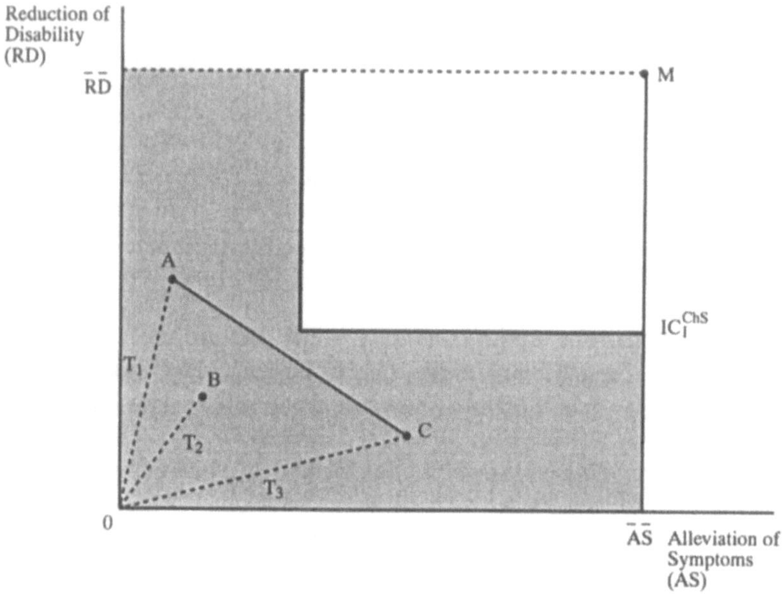

Figure 6.6 The introduction of a new treatment, or approach, for mental disorder in characteristics space (ChS)

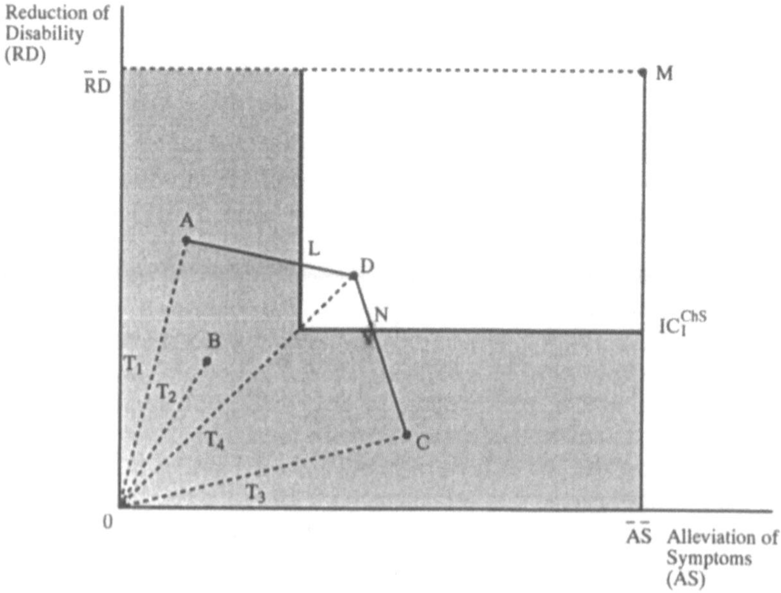

note that AC may be within IC_I^{ChS} either because treatments themselves are inefficacious or because insufficient resources have been devoted to mental health care.

Consider now the development of a new, highly successful treatment (T_4), or a new approach to mental health care. The new treatment, or new approach, is represented by the ray OD in Figure 6.6. (The rays OA, OB and OC relate to the same treatments depicted in Figure 6.5.) The point D is obtained with the same 'given' budget as that available for the other treatments. The efficiency frontier is now ADC. Since ADC passes across IC_I^{ChS}, any combinations of characteristics embodied in treatments represented by the segments LD and DN indicate that in-patient treatment has been successful and the individual no longer needs in-patient care. The result is that the individual no longer needs to be institutionalised. However, treatment combinations on segments AL and NC are such that the person would remain institutionalised as these segments of the efficiency frontier remain in the shaded area of Figure 6.6.

New treatments ought not be seen as the only hope of a happy life for people with mental disorders. Higher levels of patient satisfaction can also be attained if particularly productive approaches and treatments, available at present, are no longer constrained by an inadequate budget. A larger budget would constitute a (parallel) shift outwards of the efficiency frontier AC of Figure 6.5 or ADC of Figure 6.6. If the services are linearly homogeneous, a doubling of the budget would double the quantities of the characteristics, RD and AS, produced by the mental health services. There are many goods for which this assumption applies, e.g. twice the amount of veal will double the amount of protein, fat etc. embodied in the veal. Whether this relationship exists with services for mental disorders is an empirical matter that would need to be determined.

The 'Imposed Indifference Curve' in Becker-Type Commodity Space (CmS)

It is helpful now to cast the Lancastrian approach in a broader context. In effect, institutionalised treatment involves more than the consumption of characteristics AS and RD. It is useful to consider institutionalised care not only in terms of treatments for mental disorders, as depicted in Figure 6.6, but also in terms of the consumption of all other commodities such as the provision of meals, shelter, warmth, entertainment, companionship, etc. This is so because once an individual becomes a resident of a psychiatric hospital, this status largely determines the consumption of such other commodities. In other words, the institution is engaged in the joint production of treatment, meals, shelter, companionship, etc.

In these circumstances, it is appropriate to **adapt** the conception given in Figure 5.2 to Becker-type commodity space, assuming once again the existence of a natural ordering of preferences, as discussed in Chapter 5.[2] To that model from Chapter 5, the notion of in-patients who are admitted involuntarily is added, as shown by the 'imposed indifference curve' IC_I^{Cms} in Figure 6.7.[3] Note that the indifference curves in Figure 6.7 relate now to utility, and the arguments that enter the utility function are 'mental health' and 'all other commodities'. $\overline{MH}_1$ and $\overline{AOC}_1$ are the levels that society regards as the minima of mental health and all other commodities that are 'acceptable'.[4] In other words, an imposed indifference curve', IC_I, can be incorporated also in Becker-type commodity space, IC_I^{Cms}, depicted in Figure 6.7, as well as the characteristics space considered in the previous Figures.

As before, a lexical relationship exists with respect to the two Becker-type commodities. As depicted in Figure 6.7, a person with a utility level of U_1 will be institutionalised, irrespective of the combinations of the two commodities. However, this is not true of a person with a utility level of U_2. Combinations of the commodities on the segment PQ of U_2 will not indicate institutionalisation, whereas combinations on the other two segments of U_2, being in the shaded region of the Figure, will indicate institutionalisation.

Attention is now directed to a consideration of what this conceptual framework implies in terms of the demand for mental health care.

Imposed Preferences in Hicksian Goods Space (HGS)

The institutionalisation of a person for treatment is effectively an action taken to specify the person's utilisation of mental health care, i.e. imposing a level of mental health treatment which the person is perceived to 'need'. Let us consider imposed preferences in price-quantity space.

The demand for in-patient psychiatric care Recall that, in regard to general health, a person's demand for health services is determined, *inter alia*, by his/her health status. See Feldstein (1983) and Folland, Goodman and Stano (1997).

---

2 Note that Figure 5.2 has 'Mental Health Care', a marketable good/service, on the X-axis, and 'All Other Commodities' on the Y-axis. Thus, this Figure depicts classic (Hicksian) goods space, and the variable on the Y-axis is obtained by invoking the composite commodity theorem, associated with Hicks (1946). However, in the present context, attention is focussed not on marketable goods but on Becker-type 'commodities'; it is for this reason that the term 'Becker-type' is used to describe the nature of the 'commodities' being considered here (Becker, 1965). The implication of this distinction is that 'mental health', conceived of as a Becker-type 'commodity', will appear on the X-axis of Figure 6.7, which will be considered shortly.

3 This concept, as before, produces an 'acceptable' region and a socially 'unacceptable' region, where the latter is indicated by the shaded area.

4 Society's requirements about minimal consumption of **particular** 'other commodities' such as food are not depicted in Figure 6.7, but this arises because additional commodities cannot be incorporated in the two-dimensional space of such a Figure.

Figure 6.7 Institutionalised treatment of mental disorder in Becker-type commodity space (CmS)

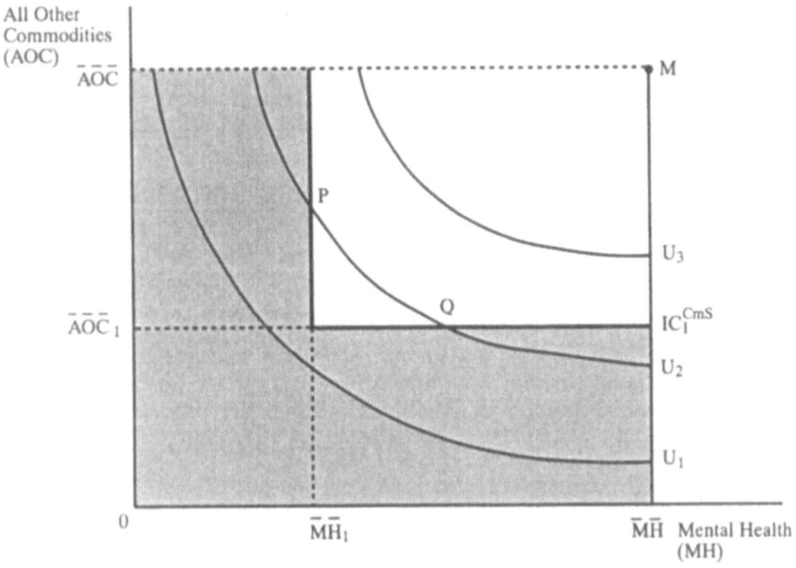

In regard to in-patient psychiatric care, the quantity demanded of in-patient psychiatric care ($Q_{I\text{-}PPC}$) may be said to be a function of the following: the price of in-patient psychiatric care ($P_{I\text{-}PPC}$); the price of substitutes/complements ($P_{S/C}$); income (Y); mental health status (MHS);[5] and other relevant variables (r,s,t,...). Thus, the demand equation may be written as follows:

$$Q_{I\text{-}PPC} = f\,(\,P_{I\text{-}PPC}, P_{S/C}, Y, MHS, r, s, t, \ldots\,). \tag{6.1}$$

Consider Figure 6.8 in which DD is the demand curve for in-patient psychiatric care exhibited by an individual, where 'in-patient treatment' is a bundle of services including shelter, food, clothing, bathing/toiletting, care, medication and consultations with a visiting psychiatrist. Given a price of OP_1 of in-patient psychiatric care, this person chooses a quantity demanded OQ_1 of in-patient psychiatric treatment. (There are cases, of course, where the quantity of in-patient psychiatric treatment consumed is zero!)

5 Note that when MHS is high, then the quantity demanded of in-patient care may be zero; MHS is a variable that will shift the demand curve.

Low mental health status and low OQ_1 Consider now the case when 'society' observes that the mental health status of a person is indicated by MHS_1, a low level, as in Figure 6.4. In that Figure the level of mental health status is everywhere below the 'imposed indifference curve', i.e. the levels of AS and RD are viewed as too low or else 'socially inappropriate'. In symbols, when

$$Q_{I\text{-}PPC} = f(P_{I\text{-}PPC}, P_{S/C}, Y, MHS_1, r,s,t, \ldots) < O\bar{Q}, \qquad (6.2)$$

then institutionalisation will occur (where $O\bar{Q}$ is society's judgement of 'need' for in-patient psychiatric care, as indicated in Figure 6.8).

If 'society' regards the consumption of OQ_1 in-patient services as too low, then a person's preferences are set aside, i.e. over-ridden, and society's preferences are imposed. This is often a murky decision, as previously discussed, involving lawyers, medical practitioners, neighbours, police and family. What is involved in this process is the view that $O\bar{Q}$ is the 'appropriate' quantity of in-patient psychiatric care that this person 'needs'. In other words, the quantity demanded by the individual for in-patient treatment and care, *viz.* OQ_1, is regarded as inappropriate.

In the institutional context of OECD-type countries (i.e. not developing countries such as Indonesia or India), $O\bar{Q}$ will be provided, **irrespective of the price.** That is, if the price is OP_1, then $O\bar{Q}$ will be provided; if the price is OP_2, $O\bar{Q}$ will still be provided. Given that 'society' will provide $O\bar{Q}$ **irrespective of the price**, then a locus of points can be specified in the price-quantity space of Figure 6.8. This locus of points is indicated by $\bar{Q}\bar{N}$.

Figure 6.8 The demand and the 'need' for in-patient treatment and care

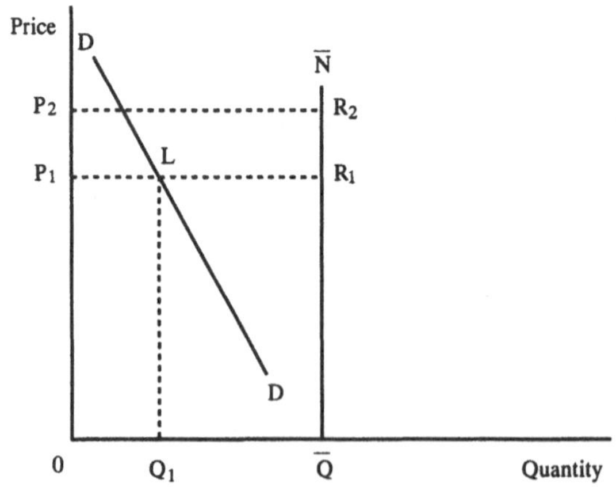

It must be emphasised that $\bar{Q}\bar{N}$ is not a demand curve. Feldstein uses the term, 'need curve' (Feldstein, 1983, p.79) to describe the relationship depicted by $\bar{Q}\bar{N}$.[6] Note that institutionalised treatment also imposes a rationed amount of all other commodities, if the individual has no other sources of consumption of all other commodities. Hence, a 'need curve' for all other consumption would exist as well. It is relevant to point out that a person subject to mental disorder may exhibit a zero demand for in-patient psychiatric care. In this case, the person's demand curve, DD in Figure 6.8, will coincide with the Y-axis.[7]

The complexity of other relevant factors affecting low OQ_1 Consider now the complexity of other possible factors that might be relevant explanatory variables in a demand equation. This issue is important as the total quantity of psychiatric treatment demanded is a heterogeneous phenomenon, and the demand for psychiatric care is, empirically, likely to be difficult to estimate.

First, instances are common of people with zero demand for in-patient psychiatric care. Because of stigma, class issues, family expectations, inter-country differences, cultural factors, and so on, many individuals do not have a demand curve for (in- or out-patient) psychiatric care. This type of zero demand for (in-patient) psychiatric care is not unlike that of vegetarians who do not have a demand curve for T-bone steaks, or non-smokers who have no demand for cigarettes.

Second, a group of so-called 'worried well' (at the other end of the spectrum) regards visits for psychiatric counselling, and even in-patient care at a private facility, as a status symbol. Recall the middle set and the outer expanses of Figure 1.1.

Lastly, recall from Figure 1.1 the core group of individuals with one of the diagnoses of serious mental illnesses and disorders. Complexity exists in interpreting low or zero demand in this group. In some instances, the illness causes individuals to lose insight and these individuals perceive themselves as not being ill, i.e. having zero demand for psychiatric care. However, some may have zero demand for psychiatric care because effective treatment does not exist. Other individuals are in gaol and, if in a state of apathy, do not access treatment. In many instances, a low quantity of psychiatric care

---

6 It is useful to observe the different expenditures that are involved in the two decision-making contexts. If the individual makes his or her own decision to consume OQ_1 in-patient psychiatric care, then expenditure will be indicated by OP_1LQ_1. However, if government makes the decision that $O\bar{Q}$ **should** be consumed, and the price is OP_1 per unit, then total expenditure will be $OP_1R_1\bar{Q}$. If the price is OP_2 per unit, then the expenditure associated with providing $O\bar{Q}$ will be $OP_2R_2\bar{Q}$.

7 In this case, the contrast between the expenditures on in-patient psychiatric care in the two decision-making contexts will be more stark, as expenditure in the former context will be zero.

demanded arises because the income of many of these individuals is insufficient to command the resources they require to overcome their disabilities. This latter group will be considered shortly.

The variation in this range of instances needs to be differentiated. A zero demand curve is one that coincides with the Y-axis, and will be encountered shortly as DO in Figure 6.9(b). In the context of revealed preference, DD is quite an accurate representation of the demand curve for in-patient care for many individuals.

Zero demand for in-patient psychiatric care and institutionalisation How, then, can the explanations in this Sub-section and Figure 6.8 relate to the previous Sections, and what is the implication? Figure 6.9 presents the case where, irrespective of the price of in-patient psychiatric care and the level of the budget, some people choose zero in-patient psychiatric care although the view of 'society' is that these people 'should' be consuming at least some in-patient psychiatric care. The top part of Figure 6.9 presents goods space, with in-patient psychiatric care on the X-axis, and a (Hicksian) composite commodity, All Other Commodities, on the Y-axis. The person's preferences are indicated by the indifference map $I_1, I_2, I_3, \ldots, I_n$. BC represents the consumer's budget constraint. Given the consumer's preferences and the budget, the optimal outcome is indicated by the 'corner solution' at the point B, and the consumer purchases zero in-patient psychiatric care, thus allocating all of his/her income to 'All Other Commodities'. Figure 6.9(b) presents the price-quantity space for in-patient psychiatric care and, as usual, the demand curve for the commodity can be derived from goods space. In this case, the demand curve, DO, coincides with the Y-axis and the consumer purchases zero in-patient psychiatric care.

This outcome may not be agreeable to the consumer's neighbours who, for various reasons associated with the person's behaviour, call the police or a relevant psychiatric assessment team. The latter take the view that 'society' can over-ride the consumer's preferences and impose a different set of circumstances on the consumer, as indicated by the 'imposed indifference curve' in Hicksian goods space, IC_I^{HGS} in Figure 6.9(a). The key characteristic of this imposed indifference curve is that it involves the compulsory consumption of in-patient psychiatric care, i.e. the person is deprived of his or her liberty and is institutionalised. Note that the need curve, $N\bar{Q}$ in Figure 6.9(b), is derived from this imposed indifference curve in Figure 6.9(a).[8]

Attention is now directed to an implication of the bureaucratic or non-market allocation mechanism that is associated with the need curve in Figures 6.8 and 6.9. If the average cost of in-patient psychiatric care is OP_2 and $O\bar{Q}$ is compulsorily consumed, then the expenditure associated with this decision to

---

8 The implicit assumption here is that separability applies to in-patient psychiatric care and other mental health services.

Figure 6.9 Zero demand for in-patient psychiatric care and institutionalisation

(a)

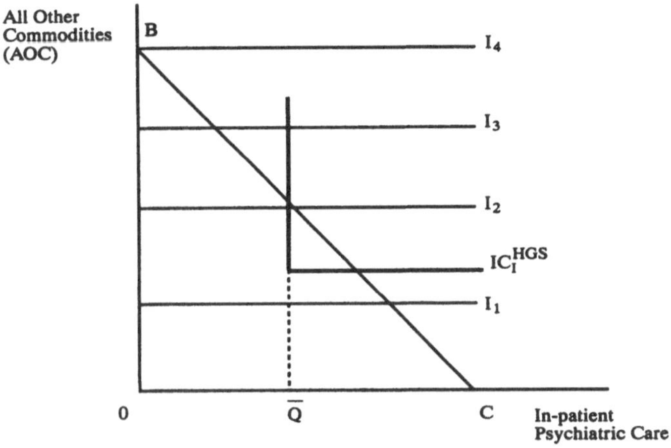

(b)

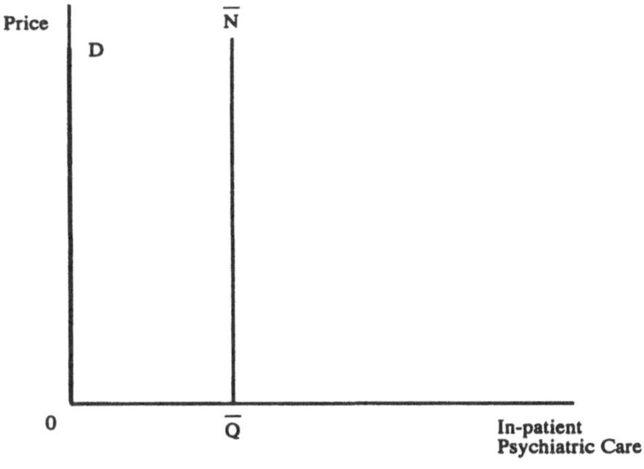

institutionalise the person is indicated by the area $OP_2R_2\bar{Q}$ in Figure 6.8. A similar area is implicit in Figure 6.9(b) but is not indicated because more notation would complicate the diagram. The significance of this bureaucratic process is that the expenditure area in Figure 6.9(b) is not associated with a budget constraint in Figure 6.9(a): bureaucratic processes imply a single 'budget point' in Figure 6.9(a), not a budget constraint (i.e. a line). Whereas a budget constraint has a slope and this slope reflects the relative price ratio, a 'budget point' has an infinite number of relative prices (because it is a point) and one cannot conceive of a determinant outcome. The absence of a (government) budget constraint in the space of Figure 6.9(a) is simply a manifestation of implementing a non-market process.

Income as a determinant of in-patient psychiatric care Given that attention is being directed at present to various dimensions of zero consumption of mental health services, it is relevant to consider another variable. It was pointed out, in the discussion of Equation (6.1), that income was a determinant of the consumption of in-patient psychiatric care. Figure 6.10 presents the case of two people who have the **same preferences**, as indicated by the same indifference map, $I_1, \ldots, I_4$, for In-patient Psychiatric Care and a Hicksian composite commodity, All Other Commodities. This implies that the two people have the same mental health status. However, these two people differ in terms of income, the two budget constraints being B_1C_1 and B_2C_2. Note that these two budget constraints are parallel, thus indicating that the two consumers face the same relative prices.

Figure 6.10 The importance of income as a determinant of the consumption of in-patient psychiatric care

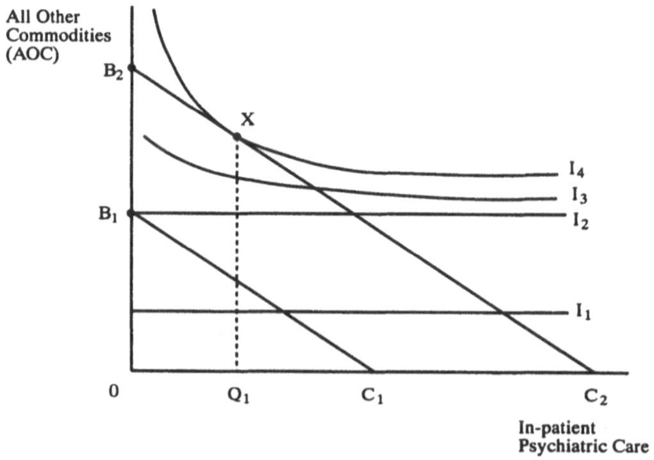

For Person 1, with the low income, the optimal point of consumption is the 'corner solution' where I_2 is tangential to B_1C_1 at the point B_1. This means that Person 1 allocates all of his/her (low) income to All Other Commodities and zero income to In-patient Psychiatric Care. On the other hand, Person 2 with his/her higher income will consume at point X, where indifference curve I_4 is tangential to B_2C_2. This means that Person 2 will consume OQ_1 units of in-patient psychiatric care, thus splitting his/her income between this commodity and All Other Commodities.

The Demand for Mental Health Care and the Utilisation of Services

The focus of this Chapter broadens at this point to a level of conceptualising mental health care: the perspective is that of a bird's eye view. In this Section, the interactions among fundamental economic relationships that determine a person's well-being are considered, with mental health status explicitly acknowledged. These interactions are shown by using various notions that

Figure 6.11 The household treatment of mental health

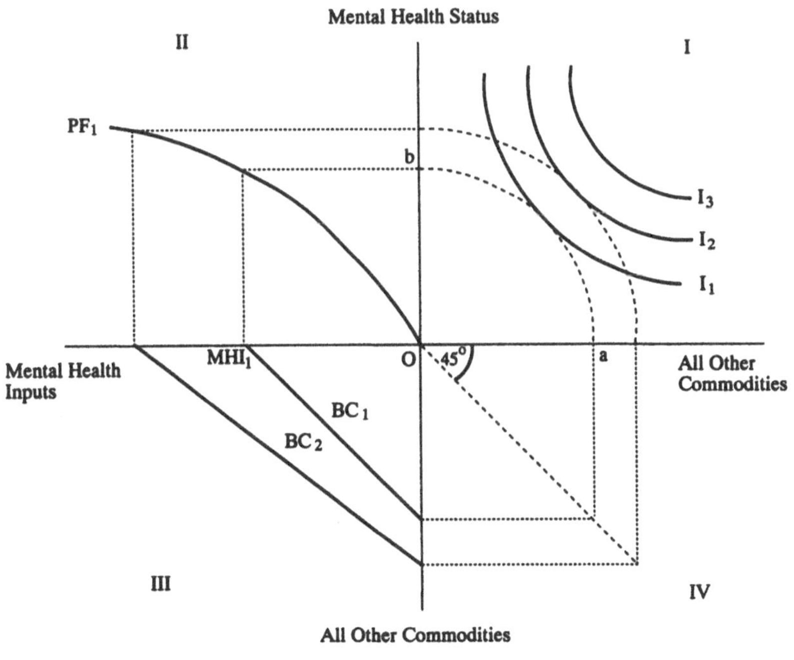

Source: Adapted from Wagstaff (1986).

have been developed in previous Sections, as well as in Chapter 5. Recall that one focus of Chapters 5 and 6 has been to conceptualise the multi-dimensionality of a person's preferences for mental health care, in the context that combinations of mental health care and other desirable commodities maximise the well-being of people having a need for mental health care. Having addressed preferences, it is necessary to address the problem that people's preferences over the goods and services, which are capable of maximising their well-being, are constrained. That is, budgetary (or financial), as well as technological (e.g. medically possible), constraints limit the maximisation of people's preferences. Hence, this Section depicts, at a conceptual level, the previous notions about preferences interacting with the constraints. This interaction makes possible explanations about the demand for mental health care. A 'four-quadrant diagram' is useful for conceptualising the demand for mental health care, and the concept is developed below. The four-quadrant diagram developed here follows Wagstaff's model (1986), itself a development of Grossman's model of household production. Note that this four-quadrant diagram is neither unique, as an economic technique, nor the only one (i.e. other than Wagstaff's) found in the economics of health care. For example, see Folland, Goodman and Stano (1997, p. 116*ff*). However, an adapted Wagstaff approach is useful for our purposes here. Note also that in the explanations below, some background in economics is assumed. Non-economists are advised to study Wagstaff's (1986) paper, a 'user-friendly' piece, before embarking on the following text.

Individual Demand for Mental Health Care

The individual's utility maximising behaviour is analysed with the aid of Figure 6.11, a four-quadrant diagram. This diagram establishes, for example, how much 'mental health' a person will demand and how much 'mental health inputs' that person will use. It also enables predictions about the direction of changes to be made.

Quadrant I, in the north-east corner, depicts an indifference map of a person's preferences in seeking the highest possible level of well-being for himself or herself. Well-being is determined by two variables (which are commodity aggregates), *viz.* the arguments, mental health status (MHS) and other commodities consumed (which previously in Chapters 5 and 6 is referred to as the Hicksian composite 'All Other Commodities' or AOC). The highest level of well-being is indicated conceptually by the highest indifference curve, I_3 in Quadrant I.

In this four-quadrant diagram, the two main constraints upon a person's pursuit of well-being are shown by the particular information contained in Quadrants II and III. What is technologically possible in transferring mental health inputs into output (or MHS) is depicted by the mental health production function PF_1 in Quadrant II. The production function is drawn on the assumption that the production of MHS is subject to the Law of Diminishing Marginal Product but, in reality, not much is known about the shape of the mental health production function.

Quadrant III shows the relationship between the relative prices of mental health inputs and all other commodities, as discussed in regard to the conventional budget line indicated in Figure 6.9. In this diagram two 'budget constraints' BC_1 and BC_2 are depicted. Note that while these budget constraints differ, both represent the 'budget problem', which is that a person's income is spent (i.e. exhausted) by combinations of the relative prices of mental health inputs and the prices of AOC, and the quantities of these consumed.

Quadrant IV has All Other Commodities on both axes, with a '45° degree line'. This device allows the same quantity of All Other Commodities to be translated from Quadrant III back to Quadrant I. Alternatively, the information contained in Quadrant III is transferred via Quadrant II back to Quadrant I.

Hence, the four-quadrant diagram depicted here enables information derived from the budget constraint and the production function to be related on the same diagram. Such information enables, for a given quantity of mental health input, say MHI_1, the determination of the quantity of MHS that will be produced **and** the quantity of AOC that can be purchased with the income remaining, given relative prices. For example, mental health input MHI_1 is associated (via the production function PF_1) with an MHS of Ob. The relevant given budget constraint, BC_1 in Quadrant III, indicates the quantity of AOC that can be purchased with the person's income remaining. This is translated, via Quadrant IV, back to Quadrant I as the quantity of AOC consumed, e.g. quantity Oa of AOC. In this manner, a transformation curve, such as *ab*, can be drawn in Quadrant I. The indifference curve I_1 tangential to the transformation curve *ab* indicates the equilibrium quantity of MHS and AOC arising for this person.

Note that the other budget constraint BC_2 is drawn further out from the origin in Quadrant III, which shows a higher income level, and with a different slope from BC_1 which indicates a change in the relativity of prices for MHI and AOC. This higher budget involves production at a point further out on PF_1 in Quadrant II, and a new transformation curve (further out from the origin) in Quadrant I.

Some Applications

Application 1: In-Patient Status

Figure 6.12 shows the situation of an institutionalised individual who has no source of income. Being involuntarily committed to this institution, the individual must consume health inputs OH whilst the institution determines the amount OC of other goods that this individual may consume. The 'budget line' can be depicted as point I, determined bureaucratically. In other words,

Figure 6.12 Some applications

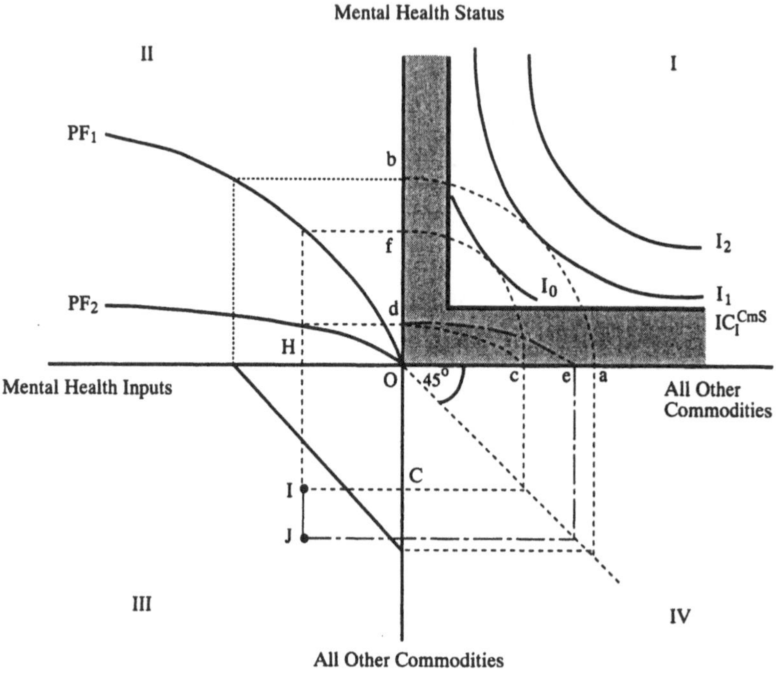

the expenditure associated with the provision of mental health inputs and All Other Commodities (predominantly accommodation and meals) is not determined by the consumer: these decisions are taken by the institution's staff. Unfortunately, treatment is producing little effect on his or her mental health status, as depicted by the shape of the production function, PF_2, in Quadrant II. PF_2 is translated into the transformation curve *cd* (Quadrant I) which is within the shaded area created by the 'imposed indifference curve' IC_I^{CmS}. Hence, the individual remains 'inside' (and inside the 'imposed indifference curve' IC_I^{CmS}).

Application 2: Income Support for In-Patients

Imagine a situation wherein government legislates that individuals in psychiatric institutions are eligible for income support, via a routinely-paid pension or allowance, or some type of intermittent grant. A determined proportion of this income support has to be paid to the psychiatric institution in the form of a nominal maintenance fee, the remainder of which the in-patient has for personal income. In effect, the individual receives an increase in income. The main effect of this policy is to transfer that part of **expenditure associated with the institutionalised stay from the institution** (which is possibly run by a local or state government) **to a provider of income support** (which is possibly the central government). Even though this individual is still required to consume CO of All Other Commodities (AOC) in Figure 6.12, he or she nevertheless has a small surplus to spend as desired, perhaps at the hospital canteen. Hence, point I extends out to J in Figure 6.12. The effect of this increase in income is, essentially, upon AOC: there is no effect on mental health status, given that there is neither a shift in the position of the mental health production function, nor a shift in the consumer's location on that function. Hence, the transformation curve *cd* pivots outwards to *ed*, the effect being confined to an increase in AOC. Given that the new transformation curve lies entirely within the shaded region of Quadrant I of Figure 6.12, the individual is unfortunately not in a state of mind to be released and his or her optimal point is still inside the 'imposed indifference curve' IC_I^{CmS}.

Application 3: The Discovery of Lithium Salts as a Medication

It has been pointed out in Chapter 5 that there have been some major innovations in the treatment of a number of diseases/conditions, including depression. The point of this work has been to indicate that, given the improved health outcome associated with these innovations, the relative prices of some medications have been falling. The analysis presented here indicates the beneficial effect of innovation in therapy, doing so in a somewhat different way, as follows. The discovery of psychotropic medication in the late 1940s and the 1950s had, for particular individuals, beneficial effects. The example chosen to illustrate this case is an 'old' innovation in medication, *viz.* lithium. Lithium, being especially successful in easing the mood swings of individuals with bipolar disorder, enables particular individuals to live quite normal lives in the community.

Consider the circumstances just analysed. The production function PF_2 is a manifestation of the essentially inefficacious pre-lithium technology for treating bipolar disorder. PF_1, which incorporates treatment with lithium medication, represents a massive shift in the production of mental health status derived from mental health inputs. Given the application of the same quantity of mental health inputs (albeit with a substitution of lithium for other drugs), the person now obtains *Of* mental health status, compared with *Od*, the amount obtainable given the former technology. This in turn creates a new transformation curve, *fc* in Quadrant I. Note that this new transformation curve involves a pivot out from the point *c* on the 'old' transformation curve, *cd*.[9] Note also that a segment of *cf* is north-east of the imposed indifference

9 This assumes that the person being considered here has no income. This is not an important assumption: if an assumption were invoked that the person had a residual income (from a disability support pension, say), then the relevant 'old' transformation curve would be *de*.

curve IC_I^{CmS}. If the person is on this segment then he or she will be discharged from the institution. This would involve a point of tangency between cf and an indifference curve, I_0, in Quadrant I.

Application 4: Individual Preferences over Side Effects of Treatment

Few treatments have a 100 per cent success rate with no side effects. Thus, it is common for individuals to 'trade-off' the efficacy of treatments with the side effects that treatment induces. The example here concerns the side effects some individuals may face from medication.

Not all individuals who suffer bipolar disorder continue with a course of lithium. While, for some, it is a 'miracle' drug, others, often highly creative individuals such as poets, writers and artists, find themselves losing much of their creative energies that come into play at various stages of the mood swings. In these circumstances, individuals may opt for a lower mental health status and decline medication, i.e. opt for an indifference curve nearer the origin in Quadrant I in Figure 6.12. On the other hand, they may be able to exercise a trade-off, on the same mental health indifference curve, over choices regarding the treatment they undergo, i.e. between a lesser alleviation of unpleasant symptoms (by refusing lithium for mood swings) for lesser disability, which effectively would encourage more creative ability.

Often the achievement of this 'happy medium' entails a price that has to be paid by the consumer and possibly relatives and friends too. All people concerned have to live with the considerable uncertainty as to the outcome of such individuals' experimental searches for the inputs that are needed for a better level of well-being.

Summary and Conclusion

The purpose of this Chapter has been to clarify the outputs of mental health care, the services being conceptualised as multi-dimensional. In this Chapter, people's preferences are also expressed in multi-dimensional space.

When utility is most simply defined in economics, it is synonymous with economic welfare, happiness or satisfaction, as outlined in Chapter 1. Another of its meanings, also outlined in Chapter 1, is that an individual derives utility from a good or service, or event, if he or she prefers it to exist rather than not to exist. When an individual derives more utility from good X than from good Y, the economic connotation is that the person prefers good X to good Y. Utility, in its ordinal meaning, has explanatory power, given the present state of knowledge of economic phenomena. It is this interpretation that is employed in Chapters 5 and 6, with the qualification that only one aspect of Sen's approach to the standard of living, briefly explained in Chapter 1, is being addressed in these Chapters.

Initially, a distinction was made in Chapter 5 between the need for care and the demand for care, specifically important for matters relating to resource allocation. It was then suggested that it is helpful to think of mental health as entering into the household production function as a commodity vector, following Becker (1965) and Grossman (1972a)(1972b). Preferences for mental health and for all other commodities were shown to exist in Becker-type commodity space upon the application of an appropriate separability function involving two-stage budgetting. This clarification enabled the description of various notions. It helped explain the relationship between mental health care inputs and the output of the mental health care sector. Also, it enabled a clarification of implications arising from the rationality assumption, basic to the approach at hand. In particular, an explanation was possible, within characteristics space, of preference behaviour relating to two mental health sub-vectors: symptom alleviation and disability reduction.

This approach was useful for explaining individuals' preferences regarding voluntary in-patient care, or ambulatory care. It was then used in Chapter 6 to show what it means, in an economic sense, when society 'draws the line' and an individual is involuntarily committed to in-patient treatment/care. The introduction of an 'imposed indifference curve' to the analysis enabled this clarification. By connecting the notion of indifference curves and mental health care production functions, after Wagstaff (1986), an economic explanation was given as to why some individuals are, or remain, institutionalised: it may be due to the shape and position of the mental health care production function itself or it may be due to society allocating insufficient resources to mental health care. Of course, it could also mean that society's 'imposed indifference curve' is inappropriately placed, i.e. unjust in terms of a person's liberty, but this is a legal issue beyond the scope of this study.

This Chapter focussed further on the 'imposed indifference curve' as a conceptualisation of the nature of government response to mental health care. Also in Chapter 6, an implication regarding the role of the government's agents or 'gatekeepers' to mental health care, *viz.* the medical profession, was considered.

An alternative terminology could be applied to some of the concepts employed in this Chapter. The arguments herein have been in terms of governments 'imposing an indifference curve' which specifies minimum amounts of mental health, mental health care services, or particular aspects of daily living (to do with individuals' behaviours or their functioning); and governments intervening if a person's consumption of these phenomena fall below those stated minimum quantities. An alternative way of stating this conception should be recognised. Rather than thinking of the lexicographic relationship of those minima as an 'imposed indifference curve', the relationships can be conceived of as constraints: people are free to choose their own combinations of these phenomena, subject to their consumption not being less than the government-determined minima.

Finally, it should be noted that, given the considerable attention in Chapter 5 and in the present Chapter to the notion, 'individual preferences', the intention has not been to convey an overarching libertarianism. If that were the case, the preferences of individuals who utilise mental health care would count above all else and all others. Rather the intention, in considering preferences, has been to shed light on the (economic) sense in which individuals with mental disorders do or do not have preferences, and ought or ought not have preferences. In so doing, it has been possible to clarify the nature of the outputs of mental health care.

7 The Role of Government in Mental Health Care: A Normative Analysis

Background

Historically speaking, care and provision in Western societies for 'lunatics', 'idiots', the 'mad', the 'insane', 'the mentally ill' or 'people with psychiatric illness', whatever individuals have been called at various periods in human history, have been framed within a 'pattern of long-term neglect in provision ... punctuated by periods of reform' (Lewis, 1988, p. 2). The accounts of this process of intermittent interest, e.g. Foucault (1967), Howells (1976), Lewis (1988), discuss the scope and efficacy of treatments, the settings within which individuals are treated and cared for, and the sources of funding for these measures. There are two recurrent themes in these histories: first, the normative issue of how society should have been (or now should be) responding to these individuals' own personal suffering and/or socially intolerable behaviours; and, second, the positive issue of how society has been, and is, responding.

The role of the state and the boundaries of government intervention, both from a positive, and from a normative, perspective are leading considerations that are recognised in the legal, clinical and political literatures, though the distinction between the two perspectives is not always drawn clearly by the writers. The focuses of these literatures include, respectively, the deprivation of liberty of involuntary patients, e.g. Kirby (1983); the treatment *milieu* in state institutions, e.g. English and McGarrick (1989); and the politics behind state action, e.g. Lipton (1983). On the other hand in the economic literature, there has been little explanation, either of a positive or a normative kind, of the role of government in mental health care. The economic issues associated with mental illness have some parallels with the theory of the role of government in the health care provided for physical diseases and/or conditions. However, it is what that theory does **not** explain that calls for attention. The purpose of this present Chapter is to suggest some introductory analyses of the role of government with respect to mental health care.

The Nature of Government Responses to Mental Health Care

Public Facilities

Compared with the efforts of government in the eighteenth century, government involvement in mental health care is now considerable.

It was during the nineteenth century that government undertook an unprecedented degree of responsibility for the well-being of people with mental disorders, replacing efforts and responsibility that had largely been the domain of the parish and the family. However, an historical overview of the facilities serving the needs of the mentally ill and their families reveals in the facilities themselves a 'deviance' in, and haphazardness about, their usefulness. This is ironic, given people themselves were being judged as deviant. Indeed, a prerequisite for reform in government services was for society to draw a distinction between the notion of the 'insane' and other types of (so-called) social 'deviant' such as the vagrant, the pauper, the petty criminal, the physically disabled.

In early periods in Australia, many aspects of the approach to mental illness and disorders followed British principles and practices. By the mid-nineteenth century in England, the insane were typically isolated from society. They were merely kept alive in special institutions, the now infamous 'asylums', a term far less pejorative in those times than today. In the colonial era of Australian history, insanity and criminality were closely associated in the public mind (Lewis, 1988, p. 6). There was a disposition to house the 'insane' in gaols and lock-ups, after committal to imprisonment by order of a magistrate. In the State of Queensland, for example, it was not until 1865 that the Woogaroo Lunatic Asylum was opened as a result of extreme overcrowding in the gaols. The impetus for the creation of this 'new' institution was in response to an inquiry by the imperial government into colonial hospitals and asylums, the report having denounced the gaoling of lunatics, arguing that they ought to be placed in institutions devoted to care. Unfortunately, this care did not occur at Woogaroo initially, since the asylum was staffed by prison officers, rather than nursing and medical staff; and inmates were kept in exposed yards during the day-time and confined to dark, overcrowded quarters at night. These circumstances were little different from the gaols (Evans, 1969).

It is not relevant here to trace the development and history of such facilities. Patrick (1987) has included mental health services in his historical account of services in Queensland, for example. For a report on the status of psychiatric facilities just prior to some of the current changes, see Stoller and Arscott (1955). For an historical account of institutionalised patients in the State of Victoria, see Krupinski and Stoller (1962, 1975).

The current era presents new challenges. These days, nursing staff and medical staff provide care for in-patients, and hospital conditions have vastly improved.[1] However, the problem of inadequate funding has largely persisted, an 'obvious indicator of the low priority that psychiatric services had for governments and for voters' (Lewis, 1988, p. 47). People who are deemed not sick enough to be hospitalised have access to extremely under-funded and understaffed community facilities. If needing to be hospitalised, spells as in-patients are relatively brief, although the rate of hospitalisation is likely to be different for publicly-insured patients from what it is for privately-insured patients. Community services and household resources are greatly stretched by the move to community care, however the pressure on psychiatric hospital facilities has been alleviated in the last three decades. The pressure on public facilities has been eased also by the integration of acute mental health services with physical health care services in general hospitals. For a detailed account in the Australian context, see Lewis (1988) and Patrick (1987).

In contemporary times, expenditure by the state governments is more restricted than in earlier eras. See Hart (1989) for some time series data on expenditure on mental health services. See also Whiteford, Thompson and Casey (2000). Frequently, reforms are promised when scandal erupts, but seldom does a substantial increase in budgetary allocation occur once public concern dies down.

Historically as well as constitutionally, the Commonwealth Government in Australia has had no direct responsibility for the provision of psychiatric care, except in its own Territories. Successive Commonwealth Governments have made 'limited forays' (Lewis, 1988, p. 77) into the financing of psychiatric services, with varying degrees of involvement and success. Subsidised voluntary health insurance was introduced by the Commonwealth, in the form of hospital benefits and medical benefits in 1952 and 1953 respectively. Voluntary insurance continued until 1975, when the (then) Labor Government introduced Australia's first system of universal national health insurance, Medibank. When the Australian Labor Party next returned to government, Australia's system of universal national health insurance, Medicare, came into being in 1984. For details, see Sax (1984) and Palmer and Short (1994).

Universal national health insurance has expanded considerably the role of the Commonwealth Government within psychiatric care. As with its predecessor, Medicare provides comprehensive, non means-tested entitlement to benefits to cover basic medical and general hospital costs, and this effectively amounts to subsidised visits to general practitioners (GPs) and to psychiatrists for ambulatory treatment, as well as access, free of charge, to the first 35 days of in-patient care at a general hospital. It is important to note that these schemes of public funding involved discriminatory policies for persons with medical qualifications, whether they be GPs or psychiatrists, and other health

---

1 For an account of general hospital conditions for patients with mental illnesses in British history, see Freeman (1995).

professionals (psychologists, social workers etc.) with relevant skills for the treatment of some psychiatric disorders. Australian policy on government subsidies for health services has been to give subsidies only for services provided by two professional groups, namely, medical practitioners and (the numerically small) optometrists. There has been no obvious reason given for this differential treatment. Additionally, the Pharmaceutical Benefits Scheme introduced by the Commonwealth Government in 1944 has subsidised prescribed medication.

For a detailed account of the recent period, one of the authors being the architect of Medibank, see Scotton and Macdonald (1993). See also Scotton and Macdonald (1995).

Treatment

Attention is directed briefly here to an overview of the provision of treatment. The historical variations in the approaches to mental illness have considerable bearing on an understanding, in economics, of the positive role of government.

The idea of trying to treat insanity has an unfortunate history of cruelty and misguided compassion. Barely two hundred years ago, it was believed that madness could be controlled by blood letting and purging of the bowels, by mechanical restraint or by the 'more humane' approach of psychological restraint espoused by the 'moral treatment' movement (to which reference was first made in Chapter 3). See Rosenblatt (1984) and Lewis (1988).

There have been ongoing changes in attitudes and treatments in the last hundred years. Late in the nineteenth century, these notions gradually lost ground to biological and hereditary explanations of the cause of mental illness. By the early 1900s, Freud and psychoanalysis were being discussed by Australian doctors. While the overwhelming emphasis on heredity lessened, the medical model of mental disorder gained favour, so much so that by the 1930s to 1940s, insulin therapy and electro-convulsive therapy (ECT) were widely available as an espoused means to reduce the suicide rates in institutions, and as a cure for severe depression. The next generation of physical treatments, the psychotropic drugs, arrived in the 1950s. While the policy of deinstitutionalisation in the United States was an outcome of the widespread use of psychotropic drugs in treatment, it has been said that this was a less important factor in Australia. It has been argued, perhaps naively, that factors such as earlier treatment, the presence of facilities already in existence in the community, and more sympathetic public attitudes, rather than the use of the new drugs, were key factors in the 'emptying' of the state psychiatric hospitals (Stoller, cited in Lewis, 1988, p. 56).

By the 1960s and 1970s tension was apparent between two perspectives of treatment for mental disorder: the psychodynamic, or psychological, approach; and the organic, or biological, approach to treatment. This conflict resulted, during the 1980s, in increasing disillusionment with the old biological approach.

Indeed, by the end of the 1970s, at least seven views of madness were identifiable (Bates, 1979). Attention will be directed next to each of these views, not with the purpose of offering detailed understanding of each view, but rather of giving insight into the breadth of approaches to mental illnesses in recent decades. Having an appreciation of the range of views is pertinent to an understanding of the role that government adopts in mental health care.

Bates' 'models' of madness It has been suggested by Bates (1979) that the conception commonly referred to as the classical medical 'model' regards mental illness as a biological event. Social circumstances have an effect only incidentally upon mental illness. This view of madness rests on the key notion that what individuals suffer is an illness, like any other illness. Existing in parallel with this view is another medical view that acknowledges the contribution of social influences upon the patient in causing mental disorder and, thereby, admits stigma into the experience of mental illness. A third view, apparent more within community psychiatry, blames social issues or circumstances for the major contribution to mental disorder. Fourth, an 'anti-psychiatry' view owes allegiance to Laing (1965), Cooper (1970) and Szasz (1961). Laing is recognised for his denial of the reality of mental illness. He argues that psychiatry amounts to a political activity to support the interests of the powerful and to aid the oppression of weaker members of society. Along with the 'liberationists' (like Laing and Cooper), Bates (1979) looks at the argument that protesters against political and social oppression are essentially those who are labelled 'ill'. Both the anti-psychiatry and liberationist views hold to an opinion that it is society, not the patient, which needs to change.

Bates (1979) describes an educational view of madness. This perspective is best understood in terms of the purposes of cognitive behaviour therapy, practised by many psychologists. With cognitive behaviour therapy, 'patients' are people who have learned inappropriate behaviours that need to be unlearned. Perhaps the most useful contribution of this approach is that it recognises the human ability to adapt, and indeed mal-adapt, to the ongoing presence of an illness or condition faced in life.

The approach that has its roots in the discipline of sociology is a relativistic one, namely, that madness and normality are relative concepts. For example, what is considered madness in one society is not in another.

One of the more recent views is not so concerned with defining the cause of mental disorders, as with suggesting that fellow sufferers and former sufferers are the source of the best long-term care. According to Bates, the 'self-help' approach asserts that lay people should not only offer mutual aid, but should also acquire the knowledge needed to regain a sense of control over their own lives. The work of Illich (1976) has been influential among some of the 'self-help' school.

The present approach Contemporary psychiatric practice is characterised by eclecticism. A 'bio-psycho-social' view has replaced the former medical approach. This view looks to the social, psychological and behavioural aspects of mental disorder, with diagnosis remaining in the hands of a psychiatrist who is also the director of a team-based plan of treatment.

In Australia, this contemporary eclecticism is evident in the community clinics of the relevant state government departments and in the private psychiatric hospitals. It is less evident in the resource-stretched public hospital facilities. In the private workshops of GPs, psychiatrists and psychologists, each practitioner delineates his or her own type of product.

A structural, or institutional, feature of the Medibank system introduced in 1975, and also embedded in the Medicare system of health funding implemented in 1984, is that the Commonwealth is subsidising the current models of treatment of mental disorder, whichever ones are being implemented in practice. On the one hand, access for individuals to psychiatric treatment is widened but, on the other hand, subsidisation limits individuals' treatment choices by constraining the expansion of the 'territory' of other professional groups. It is unlikely that psychologists and psychiatric social workers will be successful in the immediate future in their attempts to secure listings in the *Medicare Benefits Schedule Book*. See Medicare Benefits Review Committee (1985). The analysis of these issues is beyond the scope of this study.

In view of the range of opinions about mental illness outlined in this and the previous Sub-section, it is not a trivial concern when government makes decisions to subsidise particular treatment settings or practices.

The Characteristics of the Public Sector

The Nature of Mental Health Facilities

Initially, present arrangements for mental health care facilities that were mentioned in the previous Section will be summarised here in Table 7.1. This Table indicates that the production of mental health care involves one, or a combination, of the following elements: deprivation of liberty, accommodation, treatment, medical/nursing care, personal/familial support. The Table classifies these five production characteristics according to three residential settings, and the levels of care associated with each type of accommodation. At this point, it is assumed that the characteristics presented in the Table do not necessarily imply public or private provision. In fact, for the moment, they are best considered as mental health care outputs *per se*, regardless of which sector provides them.

The Table can be read in either of two ways. By considering the entries in any column, one can determine the characteristics of a particular service provided. For example, ambulatory care does not involve deprivation of liberty, does not involve the provision of accommodation etc. Alternatively, by concentrating on the entries in a particular row, one can quickly determine the type of service that 'embeds' or provides a particular characteristic. For example, medical/nursing care is limited in both ambulatory and hostel care, but is available with in-patient care. It should be noted that the important characteristic, 'personal/familial support', is associated, in complex ways, with all three types of care. This Table depicts the general contemporary landscape of mental health care in Australia.

Table 7.1 Characteristics of services for individuals with mental disorders

	Type of Service by Residential Status Provided at:		
Characteristics of Services	Home (Ambulatory care)	Hospital (In-patient care)	Hostel (Hostel care)
Deprivation of liberty	No	Yes (where required)	No
Accommodation	Available	Provided	Provided
Treatments	Available	Provided	Available
Medical/nursing care	Limited	Yes	Limited
Personal/familial support	Widely varied	Limited	Limited

Note: It is recognised that this Table does not account for, or recognise, those persons with mental illness who are homeless or 'on the street'. The existence of such people would be overlooked in a Table such as this.

The Public Sector

From the historical accounts of the previous Sections of this Chapter, it is apparent that the original role of government was understood only in terms of deprivation of liberty, since decent accommodation was seldom provided and the treatments available were not efficacious.

Treatment and care increasingly came under the umbrella of government, once the institutional setting of state psychiatric hospitals provided the accepted mode for managing 'madness'. The hospital continued, until recent decades, to be the traditional setting in which accommodation, treatment and care and, for some, the deprivation of liberty occurred. That is, psychiatric hospitals have been (and are) characterised by joint production.

The current era of deinstitutionalisation has predominantly involved the privatisation of accommodation, care and home support, with treatment given on an ambulatory basis at public clinics. In the US and Canada, many European countries and Australia, individuals who are quite seriously ill, though not dangerous, have been discharged from hospitals, having to revert to community life.

Particular patients, a minority, still can be detained against their wishes. The matter of whether this is a (Samuelsonian) public good will be considered later in this Chapter. A few, a very few, patients in state psychiatric hospitals are there on an involuntary basis. Additionally, it is thought that a proportion of individuals with a mental disorder continue to face detention in the prison system rather than receiving proper psychiatric treatment and care.

Now one other type of facility, not uniquely public, is indicated in Table 7.1. Supervised hostels provide a type of 'half-way house' facility before patients' relocation in the community. These are facilities for limited-term care. Relatively little government-provided hostel accommodation is available for individuals suffering with long-term or chronic illness, except in instances where an individual has a physical or intellectual disability.

A Normative Analysis of the Role of Government

The following Sections of this Chapter will examine the economic rationale for the role of government generally. Attention will then turn to some of the economic principles of efficient resource use in the public allocation of mental health care.[2]

In defining a role for government generally, two arguments can be invoked: market failure and the merit good. On the grounds of allocative inefficiencies arising in the presence of market failure, it is necessary to show, first, that the market does not satisfy the conditions under which Pareto optimality can occur; and, second, that the costs of government intervention to alleviate the costs of the market failure are smaller than the market failure itself. Note that it is not uncommon to find the so-called 'merit good argument', first advocated by Musgrave (1959), being applied to mental health care.

In this Section, the grounds for each of these rationales will be considered, but it is helpful, first, to consider an important question. Into what is government intervening?

The Avenues for Government Intervention

In matters of mental health care, economists are prone to ask what it is about the behaviour of an individual with a mental disorder that presents economic grounds for government intervention. This naturally can have a normative implication but, in the first instance, the purpose is merely to clarify the economic grounds.

If society believes it knows what is best for individuals with mental disorders, then 'society's' preferences will over-ride individual preferences

---

2 Attention here is directed to the allocative role of government. Stabilisation and distribution are two other functions of government in the framework of Musgrave (1959).

in all cases, and arguments for government intervention, in order to provide goods deemed to be merit goods, will pertain. This matter will be considered again later.

Can there be, however, any instances when individual preferences count in regard to mental disorder? Some people may say 'no'. And yet, unless it is made quite clear why the state is intervening, the result is that the public sector provides a role in mental health care for reasons that, regrettably, are not made transparent.

The first point to note is that only the most seriously ill people suffer extreme preference dysfunction. That is, these individuals are incapable, in their state, of carrying out the mental functions necessary to exercise preferences in the most basic manner. In this condition, it is likely that government will undertake guardianship.

Not all individuals are, however, as extremely indisposed as this. With respect to other persons, there are two issues raised in Chapters 5 and 6 that ought to be examined in regard to aberrations in their preferences. These issues will now be addressed.

The range of impairment in preference capacity The thrust of the argument in Chapters 5 and 6 was that the preference functioning **capacity** of some individuals is impaired in itself. Put otherwise, preferences cannot be ordered, subject to a budget constraint, to allow such individuals the chance to achieve an optimal choice decision. For example, a person with schizophrenia often suffers impaired capacity for planning. It is important to note in these instances that the person's preferences are not necessarily irrational, *per se*. Rather, it is that the preferences cannot be expressed or exercised.

Another aspect of the aberrations that arise in the preference-forming capacities in individuals is related to how illness manifests itself across the passage of time. For example, it is not at all uncommon for suffering individuals to wish to be dead rather than alive, but most individuals, once restored to health, are glad to have been kept alive. At this point it is relevant to recall Chapter 5 where the transitivity axiom of consumer behaviour was stated. This (just mentioned) example of preference reversal raises the issue of violation of the transitivity axiom. In this instance, the preference reversal arises to the extent that ill-health progresses through various stages. See also Schwartz and Griffin (1986, p. 140 *ff*).

Impairment in preference capacity also affects care-givers. Strain can arise whether those others are employed care-givers, such as nurses or social workers, or whether they are family care-givers. Part of the strain is due to the nature of the preferences of the disordered individual. The other part of the strain is due to a shortfall in the procedures for providing adequate care in the presence of this problem. Care-giving spouses and daughters of elderly people suffering advanced stages of Alzheimer's Disease, for example, are known to face extreme strain due to this problem (Power, 1989). Such cases of impaired preference functioning capacity and its effects imply that there is a range of significantly differing economic rationales for government involvement and, thus, for the type of care and treatment individuals receive.

A qualification is pertinent at this point. The references, above, to the axioms of utility theory are not to suggest that these axioms serve as incontrovertible yardsticks of rationality; medical psychology indicates their limitations in describing consumer decision-making (Schwartz and Griffin, 1986).

Socially unacceptable preferences One other point made in Chapter 6 refers to the situation where an individual's goals are socially unacceptable.[3] An example in this context is of a seriously ill individual whose goal is to consume no mental health care, in other words, absolutely zero mental health care. Individuals suffering a mental disorder frequently live in an unreal world. Some of the goals that are expressed through a mental health utility function such as in Equation (5.3) in Chapter 5 are an expression of this unreal world. Hence, socially unacceptable goals frequently are symptomatic of serious mental disorder. Such a situation is represented by 'society' preferring a different set of indifference curves from those of the individual.[4]

The question arises as to which preferences will be socially tolerated. On a spectrum of socially acceptable goals, at one extreme the utility functions of seriously ill individuals may incorporate goals that are socially intolerable, for example, doing violence to oneself or others. At the other end of the spectrum there exist the individual differences which arise between individuals merely over matters of lifestyle, or taste, or manners. The less an individual's utility function matches a social norm, the greater the stress, felt either by the individual or by others in the community, from externalities arising from interdependent utility functions. Between the two ends of the spectrum is a murky area with regard to mental disorders, wherein some of an individual's goals are deemed socially unacceptable. In the light of these points, it would seem important to distinguish between an economic rationale for government, based on the presence of socially unacceptable preferences, and such a rationale based on the presence of impaired preference capacity.

One of the duties of the 'gatekeepers' to the public system of care, say, medical practitioners, is to serve as delegates for society's decision-making over which individuals are to use what public facilities. The implication of the argument of this Section is that an important distinction needs to be made

---

3 An 'unacceptable goal' is really just an extreme or polar case of 'unacceptable preferences'.

4 This is exemplified in the widespread, everyday use of vocabulary relating to mental disorders which is used to describe attitudes or behaviours that are disapproved or disagreed with, as in such words as 'mad', 'crazy', 'irrational', 'bizarre' (Edwards, 1975, cited in Lewis, 1988, p. 226).

between their role as clinicians and their role as society's delegates in decision-making about the use of resources. Guidelines for hospitalisation of patients with chronic mental disorders, as published in the clinical literature (e.g. Glick *et al.*, 1984), do not spell out this fundamentally important distinction.

Market Failure

In the previous Sub-section the avenues of government intervention were broadly explored. In this Sub-section the economic grounds for government intervention are considered. With respect to health care, there are several aspects of the arguments for government intervention based on market failure. The aspects most relevant to mental health care include the public good argument, the presence of externalities and the problem of informational asymmetries. In the following paragraphs two of these arguments for the role of government are examined: the presence of a public good and the presence of externalities. Attention then turns to a brief examination of the 'merit good' argument as a justification for the role of government. This topic is examined because government intervention in mental health care raises issues which appear to suggest that mental health care is a merit good.

The 'public good' argument Public goods are distinguished by the degree to which two defining characteristics are present in a good or service: first, whether or not the good is 'excludable'; and second, whether or not the good is 'rival' in consumption (Samuelson, 1954, 1955). Goods are public when other people cannot be prevented from using the good, i.e. the good is characterised by non-excludability. Second, goods are public in instances where the good is not only non-excludable by nature, but also non-rival, that is, one person's use of the good does not diminish another person's enjoyment of it. Because public goods are characterised by non-excludability, the free-rider problem is present: this prevents the private market from supplying such goods and services in appropriate quantities. The free-rider problem arises because a person can receive the benefit of a good but can avoid paying for it. With public goods, due to the presence of externalities, a price cannot be attached to the good, although it has value. Hence, a provider of a public good faces the problem that people are better off enjoying the benefit that the good gives, and yet a price for the good cannot be effectively charged. Because of the free rider problem, the level of output is under-, or even non-, provided in terms of Pareto optimality.[5]

Mental health care, across the spectrum of treatment, care, accommodation and so forth, is not a pure public good. A degree of excludability and of rivalry in consumption is evident.

---

5 These characteristics aside, it is not a foregone conclusion that a public good *necessarily* be provided by the public rather than the private sector. The classic public good argument leads to a conclusion of public funding. Whether this involves public or private production is a separate matter. Musgrave (1959) makes this quite clear.

There is an obvious exception. When a person is deprived of liberty, he or she is placed in an institution. The consequent non-excludable nature of deprivation of liberty means this aspect of mental health care is public, by nature. This is because it is simply not socially feasible to exclude an extremely psychotic individual who is, say, suicidal or homicidal, from mental health care on the grounds of a free rider argument. In the production of deprivation of liberty, however, 'jointness' is involved. This is because, when a person is detained, the subsequent need to provide food, accommodation etc. arises. Now, accommodation and food are private goods, on the grounds of the possible exclusion of individuals from their consumption and also because the addition of extra individuals depletes each person's consumption (due to crowding).

How then can the present role of government, as indicated previously in Table 7.1, be reconciled with a public good argument? There is a paradox: treatment, care, accommodation and personal/familial support of contemporary times have the characteristics of private goods; but society may, however, require a particular standard or quality of care. An externality now can be recognised. In order to explain this, consider first describing 'quality of care' in terms of the presence in the good of particular characteristics that are seen to be desirable. See the Appendix to Chapter 5. Now, Samuelson (1969) has defined a publicly provided good as a good which 'enters two or more persons' utility' (p. 108). When a 'quality of care' externality is acknowledged, then not just deprivation of liberty but the joint provision of treatment, care, accommodation and personal/familial support behaves as a public good. In the following paragraphs, the externality argument is examined further.

The externality argument The presence of externalities in mental health care was discussed earlier in Chapter 3. Recall that when private benefits do not equate with social benefits, and private costs do not equate with social costs, these spillover effects mean that the market solution is less than Pareto optimal. This distinction was first made by Pigou (1932), and the subsequent literature is huge. See, for example, Meade (1952) and Mishan (1981).

For example, it can be proposed that individuals care about each other in the following specific sense. Individuals care that other individuals are not getting enough treatment or care in their state of ill-health. In this sense, an externality exists (Culyer, 1980). Of course, the quality of care which individuals may expect to be available for themselves, should the need arise, is very likely to differ from that quality which is demanded in response to a caring externality (Pauly, 1981).[6]

6 Individuals are also said to have an option demand for hospitals (Weisbrod, 1964), in that they have a continuing demand for the prompt availability of hospital services, if and when the need arises (Stevens, 1968, p. 244). This notion could also be cast in the expected utility framework, i.e. the value of a hospital is the sum of the utility an individual will receive from the service it renders times the probability that the individual will want the service (Mills, 1968, p. 250).

On wider grounds, it may be argued that an externality arises from the fact that individuals in society feel concerned that care-givers, say in the home, are exhausted; or that family life is breaking down due to the demanding circumstances of looking after a family member with a severe mental disorder. Both of these spillover effects constitute a divergence between the private marginal valuation curve and the social marginal valuation curve.

An externality of another kind exists: stigma. On even wider grounds this results because some individuals are affronted by particularly odd or different behaviours of particular individuals. Put otherwise, the essence of stigma is effectively an externality. The emotional problems arising from mental illness are greatly aggravated by stigma (Goffman, 1963). Goffman's (1963) analysis (cited in Small, 1996) suggests that 'considerable emotional management is usually necessary for people to maintain a sense of dignity and self-worth in the face of public antagonism and avoidance. Furthermore, to the extent that such efforts are successful, he or she often requires the support of additional emotion work from significant others and professionals who are expert on the stigmatised condition, whom Goffman (1963) labels, respectively, the "intimate wise" and the "professional wise" ' (Small, 1996, p. 271).[7]

Individuals may also suffer spillover effects of what they perceive to be the ignorance of others as to how to be happy living in their life circumstances. This externality is better understood in terms of the discussion of merit goods in the Sub-section following.

Even more examples of externalities could be suggested here. The point, though, is this: with respect to the role of government in any of these cases, a divergence *per se* between social and private costs or between social and private benefits does not constitute enough grounds for government involvement. Rather, the grounds are that there is a divergence at the margin between the sum of internal and external benefits and the sum of internal and external costs. See Coase (1960).

The 'Merit Good' Argument

Can the role of government be justified on the grounds that mental health care is a merit good? Before such a question can be addressed, some preliminary comments are needed. The notion that merit goods provide a justification for the role of government was first suggested by Musgrave (1959). This concept has induced a somewhat spirited debate as to its appropriateness, in Musgrave's normative framework of the public sector. For a survey, see Head (1966).

---

7 Although stigma is a relevant term to use in this context, it does not entirely capture the reciprocal nature of this particular externality. A mentally ill person can feel uncomfortable, or embarrassed, when well people notice the person's strange behaviours while, simultaneously, the well people can feel discomfort over the strange ways of a mentally ill person.

However, the concept has been interpreted in several quite different ways, making a single, adequate definition of the merit good quite difficult to provide.

Some definitions imply paternalism. This is the concept that a particular good may be deemed so intrinsically worthwhile that an informed group of individuals is justified in imposing its decisions/preferences on others. For example, in regard to particular goods such as education, housing, particular foods, etc., individual preferences are so distorted as to make it necessary to override consumer preferences. In such instances, the intervening group usually seeks to impose a minimum or maximum level of consumption of these goods on all members of society.

Other types of definitions are not of the paternalistic kind and yet still encompass the notion that a norm other than consumer sovereignty applies. Six situations, considered by Musgrave (1987), are summarised below.

First, the notion of the merit good cuts across the distinction between public goods and private goods. Consumer sovereignty is relevant regarding the public goods and private goods, but is inapplicable with regard to merit goods. Second, Musgrave suggests various instances where rational behaviour is impeded, due either to pathological factors, as in acute psychoses; or to imperfect information, say, where prior to an event the initiator of the event presumes to know that people's preferences will be favourable after the event, though not before; or else finally in situations where there is oversight or myopia. In these instances, Musgrave points out that 'the *implementation* of individual preferences is affected, but *without questioning their dominance* at the *normative* level' (Musgrave, 1987, p. 452). In other words, consumer sovereignty applies in principle still, but temporarily is not exercised.

Next, Musgrave considers whether fashion, or general societal influence, negates individual preferences. He argues that this is not so. While acknowledging that social influences encroach on individual preferences, a range of individual responses exists in spite of social influence. Musgrave argues that it is inappropriate to equate the concept of merit goods with fashion.

Fourth, Musgrave raises the situation where individuals adopt community values even though, individually, their preferences differ. Common values effectively act as a restraint upon individual preferences. Examples of this include concern about historical sites or endangered species, respect for national holidays or for national beliefs, as well as restrictions on activities that offend human dignity, like prostitution or drug abuse. Such 'community values' are, according to Musgrave, the product of the historical processes wherein individuals interact with one another, resulting in common values being formed and being passed on over time. Musgrave sees such situations as clear justification for the existence of the merit good. A trend towards greater concern about the well-being of people with mental illnesses and disorders is apparent in recent centuries, which is at least partly due to a slow, positive change in community values about mental illness.

A fifth concern relates to issues of distribution and of redistribution. In matters of charitable giving, redistribution may occur in kind, rather than in cash. The donor, having altruistic motivations, imposes some preferences upon the recipient, if the donor has some particular meritorious good in mind for the recipient. A donor may, for example, want the treatment of mental illness for recipients. Where society wishes to ensure that minimum standards in well-being are met, it may do so by providing a minimum bundle of goods and services to an individual rather than by giving the equivalent in terms of a minimum sustainable income, to be spent as the recipient wishes. Such goods singled out for distribution may be termed merit goods.

These five interpretations of merit goods involve a digression away from the norm of consumer sovereignty. The sixth instance given by Musgrave is, however, one that interprets merit goods in the context of preferences, but preferences of a different kind from the preferences attached to goods for which consumer sovereignty is applicable. Merit goods have ethically superior implications, and 'demerit goods' have unethical implications. Colm (1955) offers a stronger interpretation of this idea. Individual voting behaviour reveals that a person, when dealing with political issues, operates in a frame of reference that is quite distinct from that which allocates his or her income as a consumer. In the former situation, the individual acts as a political being who is guided by his or her image of a good society. In the latter, the individual operates in a private sense, determined by self-interest, giving consideration to personal wants only. The person, as a political being, has a frame of reference that is quite distinct from that which allocates his or her income as a consumer. Colm asserts that the two approaches are fundamentally opposite, arguing for the essentially different nature of individual behaviour in the face of the government budget. Colm does not, therefore, accept the externality argument. He sees individual preference patterns as not independent of the social environment in which preferences form, i.e. individuals' and society's preference patterns are interdependent, simultaneously determined systems.

Colm's view is not without limitation. First, his view validates the existence of altruistic externalities and hence seems unnecessary. Second, his assertion of the existence of an image of the good society could result in a decision making mechanism which produces highly paternalistic mental health services because of the overriding need to contain social deviance.

It should finally be noted that it is not conceptually possible to integrate the organic view of the state, which is where the merit good argument resides, with an individualistic view of the state. This would mean that a socially 'imposed indifference curve' on an indifference map would be conceptually invalid. For a discussion of the 'individualistic' and 'organic' frameworks, see Buchanan and Tullock (1967, pp. 316-17).

What, then, is the relevance of paternalism in an economic analysis? Within an individualistic framework, the answer is that paternalism cannot be justified on normative grounds. If a positive approach is being attempted, paternalism can be acknowledged in so far as government is not concerned solely with economic objectives, at the expense of legal, moral or political ones.

Conclusion

This Chapter has been concerned with recognising the multi-faceted nature of publicly provided/financed mental health care. It has been argued that at least five elements, i.e. **characteristics**, of mental health care facilities, publicly or privately provided, can be recognised: deprivation of liberty, accommodation, treatments, medical/nursing care, and familial/personal support. Having acknowledged this, it is relevant to ask why, from an economic perspective, government intervenes.

A distinction has been drawn between government intervention on the grounds of an impairment in the preference functioning capacity of an individual, and on the grounds that an individual's goals are socially unacceptable in terms of social norms for social behaviour or personal habits.

Both of these grounds are explained, in an individualistic framework, in terms of externalities. It has been argued that it is not relevant to invoke a broad 'public good' argument for mental health care. Furthermore, it has been argued that, in the individualistic framework, the presence of externalities clarifies the normative role of government. In particular, the precise economic sense in which an indifference curve should be imposed upon individuals' preferences has been considered. Also, it has been possible in this Chapter to point out the economic sense in which the medical profession acts as agent in regard to the public provision of treatment and care.

Before changing the focus in the next Chapters to community issues in mental health care, it is useful to reconsider now the broad purpose of the theoretical analyses provided here in Chapters 5, 6 and 7 about mental health care outputs and to indicate ways of approaching empirical applications. These three Chapters have provided a conceptual framework relevant to the issues in mental health care which have been under study. The central message of those Chapters is that the provision of mental health care is heterogeneous: it involves multiple outputs, and that each of these outputs is multi-dimensional, i.e. having multiple attributes or characteristics.

The analyses contained in these Chapters are likely to provoke questions from the reader about empirical applications. No empirical applications are undertaken in this study. However, the relevant concepts for empirical work are concerned with the hedonic function. For an overview, see Triplett (1987) and Streeting (1990). The hedonic function is useful wherever the price of a good or service under study is dependent upon the quantities of characteristics embodied in that good or service. Multiple regression techniques are applied in order to determine the prices of these characteristics. Essentially, the approach makes the empirical estimation of the underlying demands for heterogeneous goods or services possible.

Since possible areas of future research in the field of mental health care are suggested in Chapter 11, that Chapter is the better place for further discussion of empirical work involving hedonic pricing. See the Sub-section titled *Towards Application: Hedonic Prices and Heterogeneous Services*.

8 Mental Health Care in the Household Sector

Introduction

The purpose of this Chapter is to consider descriptive and conceptual aspects of the provision of care by 'the community', within households, for people with mental illnesses.

It is important to recognise a confusion over terminology existing in various discussions of mental health care: the confusion relates to 'deinstitutionalisation' and to 'community-based' or 'non-institutional' care. The word, deinstitutionalisation, is used rather loosely. It is used in reference both to the recent processes bringing change to mental health care and to the care itself, currently undertaken mostly in the community, i.e. non-institutionally. To an economist, there are important distinctions between these meanings. Deinstitutionalisation means something different from community-based or non-institutional care in an economic framework. 'Non-institutional', or 'community-based', care is a **way of**, or an approach to, **giving care**. This community-based approach is different in both its input combinations and outputs from 'institutional' care. It is best to reserve 'deinstitutionalisation' for referring to the political and bureaucratic **processes** that bring about the changes to the ways of delivering care.

Mental Health Care in the Household Sector

Attention is directed in this Section to describing situations where families, and other households, provide care to relatives or friends who have severe and persistent mental illnesses and disorders.

Some characteristics of mental illnesses and disorders have been outlined in Chapter 1. (The Appendices to Chapters 1 and 3 also are pertinent at this juncture.) The descriptions in Chapter 1 indicate that mental illnesses and disorders are characteristically varied in terms of diagnosis, length of illnesses, the nature of the illness episodes and levels of functional impairment. At one extreme is the group of individuals whose course of illness causes them to undergo frequent hospitalisation. Others suffer the symptoms of their conditions occasionally. Some individuals, particularly those with mood and anxiety disorders and even some who endure schizophrenia, may suffer the impairments of their condition relatively infrequently. Because of this, some of these individuals are able, more or less, to participate quite fully as members of society. Some are able to function quite effectively in labour market activities.

The diagrams in Figure 8.1 are a stylised approach to passages through the course of (life) time for four different individuals who experience a mental disorder. The approach is stylised because depictions of heterogeneous groups of illnesses and heterogeneous groups of people are being attempted. Depicted in the diagrams is the natural history of four selected illness types. They are representations of individuals not living along a figurative norm of 'well-being' for the person, although this norm could be difficult to define because of the question of where healthy personality ends and the disease begins. The first diagram depicts the case of an individual who initially is very healthy but who experiences a single episode of mental illness. The person fully recovers, enjoying in recovery a higher level of mental health than before the onset of the illness. Instances of this occur with post-natal depression or with exogenous depression arising with, say, an episode of severe grief.[1] The second diagram depicts the passage through time of a person experiencing severe mood swings, as is the case with bipolar disorder. The person's mental health settles, over time, into a less volatile state, i.e. the mood swings are more like what people normally feel but, even so, most of the person's lifetime is spent 'below par'. The passage through time in the third case represents a chronic condition (such as endogenous depression) that prohibits the person from reaching the norm in mental health for this person. In contrast, in the fourth case, a deteriorating condition is depicted such as Alzheimer's Disease or some sub-sets within the schizophrenia diagnosis.

Historically speaking, of the group of individuals capable of being productive, a few, indeed very few, have made superior contributions to society. Lefley (1996) lists Beethoven, William Blake, Samuel Coleridge, Leonardo da Vinci, Herman Melville, Sylvia Plath, Robert Schumann, Anne Sexton, Virginia Woolf and Vincent van Gogh. The economics profession acknowledges John Nash.

Lefley (1996) points out that while individuals, like these just mentioned, made superior productive contributions, caring people were highly supportive of them and their endeavours. Lefley then adds that those historical situations ought not to be taken as representative of the typical population turning to family for care-giving in the present day. In order to gain further insight into more typical situations of need, attention is directed shortly to empirical and anecdotal studies of family care-giving.

---

1 For an account of the stages of the grief process, see, *inter alia*, Kubler-Ross (1975; 1981). For a biography of this remarkable lady, see Gill (1980).

Figure 8.1 Passages through time of four individuals with a mental disorder

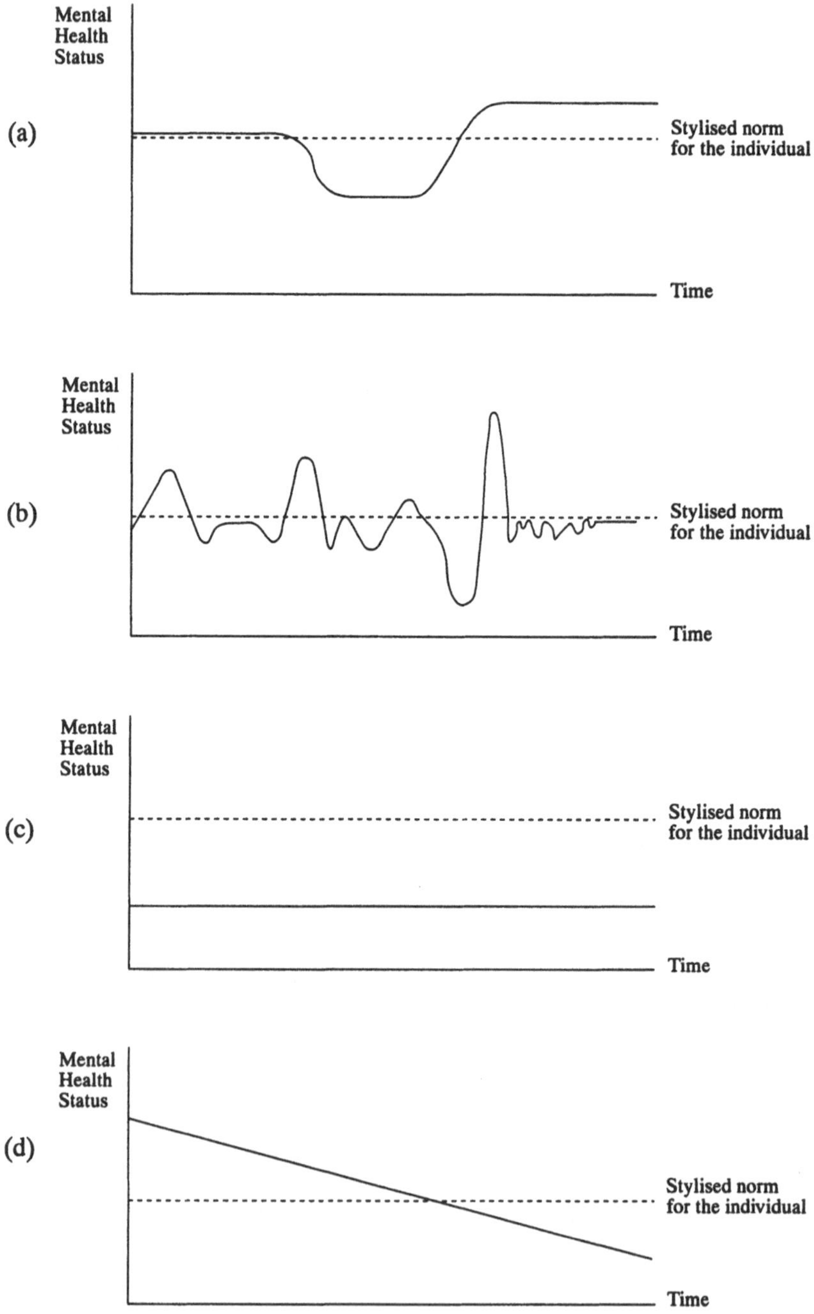

Household Care of People with Mental Illnesses

Typical care-giving by households involved with mental illness is not like that for a relative with physical or developmental disabilities. For example, it normally does not involve nursing duties, as is the case with physically ill or developmentally delayed relatives. It can involve 'hours devoted to activities of daily living... [and] ... multiple expenditures of time and energy in trying to obtain timely services from mental health, welfare and medical systems, and interactions with legal and criminal justice systems' (Lefley, 1996, pp. 6-7).

There is comparatively little known about the family care-giver, a major provider/producer of mental health care. Lefley comments that the larger portion, by far, of the current literature on care-giving has been concerned, as in the past, with the notion that families are a pathogenic factor in the illness of the relative. The literature has, thus, largely ignored conceptualising the family members in the role of nurturing and caring. The following is an additional excerpt from Lefley (1996). It elaborates the experiences of families living with mental illness. Her descriptions stand out in a relatively sparse literature:

> Behavior management issues are ongoing tensions between mentally ill persons and their family members. Caregivers frequently have to contend with abusive or assaultive behaviors; mood swings and unpredictability; socially offensive or embarrassing situations; negative symptoms of amotivation, apathy, or anhedonia; and conflicts over money likely to be ill managed or squandered, or lost. Conflicts often arise regarding behaviors disturbing to household living. These include poor personal hygiene and offensive odors in the home, excessive smoking and fire hazards, indifference or actual damage to household property, and sleep reversal patterns that may result in pacing or loud music at odd hours of the night. Relatives' refusal to take their medication is a common area of contention...
>
> ... [A]ttentional and information-processing deficits, such as prolonged silences and delayed reactions of schizophrenia, are frustrating ... [and] tend to deprive caregivers of the rewards of human interaction and reciprocity. Perhaps the most devastating stressor for caregivers of persons with mental illness is learning to cope with their relative's own suffering over an impoverished life of their own lack of skills, impaired productivity, and poor future prospects...
>
> ... [A]mong caregivers, there is almost ubiquitous guilt about hospitalizing a mentally ill relative, even under conditions of assault, florid symptomatology, or flagrant self-neglect. And indeed, when patients recover, there is strong likelihood of anger and recrimination toward caregivers for having done that which was necessary and potentially lifesaving at the time. ...Caregivers must learn to deal both with the patient's behaviors and with their own reactions, to distinguish between volitional and nonvolitional behavior, to recognize and deal with manipulation, and to know how and when to set limits (Lefley, 1996, pp. 69-71).

A further problem encountered by care-givers arises because of a pervasive inability of the relative with a psychiatric disorder: that is, the inability to do what it takes to perceive his or her own reality adequately, merely to live day-to-day life. Such a disability is an elusive and nebulous limitation for such persons themselves, and for care-givers. Indeed, not to possess an ability to perceive and process information about reality is a most disabling factor in mental illness. The absence of this ability has implications for performing tasks of personal care and decision-making as well as other tasks like shopping, banking and attending to mail. (Most of us, at least sometimes, have trouble with perceiving reality optimally; but the capacity to do so exists, i.e. to an extent that is in the range of 'normal').

The inability described in the previous paragraph may not be a static phenomenon. It can vary over time. It is likely to vary with the individual's current capacity for managing life. Such capacities are subject to stress levels, to the day-to-day variations in physical and emotional capacities, and in the fluctuations in the levels of a day's demands. Care-givers regularly assist their relatives in clarifying their own reality, but need to make fine judgements as to when it is appropriate to impose their values on the values of another adult, albeit someone with a psychiatric condition. Such a role is particularly difficult for parents of adult children. Moreover, care-givers need to adopt such a role without escalating stress. Individuals with a psychiatric illness are particularly unable to manage stress. In other words, most suffer a low stress threshold.

Care-givers of a relative with a psychiatric disorder can be involved in complex conversation with the relative, skilfully being the 'necessary contradiction', balancing in the relative the reality that clouds over so regularly. When care-giving people repeatedly help to clarify the reality of an individual with a psychiatric disorder, that individual may be able to function in the tasks of his/her daily living more often. Thereby, family members can become skilled in techniques of interaction and conversation that help the relative reconstruct a reality. Because the people with a psychiatric disorder do not possess the capacity to do this for themselves, or at least to sustain it, care-givers engage in this role repetitively and regularly.

For documentation of professional support given to family care-giving, see Leff (1996).

The Household

The present institutional arrangements in mental health care assign lesser importance to the hospital as a setting for care and treatment of mental illnesses, and far greater significance to other institutions and other settings for care and treatment. The health care literature mostly refers to these other institutions and settings as occurring in 'the community'. It is helpful in an economic study to consider the terms, 'community' and 'household'.

In the economics literature the term 'household' is employed, whereas in the various literatures dealing with psychiatric services and issues, the term 'community' is commonplace. In this context it is relevant to shed light on the degree of commonality between these terms. Some aspects of the nature of mental health care arising in the household and the household sector are then considered.

A 'sector', in economics, is a group of decision-making units which share a common motivation that differentiates this group from another. The distinguishing economic activity in the household sector is that of individuals maximising utility subject to the household's income. (The other major sectors are the business firms sector, the government sector and the foreign sector, and the same individuals in households can be found undertaking various other types of economic activity that occur in the other sectors.)

The individual as a 'decision-making unit', to which reference was made in the previous paragraph, reflects a simplification undertaken in economics. The simplification enables a focus on the choice-making behaviour of the individual and, also, the household.[2] In so far as the household, as an entity comprising individuals, can be represented by a single utility function, then the choices in which the household engages so as to maximise utility can be examined. In the present context, household utility is at least partially determined by the need for mental health care.

Now in the introduction to conventional first-year courses in Macroeconomics where students are being introduced to the Circular Flow Model of Income (e.g. McTaggart *et al.*, 1999; Waud *et al.*, 1996), students are reminded of a seemingly self-evident notion: the household sector comprises consumers and the firms sector comprises producers. Firms combine economic resources of land, labour, capital and entrepreneurship to produce goods and services, which then are sold to households. Such a basic distinction between the consuming sector and the producing sector enables a fundamental assumption for macroeconomic modelling. For macroeconomic applications, **distinguishing economic motivations** underlie the economic activity of each sector.

The limitation of the simple distinction about motivation, just stated, is readily apparent. It is too simplistic an assumption, for some applications, to define the household simply as a consuming unit. Households undertake another activity, production. The limitation, described above, is significant in the context of households being the place of care for many individuals with psychiatric illnesses. The conceptual framework of households as places of work and production, not just consumption, is found in Becker's seminal paper (1965). (His conception was employed in Chapters 5 and 6, taking another perspective.)

Care performed in households has economic meaning from two perspectives. One aspect involves the concept that household work has value

---

2 The reality of the assumption of the household as an entity represented by a single utility function is debated elsewhere (e.g. Berk, 1987).

because it involves an opportunity cost. The opportunity cost of household work, namely the value of the next best alternative foregone by the work having been done 'in house', is provided by the market, sometimes.

The second aspect is that, though labour is unpaid, this work is combined with household capital 'to add value to the intermediate inputs of materials and energy purchased by households from the market' (Ironmonger, 1994, p. 48). Ironmonger is referring here to such household activity as, for example, meal preparation. Meal preparation by households involves the purchase of grocery items. Subsequently, household labour and household capital are employed, along with the purchased (or home-grown) food. The outcome is meals.

It is in this general context, then, that the provision of services to the psychiatrically ill can be given in the household (in economic terminology) or in the community (in other terminology). Since the deinstitutionalisation movement, the relative importance of this location/institution has increased.

The Economics of Household Care-Giving

Household production occurs in diverse ways. One aspect of household production, 'housework' in colloquial language, mostly refers to the effort involved in satisfying basic human needs in the home for meals, shelter, recreation, care services (such as activities of daily living and life management skills). The word, housework, is often inclusive of complex and broad interpersonal tasks such as child rearing. In the present context of the household, other sorts of care-giving are described, such as that outlined in previous Sections of this Chapter. It is not possible here to provide an authoritative account of housework, adequate to conceptualise the economics of care that is given to people with mental illness. This deserves a separate study. However, an introduction to some economic features of housework is given.

To the extent that households operate productively like small firms, then the household-firm combines market inputs, such as food purchases or employed domestic help, and time, to produce commodities such as those given in the previous paragraph (Becker, 1965). In a simplified model, substitution between time and market inputs can be examined, and it is this issue that is of prime interest in the economics of household care-giving. Brown and Preece (1987) report as follows:

> Empirical studies of the home-making process and family budgets in the US have shown that very little substitution occurs between the home-maker's time and market goods in housework. Empirically, after standardizing by family income, the employed wife uses few market goods and services outside of childcare to substitute for her own time, and both employed and full-time home-makers use the same techniques for performing housework (Brown, 1979; Strober, 1980; Berk and Berk, 1979). The main substitution tends to be between the wife's market time and her leisure time (Brown and Preece, 1987, p. 678).

The lack of substitution between housework and purchased goods and services is explained, *a priori*, according to Brown and Preece (1987), partly by the social norms governing the sorts of activities that generate family life. The other explanation is the possibility of a weak cross-elasticity of (input) demand for services provided by the home-maker and the goods and services purchased in the marketplace. That is, aside from instances where household and market services behave as substitutes and complements, could the two types of services be more or less unrelated? Brown and Preece argue that '[t]he home economy specializes in producing mothering and nurturing of family members, along with personalized care in providing food, clothing and shelter. The marketplace produces sophisticated medical care, advanced education, the means of transportation and communication, urban housing and the ability to pool risks, as well as mass-produced food, clothing, cars and other consumer durables' (Brown and Preece, 1987, p. 678).

The degree to which there is substitutability, complementarity or unrelatedness between the two types of service inputs, namely, household production and market production, is an empirical matter about which little is known. To know the nature of such relationships is useful for policy formation about community care, but major measurement difficulties beset empirical work. The personalised and on-call nature of the full-time homemaker's work results in troublesome estimation work on the costs of, and value of, household production. Estimates in dollar terms of household production are more difficult because of the multi-dimensional nature of the household work. A recent example of a time-use study, and the value of unpaid work in general, is Australian Bureau of Statistics (2000).

To add to the difficulty of finding shadow prices, in the real world, the household does not effectively contract to buy these services 'more impersonalized than the housewife's in the small amounts of time and at the random hours that the housewife actually performs these duties. The purchased services usually are not equivalent to the service which the housewife provides because she knows intimately the family member she is serving and takes responsibility for organizing and providing of care as it is needed' (Brown and Preece, 1987, p. 678).

Similar phenomena are reported by Franks (1990) in her empirical study of the costs borne by family members for the care provided to a relative with a mental illness. McGuire (1992) comments as follows: 'Resources are usually measured in dollars, but often even this metric is hard to apply, as in the case of many family resources devoted to the care of a mentally ill adult child (*sic*). In Franks' (1990) study of family costs, many parents answered the question of ' "how much time do you spend caring for your child?" as "24 hours a day." There is both error and truth in the response' (McGuire, 1992, p. 4).

And so it is that the estimation of the value and the cost of relations between the household economy and the market economy is elusive. Interaction nevertheless occurs, occurring as if non-dollar, time-stretched 'units of interaction' exist. Dollar estimates are better than counting the cost of care provided by households as zero, because such estimation work is difficult.

In spite of the presence of conceptual and measurement problems, some dimensions of care in the community are analysed in the following Chapters, though empirical work is not undertaken. Berk endorses efforts to understand the economic nature of household production with the following comment: '[T]he sensitizing role of recent efforts by neoclassical economists to understand family life has been extraordinarily useful. The new home economics forces one to address seriously the nature of household production and the degree to which concepts from neoclassical economics can be instructive. In other words, we are told where to look and given some initial tools to aid in that process. These are major accomplishments' (Berk, 1987, p. 677).

The Effect of Deinstitutionalisation on Households

Care in the household has become more important because of the deinstitutionalisation movement, the story behind that movement having been outlined briefly in Chapter 7 of this study. In this Sub-section, the purpose is to focus descriptively upon the effects of deinstitutionalisation on household care-giving.

Deinstitutionalisation is believed to have brought a range of consequences. The positive consequences suggested by Lefley (1996)(1997) will be outlined as follows. Independent living is possible for some people within the community, provided suitable treatment, care and support are available, and then provided these less restrictive settings offer therapeutic advantages. For some individuals, highly therapeutic results are arising also because the recent advances in psychopharmacology are combined with a range of non-clinical services, such as supported housing, case management, supported education and employment, peer-counselling, psycho-social rehabilitation and crisis respite houses run by former patients (Lefley, 1997, p. 2).

The major negative impacts of deinstitutionalisation are pervasive. The conditions in which many are living, especially those who live alone, are shameful. Lefley (1997) refers to the 'vastly inferior mental health ghettos in the community' in America. There is also evidence in Australia of similar living conditions (Human Rights and Equal Opportunity Commission, 1993). The degree, and extent, of homelessness that is occurring among individuals suffering serious mental illnesses and disorders due to deinstitutionalisation is grave (Jencks, 1994). For a view that questions the strength of the causal relationship between deinstitutionalisation and homelessness, see, for example, O'Flaherty (1996).

The other major negative consequence concerns families now engaged in care-giving activities for which they are 'unprepared, untrained and from which they have been systematically excluded in the past' (Lefley, 1997, p. 3). In the past, clinicians had minimal contact and interaction with families. Indeed, a family once would be blamed for a relative's illness; the cause of the mental illness was said to be due, at least partly, to the family being dysfunctional. Families previously were excluded by professional carers from opportunities that would have enabled giving and receiving information, insight, support and techniques for managing the illness. With greater understanding now of the biological, and other, bases of psychiatric disease, blame for illnesses is no longer assumed upon the family. It is clear now how unnecessary were the past practices of excluding families from treatment and care processes.

It is these very families who now face a key caring role. The families are not only bearing the burden of the legacy of almost total exclusion from a treatment and care role, but are now also struggling to provide their caring function adequately.

Some Empirical Insights

Lefley (1996) cites various empirical studies that provide insights, largely not of an economic nature, into family care-giving.

In North America, between one-half and two-thirds of individuals with schizophrenia are at any one time living in households, the majority at home with their families (Grossner and Conley, 1995, cited in Lefley, 1996, p. 5). Now, some families live in a mutually beneficial relationship with a relative who suffers with a psychiatric disorder. This is more common, though still not very common, when the disease has stabilised, often later in life. Whether or not the relationship is mutually beneficial, the people in these circumstances remain vulnerable. For example, the Grossner and Conley study (1995), just cited, reveals large numbers of adult care-givers who are, or soon will be, in the geriatric population.

Where relatives with psychiatric disorders live separately from their families, Clark and Drake (1994) (cited in Lefley, 1996, p. 5) study the continuing involvement by family with their relative. Where family remains involved and even where relatives live away, family members give considerable quantities of time, money and social support to their relative. It is believed that the provision of sufficient care and support is likely to impose a considerable strain upon the nuclear family. Lefley notes that, as early as the 1950s, sociologists believed that the nuclear family, with its limited adult resources for caring for dependants, provided little room for 'shock absorption and for tolerating the dependency of persons with long-term disabilities' (Lefley, 1996, p. 6).

Attention is directed now to another empirical study, by Winefield and Harvey (1994). This is a study of the needs of families giving care to a family member suffering chronic schizophrenia; and it offers useful insights into care-giving work. Winefield and Harvey undertook to survey one hundred and twenty-one family care-givers whose relative had been diagnosed, on average, 14.2 years previously. The mean age of care-givers was 56.6 years. Seventy-four per cent of care-givers were female. The average age of the relative was 37.6 years. Patients' usual place of residence was with care-givers (in 25.6 per cent of cases), in a hospital or jail (in 16.5 per cent of cases), in a hostel (28.9 per cent of cases) or independently in an apartment or house (28.8 per cent of cases). Care-givers were most frequently the parents of the patients (in 68.6 per cent of cases).

In this study of the nature of burden and care, Winefield and Harvey report a wide range of problems arising with care-giving, some of which are presented here. Limitations on relationships inside and outside of the home, restrictions on care-givers' lives and considerable stresses are reported. For example, the study reports on the worry involved in giving care. The authors began by asking carers to conceive of a scale of stress from zero to 100. They then asked the carers to specify the proportion of their total stress associated with care-giving. For all respondents, the mean was 51 per cent. Care-givers reported various problems that arise when a relative with a psychiatric illness lives with family members. The reported problems include self-centred behaviour, other irritating behaviours, personal or property damage, demands on care-givers' time and family arguments.

Care-givers were asked whether there were any benefits of having a relative live at home. Nearly fifteen per cent of care-givers said that there were no good points; 39.5 per cent of carers suggested the presence of intrinsic enjoyment of the person and benefits like having help with the chores. However, the reasons given by another 45.7 per cent of care-givers implied that their relative was at home because care-givers wished to avoid the alternative, a worse outcome, such as the patient being unhappy elsewhere.

Care-givers were asked also where they would prefer the family member to live. The family member also was asked where they would prefer to live. Winefield and Harvey report that almost half of the care-givers (45.5 per cent) preferred the patient to live in another supervised setting, although only 41 per cent of the relatives of the 45.5 per cent agreed. Such family members were described by care-givers as having relatively fewer self-care and communication skills and were more turbulent in their behaviour. Only 22.3 per cent of care-givers preferred the family member to live at home with them (and the family members were correlated with being relatively more capable of responsible behaviour). Of these, the relative shared this wish in 78 per cent of the cases. Seventy-eight per cent of care-givers preferred the family member suffering the psychiatric disorder not to live with them.

For some qualitative information of tasks/work undertaken by families and friends in support of disabled people in their homes, see SANE Australia (1999).[3]

---

3 SANE Australia is a national charity helping people seriously affected by mental illness.

Summary and Conclusion

This Chapter has considered descriptive and conceptual aspects of the provision of care by 'the community', within households, for people with mental illnesses.

Household care of people with mental illness is different from the type of care given for physical or developmental disabilities. Normally, the nursing duties are minimal, and yet anecdotal evidence indicates hours of time are required in order to assist mentally ill relatives with activities of daily living.

Attention was directed next in this Chapter to conceptualising 'the community' within an economic framework. In the economics of mental health care in the current era, the household is a productive unit producing care; it not just a decision-making sector involved in consumption, which is the traditional stance of macroeconomic theory. Empirically, the increased role of the household in care-giving since deinstitutionalisation has generated a small but increasing number of economic studies that attempt ways of valuing this care given in the community, as mentioned in Chapter Four. As well, there are the types of empirical studies outlined in this Chapter which adopt a non-economic approach.

Economic research on how to value the time spent on household care-giving is vital. Such studies address, though, a different issue from the economics of deinsititionalisation itself, which is about production of treatment and care being shifted from government institutions into households. An approach is developed in the next two Chapters to the economics of deinstitutionalisation.

9 Multiple Inputs: The Role of Social Capital in Community-Based Strategies

Introduction

'Community-based strategies' and 'community-based services' are examples of some new terminology arising from the deinstitutionalisation movement. These recent terms refer to a grouping, or aggregation, of services provided by government, albeit from different portfolios: a whole-of-government approach. These services lie within the diverse range of service provision in mental health care involving various people, both workers in organisations (government or otherwise) and citizens in the community. The present Chapter and the following one focus on some aspects of the economics of these services and strategies.

Attention is directed, in particular, to economic issues arising with multiple inputs into mental health care from various channels within government and 'the community'. The present Chapter considers the recent theories of social capital. In order to shed light on a framework of analysis relevant to community-based services and strategies, attention then turns in the next Chapter to the concept of co-production (Ostrom, 1996), wherein inputs from government and inputs from citizens are employed.

Community-Based Services and Strategies in Australia

The Australian National Mental Health Strategy calls for a redirection of service provision away from separate psychiatric hospitals to community-based services. In the *Report* of the National Mental Health Strategy, community-based services and strategies encompass three broad groups of services:

i. 'Ambulatory services' comprising outpatient clinics (hospital and clinic based), mobile assessment and treatment teams, day programs and other services dedicated to the assessment, treatment, rehabilitation and care of people living in the community affected by mental illness or psychiatric disability who live in the community.

ii. Specialised residential services that provide beds in the community staffed by mental health professionals on a 24 hour a day basis. These services, designed for people with significant disability and dependency needs, aim to replace many of the functions traditionally performed by long-stay psychiatric hospitals. They include residential services established as specialised psychogeriatric nursing homes for older people with mental illness, or dementia with severe behavioural disturbance.

iii. Services by not-for-profit non-government organisations, funded by governments, to provide support services for people with a psychiatric disability arising from a mental illness. These services include a wide range of accommodation, rehabilitation, recreational, social support and advocacy programs (Mental Health Branch, Commonwealth Department of Health and Aged Care, 1998, pp. 21-22).

In the above description, reference is made to residential services for severely disabled and dependent individuals. Empirical studies (described in the previous Chapter) reveal another facet of community-based services, *viz.* their insufficient quantities. Insufficient residential, and other, support for daily living means that, within this range of people with mental disorders, there are some who do not obtain the help they need and are left unsupported, although still very disabled in their daily living. These unsupported people have two types of problems. In many instances, the disability and dependency is not severe enough to qualify some individuals for access to the very limited services available. This arises because of the 'spectrum' nature of the illness. In other instances, the services defined above do not suit the requirements or disabilities of another group of individuals. In every instance, though, as Chapter 8 shows from empirical studies as well as anecdotal evidence, day-to-day life remains an almost insurmountable struggle for many, hidden individuals. Moreover, the value of the lives of these individuals to themselves, for their families and for society is greatly diminished. The empirical data outlined in Chapter 8 reveal that many individuals in this category are living with family care-givers. Others survive, due to the considerable support from family and friends, or the support given by altruistic groups and individuals. Yet others survive in abject neglect. Here, then, is a fourth group of services, those provided by individual households, as a consequence of community-based strategies, and yet not apparent from the definitions of governments, as indicated by the previous lengthy quotation.

Some Important Distinctions

The above definition of community-based services reveals the diffusion of service provision, across the range of medical services and non-medical support. The economic theory of producer behaviour is useful for clarifying various aspects of these services. The issues arising with present-day mental health care make it a difficult sector to study. In this Chapter, theories of social capital help to clarify particular aspects of economic behaviour associated with community-based strategies.

Prior to investigating social capital, it is helpful to clarify various concepts from the economics of production. These concepts are pertinent to mental health care. Many of the concepts need no clarification for economists and yet are easily misunderstood or overlooked by interested parties from outside the discipline of economics. In today's parlance, for example, it is common for the term, providers, to be used in reference not only to the many people involved in mental health care, but also to the organisations involved with mental health care. Evans (1984, Ch. 6) shows various ways in which the loose use of the term, provider, blurs important distinctions required for an understanding of the economics of producer/provider behaviour. Some of the distinctions pointed out by Evans are relevant to the present Chapter.

Technical and Economic Aspects of Production

It is fundamentally important to distinguish the technical aspects of the production process from the economic aspects of the production process. Production, as an economic study, is concerned with the process of converting, into outputs of goods and services, scarce resources or inputs that are valued by individuals living in society. Various inputs, in varying amounts, are required to produce a quantity of output or mix of outputs. The input mix required for a particular output is a technical matter, in this case pertinent to the professions of medicine, psychiatry, nursing, social work and so forth. Normally, technical matters are 'a given' to the economist.

The technical constraints of the production process can be described, at least conceptually, by a mathematical expression, termed in economic theory 'the production function'. A production function defines the relationships among the various types of inputs that can achieve a given quantity of output, or mix of outputs. It is always possible to formulate a production function at a theoretical level, and in many instances, in primary or secondary industry and even in the health sector, production functions can be determined empirically. See also Chapter 3.

Mental health production functions, however, present challenging empirical problems. Community-based strategies, of their very nature, involve multiple outputs and, hence, separate production functions are likely to exist. However, these differing services or outputs may be subject to economies of scope (Baumol, Panzar and Willig, 1982); or they may be unrelated. Economies of scope, or economies of jointness, occur whenever the production of two or more different goods costs less if produced together, i.e. jointly, than if they are produced separately. Where the outputs involve a diffuse range of medical, residential and support services, and where the outputs are processed from inputs from various channels within government and 'the community', outputs are unlikely to be separate. Rather, it is more likely for joint outputs to arise. For example, a general hospital is characterised by the joint production of medical/surgical, maternity, paediatric, emergency and psychiatric treatment outputs. A detailed treatment of the joint outputs of hospitals is found in Butler (1995). For a cost-effectiveness analysis of two alternative production processes, in the production of blood plasma, which involves joint outputs in fixed proportions, see Pink and Connelly (1999).

The technical constraints of production are, however, only one aspect of the supply decisions of a firm; an economist's attention is directed to broader supply issues. For example, the other major constraint upon production, other than the technical constraint, arises from the nature of markets. The types of markets for the firm's products and the markets in which factors of production are produced create a constraint that also influences the supply decisions of firms. (It is perhaps a curiosity for non-economists to conceive that where government or even 'the community' is the supplier of goods and services, markets are still in operation, usually implicitly.)

Together, market and technical constraints influence the supply decisions of the firm. The types of supply decisions with which economics is most concerned include the types of products supplied, the quantity of output supplied and the prices for which products are supplied (or, as in the case of the government sector, the other conditions under which products are supplied by the government sector). The economics of the production decision forms a vast area of study, and it is necessary here to make only this first and fundamental distinction, namely, that between the technical and the economic aspects of production.

Service Providers in Mental Health Care

A second distinction must be made because of confusion caused by a tendency to transfer a neologism which is used in the health care literature for workers in the health field, namely, 'service provider', to economic matters. The concept to which it is being applied has a very precisely defined use in economics. Definitional problems arise in the use of the term, service provider, when referring to inputs of production.

Inputs are conventionally classified into three groups: labour and skill inputs; inputs arising from the services of capital equipment; and finally material inputs, or supplies used up in production. Although mental health care is highly labour intensive, all three input types are employed in the production process. The assembly and transformation of inputs occur within organisations that more or less resemble that conceptual entity, the firm, in economic language. Hospitals, for example, are organisations that behave like firms, at least in some respects, in so far as various inputs are brought together and transformed to produce a valuable output. Likewise, as Evans (1984) points out, medical practices, government public health departments and private drug and equipment companies are also firms.

Herein is Evans' second important distinction. The familiar term, provider, blurs a distinction that ought to be made between the people doing work and the organisations in which they work. Specific providers and practitioners are not themselves firms. Various professional roles represent bundles of skills and capacities. These are more or less distinguishable although, as Evans puts it, 'the bundle boundaries observed in any system are to a considerable extent arbitrary ... But the services of each are all inputs to the process of health care production, whether or not the person happens to own the firm which uses those capacities. It makes no difference, from the technical point of view, whether self-employed physicians own their own firms, and hire other workers, or whether nurses own practices and hire physicians, or whether both are employed in a practice owned by the Hudson's Bay Company' (Evans, 1984, p. 115). The provision of community-based strategies is also subject to this definition.

The Economic Approach to Health Policy

All firms (whether involved in health care, mental health care or any other productive activity) interact with the constraints of their specific economic environment, in attempting to fulfil the objective/s that they pursue. This process is constantly occurring, regardless of whether the objectives are known explicitly or implicitly, or whether the environment is well understood or not. Evans lists several objectives that a firm in health care might pursue: survival, professional self-expression, profits, growth, the interests of patients or the 'public interest' (Evans, 1984, p. 116).[1]

A firm can be evaluated from a general social point of view. In reference to its behaviour and impact on its environment, the social effects of a firm's activities can be evaluated in terms of, for example, the resources it consumes, the goods and services it produces and the patterns of wealth and well-being it generates. Evaluation is a key part of policy formation. One approach of mental health policy is the moulding of the environment of the firm (which may be a provider, or it may be an organisation or it may be a strategy branch of a government health department) in order to encourage desired outcomes and discourage other outcomes. This purpose is better served by the economic evaluation of a policy that seeks to raise the output of community-based services in mental health care.

The theoretical firm, whose behaviour and outcomes are analysed in the economic theory of production, is subject to constraint, as just mentioned. Constraints arise in the presence of the firm's technology, its objectives and the market environment. Conventional theory makes it clear that these

---

1 For further discussions of the objectives of the firm in economic theory, see Putterman and Kronser (1996) and Archibald (1987, pp. 360-61).

constraints hamper discretionary behaviour. The behaviour of the firm modelled by conventional elementary theory is predictable and well-known, although within this realm of predictable behaviour modelled by theory, a spectrum of behaviours results. Firms within such a spectrum are classified as either perfectly competitive or a pure monopoly or one of the models of imperfect competition falling between the two ends of the spectrum. Each is an idealised model and a well-studied phenomenon. See, for example, Pindyck and Rubinfeld (1998).

Some fundamental characteristics of organisations and providers involved in community-based strategies are, however, quite unlike those of the well-understood firm, modelled as it was originally because of the questions historically asked of economic theory. The questions for economic theory in the present era are not all the same as those set by historical precedent. The result is that several dimensions of the behaviour of these firms (providers/organisations/strategies) are of interest both for purposes of theoretical understanding and for policy analysis.

Economic Theory and Community-Based Strategies

Organisations providing community-based services depart from those modelled in the conventional theory of the firm in that community-based services have objectives that are not simply those of a single-objective firm in the private sector, conventionally maximising profit in a constrained environment. Rather, it is likely that organisations involved in community-based strategies pursue a range of objectives. Although the pursuit of such objectives is likely to be constrained by its technological environment and by its market environment, the environments differ also from the textbook models in complex ways. Some of these points of difference will now be considered.

First, while treatment technology for some of the psychiatric illnesses is quite advanced in effectiveness, this is not true for all the diagnoses of psychiatric illness. Both misdiagnosis and poor management of patients suffering with a major depressive disorder are well-documented as a common occurrence and a difficult problem to rectify in general practice (Eisenberg, 1992). McCoombs *et al.* (1990, cited in Jönsson and Rosenbaum, 1993) document 'patterns of anti-depressant use by the California Medicaid population receiving treatment primarily from general practitioners. The results indicate as many as two-thirds of all patients using antidepressants were under treatment for problems other than depression or were being dosed sub-optimally.'

The results of McCoombs *et al.* just mentioned suggest that the standard antidepressants were either not particularly effective, were not being consumed at recognised therapeutic doses for customary lengths of therapy, or were not being used correctly by community-based physicians. Also, McCoombs *et al.* report that treatment failure for major depressive disorders was estimated to cost approximately $1000 per patient in additional health care services during the first year after the commencement of therapy. The costs mainly accrued in the first six months, and were concentrated in hospital in-patient services.

Second, the economic behaviour associated with community-based strategies is likely to be at least partly explained by models that incorporate the household production function. See Chapter 8.

Third, the rationing of services providing mental health care has formed a sector that has been, from the 1850s until recently, highly regulated. Some economists (McGuire, 1985; Frank, 1990) argue that until the 1970s the sector effectively was socialised or dominated by government-provided services. For example, within the allocations of government budgets, medical practitioners and bureaucrats decided who was to be admitted for treatment, the kind of treatment to be provided, and how long patients were to remain hospitalised. An added layer of rationing occurred via the judicial system. In the United States, for example, precedent-setting court decisions effectively set levels of inputs for the production of services. Moreover, statutes relating to commital served to decide which individuals were to (or be forced to) receive treatment. The present transformations in service provision have resulted in care mostly occurring outside the hospital setting. In Australia, there has been a gradual expansion in private psychiatry practice, and a shift in the payment mechanism for psychiatrists and other mental health practitioners from employment in the public sector to the funding of private psychiatrists by way of the *Medicare Benefits Schedule* (Mental Health Branch, Commonwealth Department of Health and Family Services, 1997, pp. 81-82). Effectively, mental health care can no longer be regarded as 'socialised' in Australia.

Fourth, the simplified model is of a single-output firm employing in the short run two inputs, a variable input, labour, and a fixed input, capital. The multiple inputs, employed to provide mental health care in the context of community-based services, are drawn from various channels within the government and 'the community'. Attention will be directed further to this fourth issue in a discussion of theories of social capital.

Social Capital

Social capital originates from social relationships. Put otherwise, social capital accrues when individuals relate socially. The term was first used by an American geographer, Jane Jacobs (1962), and was formalised in the late 1970s and 1980s by Glenn Loury, an economist, in regard to racial income differences. Social capital describes 'the set of resources that inhere in family relations and in community social organisation and that are useful for the cognitive or social development of a child or young person' (Loury, 1977, 1987, cited in Coleman, 1990, p. 300). This statement implies that human capital cannot be expanded if social capital is inadequate. The recent theories of social capital predict an intrinsic role for social relationships in individuals' capacities to function effectively. Social relationships are not merely a pleasurable adjunct to the pursuit and achievement of outcomes by individuals.

The individualistic framework of analysis of neo-classical economic theory has led, over time, to several 'unanswered questions' for social science. For example, an issue that traditionally is not addressed is why people have particular preferences. It is conceivable that the socio-economic structure or environment has a role to play in determining people's preferences. A recent paper by Bowles (1998) surveys this relatively new literature on endogenous preferences. (Some of these questions are apparent in the Sub-sections following.) There are many attempts in the literature to reformulate economic theory in order to incorporate social relations, for example, the New Institutional Economics (North, 1990; Rutherford, 1994; Hodgson, 1998). For this Section, three accounts of social capital are presented, those of Coleman (1988, 1990), Putnam (1993a, 1993b, 1996) and Becker (1974, reprinted in Becker, 1996). Attention will then turn in Chapter 10 to address issues concerning the relationship between social capital and government. In particular, the issue of whether these phenomena are substitutes or complements is considered in that Chapter.

The Account of Social Capital by James Coleman

Coleman's approach to social capital was influenced by an economic sociologist, Mark Granovetter who, as Coleman puts it, recognised 'the importance of concrete personal relations and networks of relations – what he (Granovetter) calls the embeddedness of economic transactions in social relations – in generating trust, in establishing expectations, and in creating and enforcing norms' (Granovetter, 1985, cited in Coleman, 1990, p. 302).[2]

In Coleman's perspective, 'Granovetter's notion of embeddedness may be seen as an attempt to introduce into the analysis of economic systems social and organisational relations, not merely as a structure that springs into place to fulfill an economic function, but as a structure with history and continuity that give it an independent impact on the functioning of a system' (Coleman, 1990, p. 302).

Elsewhere, Coleman's emphasis upon the intrinsic contribution of social capital is acknowledged: 'In Coleman's account social capital is an inherent aspect and – most significantly – an unintended outcome of the institutionalisation of social relationships in "social structure" ' (Harriss and

---

2 For a more general account of the role of trust in the creation of prosperity, see Fukuyama (1995).

De Renzio, 1997, p. 922).[3] Another statement by Coleman conceptualises social capital in the following manner:

> *Social capital is defined by its function.* It is not a single entity, but a variety of different entities having two characteristics in common: They all *consist of some aspect of social structure, and they facilitate certain actions of the individuals who are within the structure.* Like other forms of capital, social capital is *productive*, making possible the attainment of certain ends that would not be attainable in its absence. Like physical and human capital, social capital is not completely fungible with respect to specific activities. A given form of social capital that is valuable in facilitating certain actions may be useless or even harmful for others. *Unlike other forms of capital, social capital inheres in the structure of relations between persons and among persons.* It is lodged neither in individuals nor in physical implements of production (Coleman, 1990, p. 302) (emphasis added).[4]

It is apparent in the above statement that Coleman sees social capital as one of three forms of capital that serve productive purposes, the other two forms being physical capital and human capital.[5] In Coleman's conception, physical capital is created by changing materials so as to make equipment that enables production, and so too is human capital created by changing individuals by giving them skills and capabilities that enable them to act in new ways. Likewise, argues Coleman, social capital arises when the relations among persons change in ways that facilitate action.

Coleman gives four examples of social capital. Each of the circumstances differs considerably and the implications of these circumstances are also varying. The first example is of university student activism in South Korea. Coleman notes that the outcome in this example, namely, organised revolt, arose from study circles formed by students who came from the same high school, town or

---

3 Reference is made in this quotation to 'institutionalisation'. In this context, it is useful to consider North's definition of institutions, namely, they are 'the rules of the game of a society, or, more informally, are the human devised constraints that structure human interaction. They are composed of formal rules (statute law, common law, regulations), informal constraints (conventions, norms of behaviour and self-imposed codes of conduct), and enforcement characteristics of both. Organisations are the players: groups of people bound by a common purpose to achieve a common objective' (North, 1995, p. 231). Note that Douglass North is distinguishing between formal and informal institutions and between institutions and organisations.

4 The following extracts from *The New Shorter Oxford English Dictionary* may be useful. 'Inhere' means 'exists as an essential, permanent, or characteristic, attribute, quality etc. of a thing; forms an element of something; belongs to the intrinsic nature of something.' 'Fungible' refers to 'a thing which precisely or acceptably replaces or is replaced by another item, especially of goods contracted for, when a particular item is not specified.' It is useful in this latter context to think of substitutes from the theory of consumer demand.

5 For an account of yet another concept of capital, *viz.*, cultural capital, see Bourdieu (1986) or Throsby (1999).

church. The study circles present the possibility that such groups constitute a resource that enabled students to move from individual protest to organised revolt. Second, the decline of trust between medical practitioners and patients in the United States along with the greater willingess to file malpractice suits when a medical service has had an adverse outcome, due to a lessening in trust, results in increased costs and reduced availability of medical care. Third, an example is given of a family, choosing to move from suburban Detroit to Jerusalem because their children could play unsupervised in a park in Jerusalem and could travel together to school on a city bus unattended by parents. In Jerusalem, adults in the vicinity look after children. Coleman argues that families in Jerusalem have available to them social capital that does not exist in Detroit. Fourth, Coleman cites various instances of the social relationships existing among merchants in Cairo's central market. Indeed, '[t]he whole market is so infused with relations (of the sort just described) that it can be seen as an organisation, no less than a department store. Alternatively, the market can be seen as consisting of a set of individual merchants, each having an extensive body of social capital on which to draw, based on relationships within the market' (Coleman, 1990, p. 304).

Coleman then examines various features of social relations that appear to constitute useful capital for individuals. First, due to the presence of obligations and expectations arising from social relations, a type of insurance is present when social capital is available, making outcomes more easily achieved. The market in Cairo, in the fourth example above, is one of many instances where social capital serves as a useful resource. Next, information is communicated through social relations. Information, a key basis for action and yet at times a costly commodity to gain, is readily available through social relations. Finally, where social capital invokes the norms and sanctions that enable an individual to proceed with an activity due, for example, to a reduction in transactions costs, then social capital has performed productively. In a community, norms that support or encourage altruism greatly facilitate the task of government to care for the indigent.

Another important feature of much social capital, according to Coleman, is that it is a public good:

> The public-good aspect of most social capital means that it is in a fundamentally different position with respect to purposive action than are most other forms of capital. Social capital is an important resource for individuals and can greatly affect their ability to act and their perceived quality of life. They have the capability of bringing such capital into being. Yet because the benefits of actions that bring social capital into being are experienced by persons other than the person so acting, *it is not (necessarily) to that person's interests to bring it into being*. The result is that most forms of social capital are created or destroyed as a by-product of other activities. Much social capital arises or disappears without anyone willing to bring it into or out of being; such capital is therefore even less recognized and taken into account in social research than its intangible character might warrant (Coleman, 1990, pp. 317-18) (emphasis in original).

Coleman addresses several other important properties of social capital that are related to its creation, maintenance and destruction, including the tendency for social capital to depreciate, if not being renewed. As time passes, 'Social relationships die out if not maintained; expectations and obligations wither over time; and norms depend on regular communication' (Coleman, 1990, p. 321).

Attention will now be directed to the second of three approaches to social capital, namely, that of Putnam.

The Account of Social Capital by Robert Putnam

Putnam, a political scientist, makes several contributions to the study of social capital (1993a; 1993b; 1995; 1996). His book, *Making Democracy Work* (1993a), is a study of the performance of regional governments in Italy since their formation in 1970. Putnam and his co-authors give empirical substance to the notion of social capital. Several of the conclusions of the study are the focus of this Sub-section. The design of the study and the empirical results are not relevant in this context.

Twenty new regional governments in Italy were established in 1970. Although all governments were structurally identical, the structure was to be established in regions that differ markedly in their social, economic and cultural settings. For example, the regions ranged from the pre-industrial to the post-industrial, from the devoted Catholic to the fervently Communist, from the feudal to the modern. The study sought to understand how the new institutions evolved in the diversity of these settings. Thereby, the study enables predictions to be made, firstly, about performance differences in democratic government and, secondly, about differences in socio-economic development.

It is argued that historical forces largely explain the regional differences (Putnam, 1993a, Ch. 5). Briefly, in the south of Italy during the Middle Ages, a feudal system was established; in the north and central regions, 'communal republicanism' evolved. Furthermore, in the south, 'social institutions reflect an adjustment to pervasive mistrust. Force and family provide a primitive substitute for civic community' (Putnam, 1993a, p. 178). The north and central regions, on the other hand, have had the benefit of a long history of networks of civic engagement and norms of generalised reciprocity, both of which are mutually reinforcing.

Putnam devised several indexes, employing these to measure factors like 'Institutional Performance', 'Traditions of Civic Involvement 1860-1920', 'Economic Modernity' and 'Civic Community' which is a proxy measure of social capital. He then estimates coefficients of correlation between these variables. Some of his conclusions follow. One of the findings supports the proposition that abundant stocks of social capital lubricate a community's ability to work together. 'Norms and networks of civic engagement'[6] appear to be a pre-requisite both for effective government, and for economic development: 'Social capital is not a substitute for effective public policy but rather a prerequisite for it, and in part, a consequence of it. Social capital, as our Italian study suggests, works through and with states and markets, not in place of them' (Putnam, 1993b, p. 7). Also, as pointed out in the previous paragraph, Putnam establishes that the basis for success or failure in regional government in Italy in the 1980s is at least partly to be found in socio-political history. Indeed, the successes and failures could have been predicted almost a century earlier from the regional patterns and traditions of civic life and involvement (1993a, p. 150).

Moreover, by applying regression analysis to civic and economic data collected for several variables, Putnam is able to show that civic involvement explains socioeconomic development; indeed (and this is actually his point) the reverse is not the case: 'A region's chances of achieving socio-economic development during this century have depended less on its initial socioeconomic endowments than on its civic endowment. Insofar as we can judge from this simple analysis, the contemporary correlation between civics and economics reflects primarily the impact of civics on economics, not the reverse' (Putnam, 1993a, p. 157).

Several factors, according to Putnam, explain why social capital supports good government and economic progress. Among many reasons, Putnam states that networks of civic engagement foster norms of reciprocity and, therein, society is helped to be more efficient. Put otherwise, just as 'money is more efficient than barter, [t]rust lubricates social life' (Putnam, 1993b, p. 3). Another factor, according to Putnam, is that networks of civic involvement assist social coordination and communication and help to spread another efficient lubricant of social life, namely, reputations.

An economic study by Knack and Keefer (1997) reached some similar conclusions to Putnam's. They constructed indicators that enable observations to be made of interpersonal trust and of norms of civic-minded behaviour and co-operation. The indicators drew data from the World Values Surveys for a sample of 29 market economies.[7] By estimating a growth equation in the style

---

6 Putnam argues that networks, norms and trust enable people to act together effectively in the pursuit of shared objectives. He refers to 'civic engagement' when he means how well, and in which areas, people are connected to community life.

7 In the World Values Surveys, the variable 'norms of civic cooperation' is measured from responses to questions about whether each of the following behaviours can always be justified, never be justified or something in between:
a) 'claiming government benefits which you are not entitled to'
b) 'avoiding a fare on public transport'
c) 'cheating on taxes if you have the chance'
d) 'keeping money you have found'
e) 'failing to report damage you've done accidentally to a parked vehicle'.
Details of the construction of these indexes are provided by Knack and Keefer (1997).

of the new endogenous growth theory (Barro and Sala-I-Martin, 1995), the study reveals that a statistically significant relationship exists between social capital and the growth of per capita GDP. On the other hand, another of Putnam's findings, concerned with a controversial hypothesis about the beneficial effect of group involvement on economic performance,[8] is refuted. Knack and Keefer's results indicate that neither the regression coefficient between group involvement and trust nor that between economic performance and group involvement is statistically significant.

Finally, Knack and Keefer also address the following question: What factors determine trust and civic norms? Their evidence shows two importance sources of trust. Low social polarisation, measured in terms of the degree of income inequality, and formal institutional rules that constrain the government from acting arbitrarily, are associated with higher levels of trust and stronger norms of civic co-operation. They also show that ethnic and linguistic divisions coincide with weakened trust and civic norms. See also the study by Easterly and Levine (1997).[9]

Apart from the important empirical contribution that Putnam makes to the understanding of social capital, his work is useful in focussing on the appropriate, albeit different, issues to be addressed by studies of social and economic phenomena. **It should be noted that the social capital concept transcends conventional conceptions of, for example, the (political) left-right dichotomy.** 'Progress on the urgent issues facing our country and our world requires ideas that bridge outdated ideological divides. Both liberals and conservatives agree on the importance of social empowerment. ... The social capital approach promises to uncover new ways of combining private social infrastructure with public policies that work, and, in turn, of using wise public policies to revitalize America's stocks of social capital' (Putnam, 1993b, p. 8). (This is not to suggest that all social scientists like this implication of 'dissolving' old conceptual frameworks.)

In the following Chapter, an analysis will be undertaken that employs the notion of 'combining private social infrastructure with public policies that work',

---

8 The controversy is over two conflicting hypotheses, one being Putnam's and the other associated with Olson (1982). Putnam's hypothesis is that group associations are favourable to economic performance; Olson's hypothesis is that there is a negative relationship between the two. Knack and Keefer's results, which support neither hypothesis, show that there is no relationship between the two variables, possibly because 'Putnam' forces counterbalance 'Olson' forces.

9 The focus of Easterly and Levine (1997) is on the effect of ethnicity, or ethnic diversity, on real per capita GDP growth. Initially, their study seeks to explain economic growth with several explanatory variables. In Table IV, pp. 1225-56, the regression co-efficients on 'ETHNIC' are negative, indicating that, as ethnic diversity rises, per capita growth falls. They suggest that the reason for this is that 'ethnically fragmented economies may find it more difficult to agree on public goods and public policies. They may also be more politically unstable' (p. 1230).

in regard to the mental health care sector. However, one other conception of social capital remains to be addressed in the present Section, that of Gary Becker.

The Account of Social Capital by Gary Becker

The economic approach to studying the actions of individuals is based on an assumption that those actions are undergirded by choices. These choices reflect efforts by individuals to maximise their utility. Economic theory has conventionally assumed that preferences are determined only by the goods and services consumed by individuals at the present time. Put otherwise, a conventional simplifying assumption is made that preferences are unrelated to past or future consumption, and are independent of the behaviour of others. Becker explains that while both of these simplifying assumptions have 'proved to be a valuable simplification for addressing many economic questions, a large number of choices in all societies depend very much on past experiences and social forces' (Becker, 1996, p. 4).

Becker's approach to addressing the oversimplification is to reformulate the utility function of conventional economic theory to incorporate other preferences. The conventional utility function is as follows:

$$U = u\,(x_t, y_t, z_t) \qquad (9.1)$$

where

U is utility
x_t is the consumption of good x in time t
y_t is the consumption of good y in time t
z_t is the consumption of good z in time t.

Becker incorporates past experiences and social experience by defining two new aspects of capital formation: '*Personal capital*, P, includes the relevant past experiences and other personal experiences that affect current and future utilities. *Social capital*, S, incorporates the influence of past actions by peers and others in an individual's social network and control system' (1996, p. 4) (emphasis in original). Becker's rewritten utility function is as follows:

$$U = u\,(x_t, y_t, z_t, P_t, S_t). \qquad (9.2)$$

Becker considers a facet of social relations which is different from the two previous approaches to social capital considered in this Section. He reflects on the social importance of recognition and acceptance, that is, the respect that others have for an individual. Therein, an influence upon consumption patterns is found:

> Consumption and other activities have a major social component partly because they take place in public. As a result, people often choose restaurants, neighborhoods, schools, books to read, political opinions, food, or leisure

> activities with an eye to pleasing peers and others in their social network. I incorporate the influences of others on a person's utility through the stock of social capital, S. ...Since this capital captures the effects of social milieu, an individual's stock of social capital depends not primarily on his own choices, but the choices of peers in the relevant network of interactions. ... This dependence of a person's social capital on the behavior of others may create important externalities (Becker, 1996, p.12).

Although the formation of the concept of social capital is thought largely to have occurred in the 1980s, it is interesting to note that an earlier paper by Becker, 'A Theory of Social Interactions', was published in 1974. It is also relevant to note that Coleman and Becker were not unknown to each other: both held academic positions at the University of Chicago. In fact, they jointly organised a multi-disciplinary seminar (Zupan, 1998).

In the previous Sub-sections, three approaches to social capital were considered. The first approach, that of Coleman, addresses the concept of social capital itself, that is, the nature of the phenomenon. Although part of Putnam's contribution has been to refine the concept of social capital further, his empirical work, if not the actual detail of it, is worthy of emulation. Putnam's results serve to shed further light upon the concept of social capital and to clarify the determinants of social capital. One of Becker's contributions in the area of social interaction, the one presented in this Section, is this: to show that the utility function can be extended to incorporate social capital so that the powerful analytic tools of conventional economic analysis can be brought to bear upon a relevant issue under study.

Summary and Conclusion

This Chapter, and the following one, together focus on some issues regarding the economics of community-based services and strategies.

The particular issue for this Chapter is the presence of multiple inputs into mental health care. The significance of this is that organisations providing community-based services differ from the single-objective, single-output firm of conventional theory.

In the Chapter, various basic concepts from economic theory about production were first reviewed. Some features of organisations providing community-based services and strategies that depart from conventional economic theory of production were noted. Indeed, conventional economic theory concerning the single-output firm originally was modelled as it was only because of the questions historically asked of economic theory. The questions for economic theory in the present era are not synonymous with those set by historical precedent.

Attention then turned to just one key point of departure, namely, that multiple inputs are, in the present era, being employed in order to provide mental health care in the context of community-based services, and they are being drawn jointly, from within both government and 'the community'.

The individualistic framework of analysis of conventional economic theory further limits any straightforward application of such theory for the issue under study; theory that incorporates the role of social relations is required instead. While various attempts exist in the literature to reformulate economic theory to take account of social relations, the most fertile concept for the present study is that of 'social capital', the notion that economic transactions are embedded in social relations. Three accounts of social capital were provided here, those of Coleman (1988, 1990), Putnam (1993a, 1993b, 1996) and Becker (1974, reprinted in Becker, 1996).

Having considered such contextual matters in this Chapter, attention turns in the next Chapter to the relationship between social capital and government. In Chapter 10, the concept of co-production of government and community inputs is employed so as to clarify some aspects of the economics of organisations that provide community-based services and strategies.

10 Co-Production and Community-Based Services

Introduction

Attention turns in this Chapter to a particular aspect of social capital, *viz.* whether actions by government augment or diminish society's stock of social capital. Franks' (1990) study of family costs associated with severe and persistent mental illness raises an important issue to which economic theory has a contribution:

> The fact that families may be providing substitute resources/goods for the formal service system is an important finding for policy makers. In a society where all resources for human services are scarce it would serve the cause of efficiency to determine how formal (governmental) and informal (family) resources could act as complements to each other rather than substitutes (Franks, 1990, pp. 16-17).

Franks (1990) continues with a reference to a model of families (Moroney, 1980, cited in Franks, 1990, p. 17). In this model, families are conceptualised as resource providers wherein 'shared responsibilities' between the family and the State are enacted. The implication of this framework is that government resources and the resources of family networks are joint inputs into care and support for a person disabled by mental illness.

There is currently another approach to public-private 'collaboration' in health and human services. 'Partnership' between public and private groups seeks 'to develop community infrastructure for assessment, planning, and evaluation of community health needs and to integrate health and human services into collaborative service networks' (Bazzoli *et al.*, 1997, p. 533). A range of groups is often in a collaborative network, including, for example, private health providers, public health departments, human service agencies, local government agencies, educational institutions, health plans and managed care organisations, and business coalitions. Mental health care has not escaped this phenomenon (Alter and Hage, 1993; Goldman *et al.*, 1992; Grusky *et al.*, 1985; Morrisey *et al.*, 1991).

The approach of the present Chapter uses economic tools of analysis. It addresses two questions that arise with the issues raised above, namely, what is the relationship between social capital and government? And, second, are these two phenomena, social capital and government, of a competitive (or of a substitute) nature, or are they of a non-competitive (or complementary) nature? While the answers to the previous two questions are empirical, a general theory of co-production (Ostrom, 1996), in which inputs from government and inputs from citizens are employed, offers a relevant framework to analyse the important issues raised by Moroney (1980) and Franks (1990).

Synergy

One way of exploring the relationship between social capital and government is to test for the presence of synergy. 'Synergy' arises from co-operation and, in particular, refers to instances when the effectiveness of co-operative action is greater than the summed effect achieved by independent action. Detecting the presence of synergy may be difficult when the nature of the synergistic relationship is quite subtle.

It is understandable that some readers may be inclined to treat the word, synergy, as a manifestation of current gibberish, along with other terms like 'total quality management', 'networking' and so forth (Geneen, 1997). However, there **is** some important **content** to the material covered by 'synergy' as used by Ostrom (1996). It should be noted also that synergy does not imply the same meaning as 'economies of scope', as defined by Baumol, Panzar and Willig (1992). This latter term involves the gains for a single firm in producing multiple outputs, whereas synergy refers to gains associated with a single output from government and private inputs.

In the literature there are two opposing hypotheses relating to synergy between government and the stock of social capital. One hypothesis arises from an argument put forward by Coleman (1990). Coleman argues that when government acts, this 'crowds out' informal networks.[1] The resulting depreciation in the stock of social capital occurs because the government activity does not provide the same range of values and functions as the activity that

---

1 'Crowding out' is borrowed from the Macroeconomics literature. In regard to expansionary fiscal policy, for example, a rise in government expenditure sometimes causes private expenditure (particularly investment spending) to fall. The same pool of funds, available through saving, is used both for the bond-financing of the budget deficit and for private investment. This pool may not expand. Rather, if a budget deficit crowds out, or offsets and competes with, an expansion occurring in the private sector, then government's attempt to stimulate Gross Domestic Product is also offset. On the other hand, 'crowding in' effects reduce the contractionary impact of a budget surplus (Jackson *et al.*, 1994; Stonecash, Gans *et al.*, 1999). 'Crowding out' has also been applied to an issue more relevant to the present monograph, namely, intrinsic motivation. In some circumstances, higher monetary remuneration (extrinsic motivation) may compete with, that is, crowd out, any intrinsic motivation to undertake an activity, or it may complement, and improve, intrinsic motivation (Frey, 1997).

arises from informal networks. The result is that the community is worse off. The government 'crowding out' effect here is, according to Coleman, just one of the classes of 'crowding out' factors causing individuals to be less dependent on one another. Two other causal factors for the phenomenon of 'crowding out' relate to rising affluence and the widening net of social security.

The descriptions of Chapter 9 reveal an opposing position. Putnam (1993) puts the case that government activities and social capital are complementary. Another way of stating the argument is as follows:

> ...there is evidence that the existence of the state and the rules it establishes and enforces can strengthen and increase the efficiency of [local organisations and institutions] and that, at least in coalition with other urban-based groups, [local organisations and institutions] can give rise to collective action increasing the power of the state (Nugent, 1993, p. 629).

The resolution of these two opposing arguments is an empirical matter. Empirical work is not undertaken here. With empirical work, though, one should ascertain whether what is measured serves to clarify the nature of the phenomenon being measured. To this end, the following Sections present a framework for testing the 'synergy hypothesis'. A concept similar to synergy, namely, co-production, is outlined in the next Section.

Co-Production

The term, co-production, refers to descriptions of joint activity in two quite separate contexts: the construction of sewerage systems in Recife in Brazil; and primary education in Nigeria (Ostrom, 1996). Co-production is defined as follows:

> By coproduction, I mean the process through which inputs used to produce a good or service are contributed by individuals who are not 'in' the same organisation. The 'regular' producer of education, health or infrastructure services is most frequently a government agency. Whether the regular producer is the only producer of these goods and services depends both on the nature of the good or service itself and on the incentives that encourage the active participation of others... Coproduction implies that citizens can play an active role in producing public goods and services of consequence to them (Ostrom, 1996, p. 1073).

Elinor Ostrom, a political scientist, writes that the concept of co-production was developed by colleagues in the Workshop in Political Theory and Policy Analysis in America in the late 1970s 'as we struggled with dominant theories of urban governance underlying policy recommendations of massive centralization' (Ostrom, 1996, p. 1079). The struggle to which she refers arose over a proposition at the time that centralising local government services would enable a more effective and efficient service because clients would be served by professional staff employed by a large bureaucratic agency. The empirical evidence was to the contrary. 'After studying police services in metropolitan areas, however, not a single instance was found where a large, centralized police department was able to provide better direct service, more equitably delivered, or at lower cost to neighborhoods inside the central city when these were carefully matched to similar neighborhoods located in surrounding jurisdictions' (Ostrom, 1996, p. 1079). These findings were replicated repeatedly over a 15-year period.

The efforts of Ostrom and her colleagues to understand these strong empirical results led to a recognition of some implicit assumptions that had been made in regard to service provision by government.

Implicit Assumptions about Government Service Provision

Ostrom (1996, p. 1079) reveals three implicit assumptions, or 'myths' in Ostrom's words. It appeared these were obfuscating a reality that the theories, which were being used at the time to describe government service provision, ought to have been clarifying.

Implicit Assumption 1: About the Composition of the Industry Providing Immediate Response Services

It had been assumed that a single producer was responsible for the services. The reality was that public agencies, such as municipalities, and private firms, such as those providing security services, were involved together in the provision of (so-named) immediate response services. Put otherwise, the security services were being provided by a public-private industry, not a bureaucratic apparatus of a single government agency.

Implicit Assumption 2: About the Nature of Service Providers

Each police and security officer has a personal stock of human capital belonging to the individual in service to the bureaucracy. The personal stock of human capital does not necessarily turn as easily as a cog in a machine. 'A motivated officer uses time in many ways that enhance the safety of a beat. An officer who is not motivated finds many ways to escape the summons of the police radio and get some sleep' (Ostrom, 1996, p. 1079). Variations in human capital, and people's motivations, must be recognised.

Implicit Assumption 3: About Jointness in Service Provision

Ostrom and her colleagues suspected that, unlike the production of goods, the production of services is not undertaken only by the service provider. Service production calls for active participation from the client, the recipient of the service. That is, the so-called service provider is not the only provider of the service. In schooling, for example, teachers depend on the cooperation of students to achieve a learning outcome. Teachers depend also on the support of parents in, say, ensuring homework is done, counting on parents to nurture in the home the interests and abilities that are fostered at school. Ostrom says: '...We developed the term "coproduction" to describe the potential relationships that could exist between the "regular" producer (street-level police officers, school teachers, or health workers) and 'clients' who want to be transformed by the service into safer, better educated, or healthier persons. Coproduction is one way that synergy between what a government does and what citizens do can occur' (Ostrom, 1996, p. 1079).

An Economic Interpretation of the Implicit Assumptions

The three implicit assumptions (above) can be understood in the light of conventional economic theory in the following manner using standard economic terminology.

Implicit Assumption 1

A single source for the budget for the production of services does not exist. Rather, different firms, public and/or private, comprise the source of funds. In conceptualising the 'total budget', it is not appropriate to conceive of funds being 'pooled' into a single source. Rather, the 'total budget' is (conceptually) the sum of the costs of the inputs provided by the different firms.

Implicit Assumption 2

The production of services can violate the assumption of production theory in economics that production is least-cost and/or efficient. 'Production functions describe what is *technically feasible* when the firm operates *efficiently;* that is, when the firm uses each combination of inputs as effectively as possible' (Pindyck and Rubinfeld, 1992, p. 168) or, as Greene (1997, p. 81) puts it, 'a production function represents some sort of ideal, the **maximum output** attainable given a set of inputs' (emphasis in original). The problem here is a situation of technical inefficiency or X-inefficiency (Leibenstein, 1966). In other words, production takes place at a point under the production possibility frontier.

Implicit Assumption 3

The time of the client and of the client's family and friends is another input in the production of services, as argued by Becker (1965). Inputs of time must be included in the 'total budget' for the activity.

Fundamental Production Theory

It is pertinent at this juncture, since inputs and the production of services are being discussed, to turn attention briefly to some elementary aspects of production theory.

Ostrom (1996) invokes production theory commenting that, 'All production involves the transformation of some set of inputs into outputs – or a production function' (p. 1079), and the diagrams presented by Ostrom use isoquants (although she does not use the term, isoquant). In the following account, two special cases of isoquants are presented. Case 1 is the situation where inputs are perfectly substitutable and Case 2 is where the inputs are used in fixed proportions. The General Case is then given, followed by a re-examination of the technically optimal, or least-cost, combination of inputs.

Case 1: Where Inputs are Perfectly Substitutable

In Figure 10.1, Q_1 and Q_2 are two straight lines, and represent isoquants for two different output levels, say, 1,000 tonnes of wheat and 2,000 tonnes of wheat. The X- and Y-axes measure inputs of labour and capital, respectively. Given that the isoquants are straight lines, the marginal rate of technical substitution (MRTS) is constant. Inputs are perfectly substitutable. Production can take place at input combinations represented by A, B or C and the output does not change. It is important to note that in this case production can take place with the use of only one input.

Case 2: Where Inputs Combine in Fixed Proportions

In Figure 10.2, the production isoquants are L-shaped since only one combination of capital and labour (OK_1 and OL_1, respectively, for quantity of output Q_1) is used. Using more capital **or** more labour does not increase the quantity of output. Output can only be increased by using more of both capital **and** labour, e.g. more of both capital (OK_2) and labour (OL_2) to produce the output associated with isoquant Q_2.

The General Case: Increasing Costs of Input Substitution

In the long run, when both labour and capital are variable, more of either input increases output. See Figure 10.3. If output is to be kept constant as more of one input is used, less of the other input is used. The MRTS is constantly changing as one moves along Q_1 and Q_2. Note that the isoquants involve a physical measure of output, say, quantity of cars produced.

The introduction of costs into the analysis of production involves at this juncture the isocost line. This is the relevant framework for determining the

Figure 10.1 Production with perfectly substitutable inputs

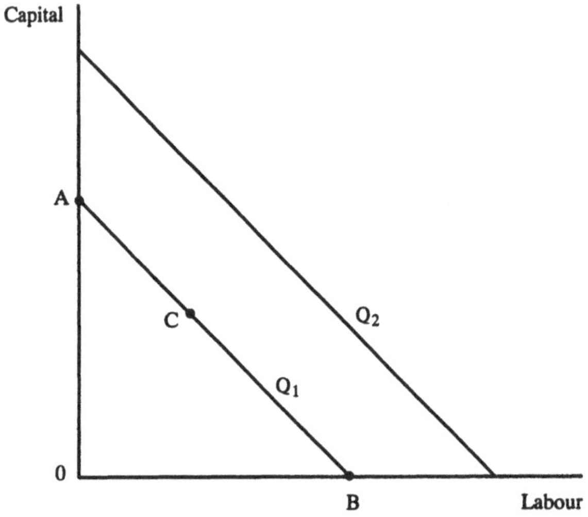

Figure 10.2 Production with inputs in fixed proportions

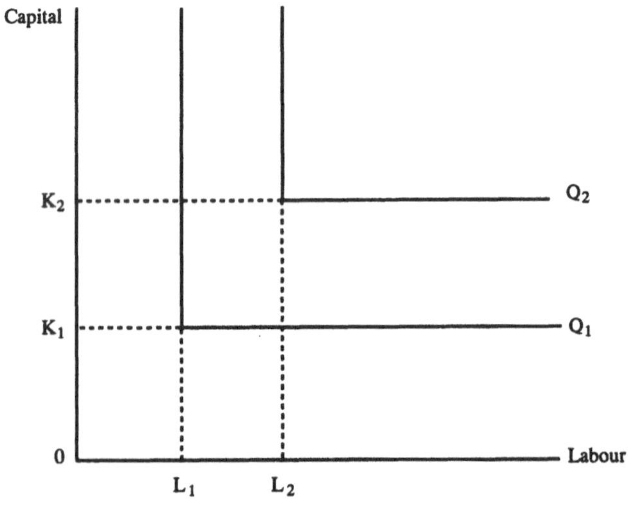

optimal combination of inputs. Total cost, in a simplified two-input framework, is the amount the firm spends on labour, plus the amount the firm spends on capital, such that

$$TC = wL + rK \tag{10.1}$$

where TC stands for Total Cost, L is the quantity of labour, K is the quantity of capital, w is the wage rate and r is the price of capital.

The isocost lines (RS and TU) in Figure 10.4 show the combinations of capital and labour that can be bought for two (given) total costs. RS is one isocost line for one level of total costs and TU is a 'higher' isocost line for a greater amount of total costs. Note that the slope of the isocost line reflects the ratio of input prices in input space.

The Least-Cost Input Combination

The optimal combination of inputs is the one where the firm minimises costs, or maximises output, subject to a constraint. This occurs when an isoquant is tangential to an isocost line. In Figure 10.5, three isocost lines are shown as RS, TU and VW. Q_1 is an isoquant. At point X, the output Q_1 will be optimally produced by employing OA units of labour and OB units of capital.

A comment about cost shares (or contributions) should be noted here. The comment to be made is this: points of tangency, such as X in Figure 10.5, imply cost sharing. At point X, the share that labour contributes to total cost is given by the ratio wL/TC, derived from Equation (10.1) above. The share that capital contributes is given by rK/TC. These two ratios can take values between

Figure 10.3 Production with increasing costs of input substitution

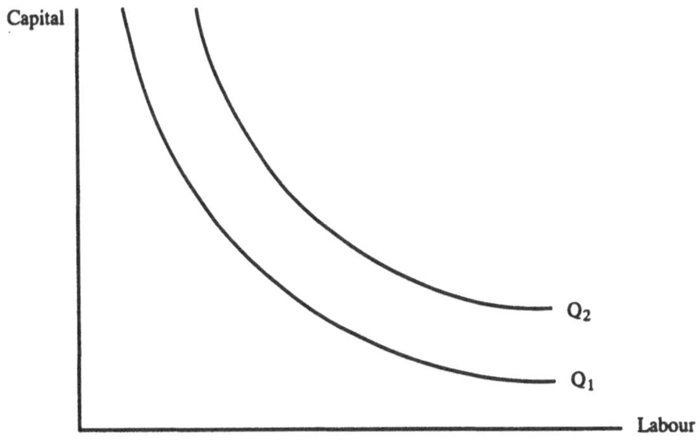

Figure 10.4 Two isocost lines in input space

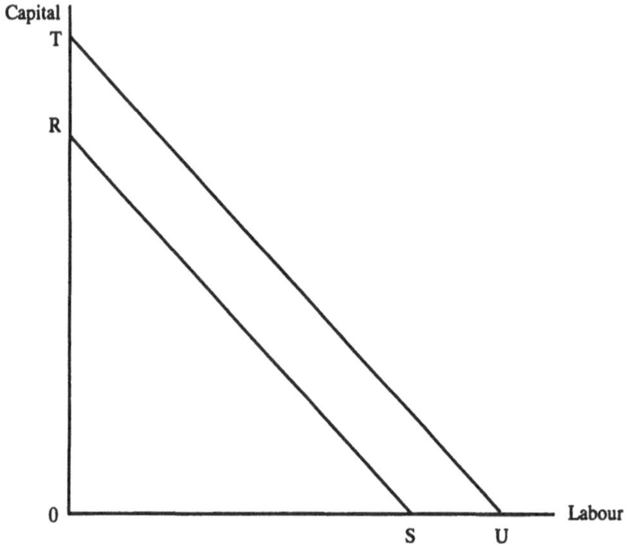

Figure 10.5 Technical efficiency in input space

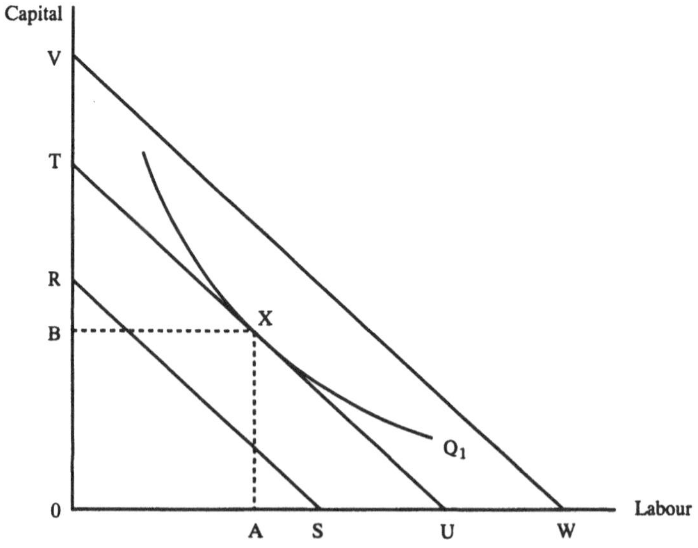

zero and unity, and these two shares will always sum to unity. Cost sharing may arise between citizens' and government inputs, not just the traditional inputs of capital and labour, a point to be considered in the following Section.

Attention can now be directed to Ostrom's analysis.

An Application of Production Theory to Co-Production

In her analysis of co-production, Ostrom (1996) applies the theory outlined briefly in the previous Section. Instead of the conventional inputs, namely, capital and labour, Ostrom models 'inputs from government' and 'inputs from citizens'.

A brief comment about this terminology is in order here. Recall that Ostrom is a political scientist and note that the term she uses, 'citizens', is a common part of the political science vocabulary. Now, mental health workers are more likely to use the term, 'the community' instead of 'citizens'. Economists, on the other hand, may refer to 'private inputs' (without wishing to imply business firms, of course). To understand the relevance of Ostrom's analysis, it is helpful to realise that the purpose here is not to emphasise the differences in terminology, differences that can often drive wedges between those disciplines that confront common problems and issues. Rather, the approach here seeks to illuminate some common ground.

In the analysis that follows, then, the relationship between two input-types is analysed using the economic theory of production in order to gain a better understanding of the nature of co-production itself, with an application later in the Chapter to deinstitutionalisation in mental health care.

The Case of No Synergy

Ostrom first considers a special case, the instance where the two input-types are strictly substitutable. In such cases, government inputs can be perfectly replaced by inputs from 'citizen-producers' (which is how Ostrom refers to them). No potential for synergy exists in the 'straight-line isoquant case' and there is nothing to be gained, in an economic sense, in looking for avenues of co-producing. Rather, it is necessary to determine whether a greater level of technical efficiency is attained either by public sector production or by citizen-production.

To illustrate the case, Ostrom gives the example of garbage collection. The alternatives are as follows: government sends a truck to collect garbage, a collective input; alternatively, citizens are required to take their own garbage to a designated location, a private input. The choice between the two alternatives will depend on 'the wage rate paid to public officials as compared to the opportunity costs facing citizens for spending their time in transport' (Ostrom, 1996, pp. 1,079-80). Assume W_{pub} = \$10/hour and W_{prv} = \$20/hour, where W_{pub} is the public wage rate and W_{prv} is the private wage rate. Assume TC = \$100. At the two 'extreme' cases, the public input will be ten hours, and private input will be five hours. In Figure 10.6(a), AB is the relevant

Figure 10.6 Perfectly substitutable contributions to an output from government and citizens

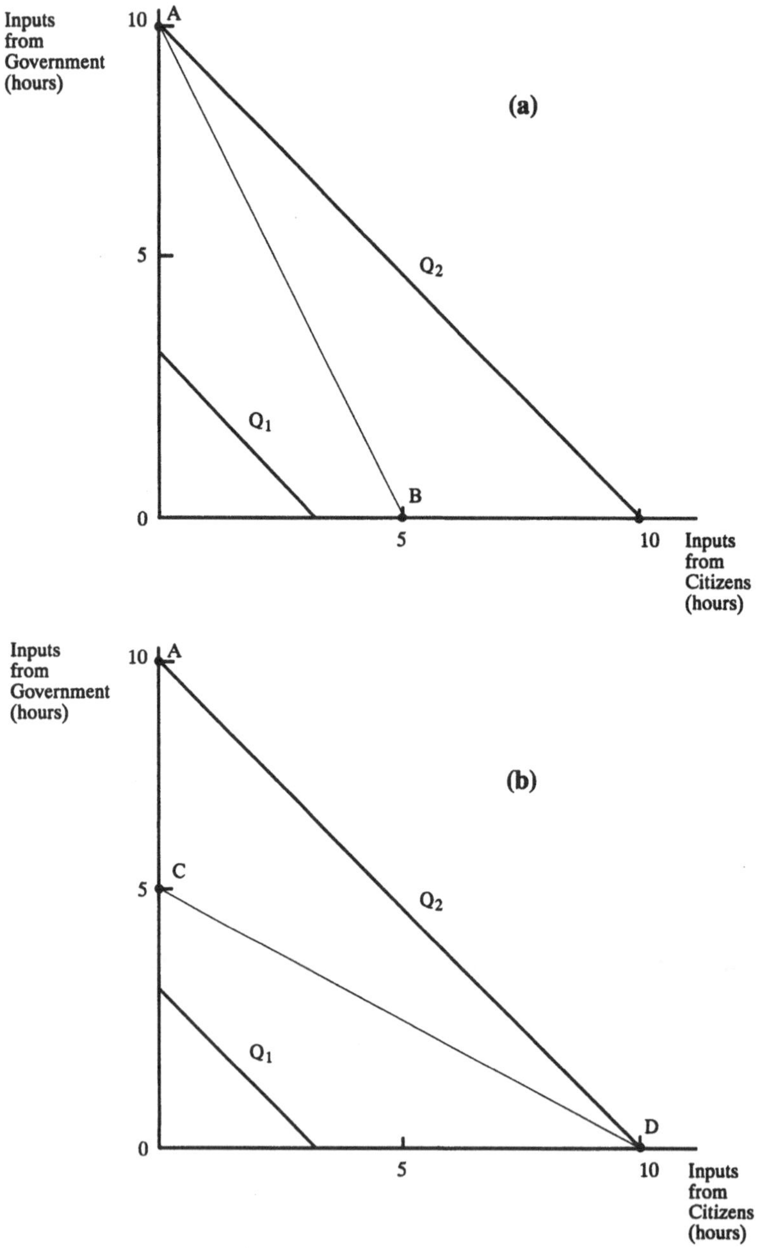

Source: Adapted from Ostrom (1996, Figure 1).

isocost line.[2] Since inputs are perfectly substitutable, the isoquants, Q_1 and Q_2, are straight lines. The point of tangency between the isoquant Q_2 and the isocost line AB is at A, a 'corner solution'. The technically efficient production of garbage services would be to have garbage collection occurring collectively.

If the wage rates are reversed, such that W_{pub} = \$20/hour and W_{prv} = \$10/hour, then the isocost line would be CD as in Figure 10.6(b). In this instance, the 'corner solution' occurs at point D, and the technically efficient production of garbage services is to have garbage collected as a private activity.

In both cases (above), there is no possibility of combining inputs from the public and private sectors. That is, no synergy exists. These two cases also imply extreme cases in cost sharing, a point that was introduced in the previous Section. In Figure 10.6(a), the cost share from government is unity, with citizens contributing a zero cost share. In Figure 10.6(b), these shares are reversed. The more general case of cost-sharing will be depicted in Figure 10.7 below.

Figure 10.7 Complementary contributions to an output from government and citizens

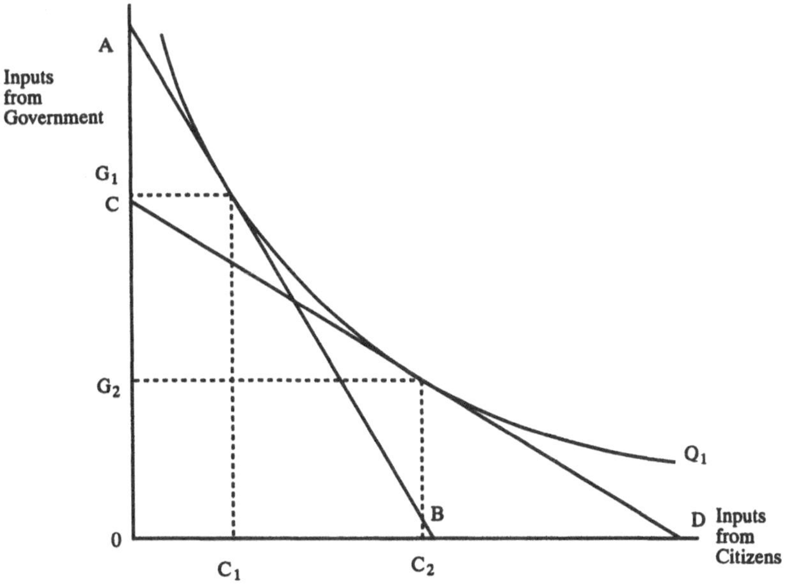

Source: Adapted from Ostrom (1996, Figure 2).

2 Ostrom uses the term 'budget constraint'. The normal term is 'isocost line' when dealing with input space.

The Case Where Synergy Exists

Synergy is present where the 'inputs from a government and citizens are complementary' (Ostrom, 1996, p. 1,080). The output is optimally produced by some combination of the input-types. Put otherwise, it is not optimal to rely just on inputs of citizens or on inputs from government. Instead, many combinations of input-types exist which achieve an identical level of output of the service. In such cases, the isoquants are downward sloping and convex to the origin, as in Figure 10.7.

Assume the instance where the public wage rate is less than the private wage rate. This wage relativity is depicted by the slope of the isocost line, AB. The optimal combination of inputs that achieves Q_1 is OG_1 of government input and OC_1 of citizen input. If the public wage rate is greater than the private wage rate, that is, the isocost line is CD, then the optimal combination of inputs to achieve Q_1 is OG_2 of government input and OC_2 of citizen input.

Ostrom then states, *a priori,* that 'Many poor regions and neighborhoods are characterized by severe underutilization of the knowledge, skills and time of residents – which means that the opportunity costs of devoting these inputs to the creation of valued public outputs are low' (Ostrom, 1996, p. 1080). Restating the notion diagrammatically, Ostrom's judgement implies that the shape of the isocost line in many developing countries is more like CD than AB in Figure 10.7.

In this Section so far, with the use of the conceptual tools of conventional production theory, light has been shed on co-production, in the manner of Ostrom (1996). Ostrom conceives of the presence / absence of synergy between two rather unconventional inputs, inputs from government and inputs from citizens. She goes on to point out that her analysis has assumed no possibility of slackness in input performance, rather 'full motivation to perform to capacity', as she puts it (p. 1080). In the following Section, the motivational disposition of workers is addressed.

The Issue of Motivation

The following account is of Ostrom's analysis of the issue of motivation, with some emendations. Ostrom illustrates her analysis with the following example from education. The account that follows will give that example and an application will then be made to mental health care.

In Figure 10.8 AB is an isocost line for a service in education, or health for that matter. Q_3 is an isoquant representing a given quantity of education or health. Isoquant Q_3 is technically feasible and OY units of government input are employed and OX units of citizens' inputs are employed. Now if health practitioners or teachers are poorly motivated, the OY units of government inputs and OX units of citizens' inputs will not produce Q_3 output but a lower level of output, say, Q_1. Put otherwise, the OY **and** OX inputs are still employed but the community does not obtain the relevant Q_3 output.

The 'waste' can be measured in two ways. By constructing a new isocost line, CD, parallel to AB and tangential to isoquant Q_1, then the measure of the 'waste' in monetary terms is either the distance AC or DB. The 'waste', measured in terms of lower education or health output, is also found by the quantitative difference between the isoquants, Q_1 and Q_3.

An examination follows where a compounding effect occurs due to spending less on education, and poor motivation. Whether education spending is reduced by government or by the community, the effect is to shift the isocost line towards the origin, thus producing a further decline in educational output. The effect is determined by the empirical value of the resulting isoquant. Figure 10.9 below now incorporates spending cuts into the previous account of poor motivation, represented in Figure 10.8. Let us begin with a total 'budget' represented by the isocost line AB: *ceteris paribus*, an optimal outcome is given by the tangency condition with isoquant Q_3, involving OY units of government inputs and OX units of private (or community) inputs. If poor motivation exists, then the educational sector will be subject to 'waste', in that, although the total budget is indicated by the isocost line, AB, the actual

Figure 10.8 Co-production in the presence of low motivation

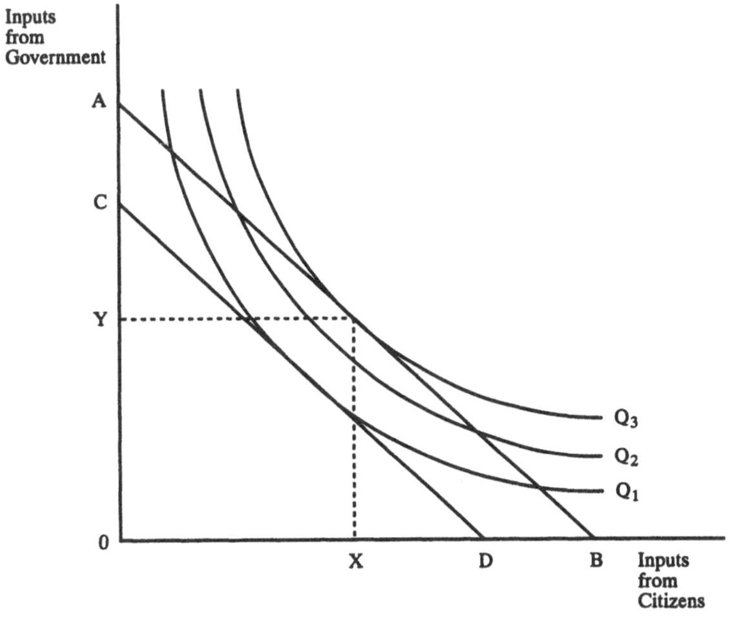

Source: Adapted from Ostrom (1996, Figure 3).

output is indicated by the (lower) isoquant Q_2. The effect of this inefficiency (arising from poor motivation) is equivalent to the effect of government inputs being reduced to OY_1 and community inputs being decreased to OX_1.

Let us now assume that the government and/or the citizens **reduce** their financial commitments to education, such that the available resources are now indicated by the isocost line CD. It is believed that the reduced budget will enable the production of education as indicated by the isoquant Q_1. The reason given for the reduced resources allocated to the educational sector may be that the teaching staff is 'slack' and students are not learning. The **effect** of this decreased financial commitment is to create another round of falling motivation or poor motivation from staff. This further decrease in motivation, induced by the reduced expenditure commitment, leads to a further decrease in educational output to Q_0. In other words, there may be a 'cumulative causation' process, or a vicious cycle at work. This concept of cumulative causation was developed by Myrdal, in the context of race relations in the US (Myrdal, 1944), and was subsequently employed to explain the disparities in regional economic growth within and between countries (Myrdal, 1957).

Figure 10.9 Poor motivation compounded by spending cuts

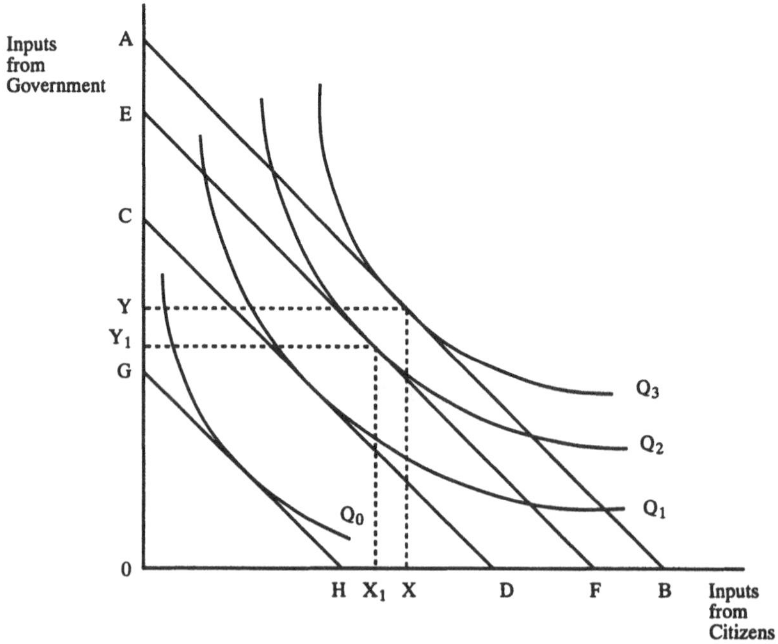

Source: Adapted from Ostrom (1996) Figure 3.

The example above has illustrated that educational output has declined from Q_3 to Q_2, then to Q_1, and then further to Q_0.

Co-Production and Community-Based Mental Health Care

Consider the shift in direction in the organisation and financing of mental health care in the US. A trend is occurring towards government acting as buyers, rather than as providers of care. This trend within the deinstitutionalisation movement raises many issues. McGuire and Riordan (1993), for example, consider the incentives and information issues that ensure the community provider serves the state interest. They regard these issues as the central problem in state contracting of mental health care, and they note the evidence that community mental health centres, when they received contracts from government with no incentive provisions, simply '*did not* target services to the seriously mentally ill' (p. 57, emphasis in original). In other words, community mental health centres 'cream-skimmed'. In the context of the move towards privatisation of government activity in mental health care, these are not trivial concerns, but the focus of this Section is upon yet another matter within community-based mental health care.

Although professional treatment alleviates some of the symptoms and disabilities, chronic problems remain, affecting the daily living of a range of individuals with serious mental illnesses. Housing, shopping, personal care, food preparation, transport, income support, banking and so on are difficult for such people. This is due largely to the illnesses intensifying the challenges in decision-making and performance of the tasks of 'getting through the day'. Previously institutionalised, this population struggles with daily living, struggling in different ways. Living in the community now, these people seem to depend rather haphazardly on its social capital, that is, on greater efforts from family, from friends, and perhaps even from passers-by, as well as from community mental health care and other government agencies, to provide care and support, and treatment.

It is highly pertinent in this context, then, to ask again: What is the relationship between social capital and government in the new community-based mental health care setting or context? Are these two entities substitutes or are they complements? With community-based mental health care, 'inputs from citizens' and 'inputs from government' are evident. The general theory of co-production presented earlier in this Chapter is employed once again here, to help shed light on the optimal input combination from citizens and government for providing the multiple outputs of treatment, care and support for individuals with mental illnesses and disabilities.

Figure 10.10 Perfectly substitutable inputs from government and citizens for providing mental health care

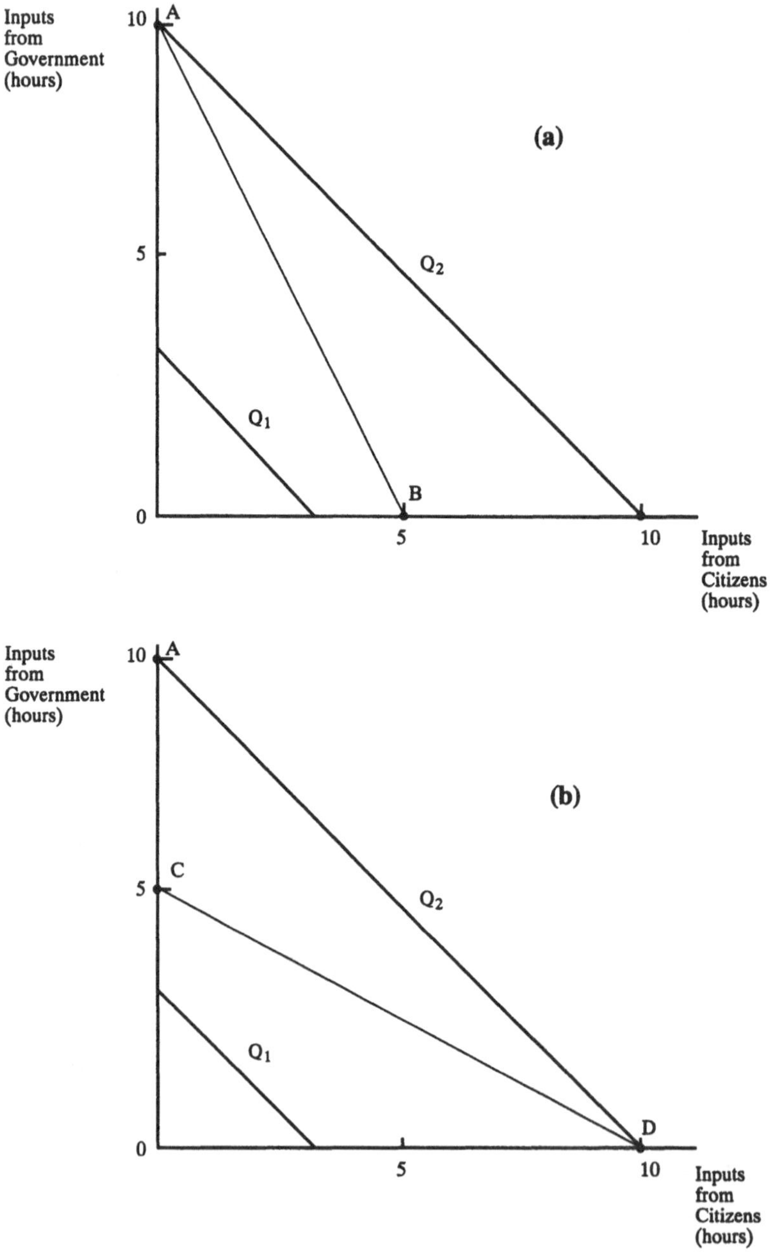

Source: Adapted from Ostrom (1996, Figure 1).

The Case of No Synergy

Consider first a limiting case, an instance where the two input-types, given in the previous Section, are perfectly substitutable. In the limiting case, government inputs can be perfectly replaced by inputs from 'citizen-producers'. In this 'straight-line isoquant case', no potential for synergy exists. There is nothing to be gained, in an economic sense, in looking for avenues of co-producing. Rather, it is necessary to determine whether a greater level of technical efficiency is attained either by public sector production or by citizen-production.

To illustrate the case, suppose the two following alternatives exist. Either, government monopolises the provision of services of mental health care, say, within the walls of a hospital; or citizens take into their homes and community their own relatives, friends and patients, caring for them. They draw solely upon citizen inputs. Suppose the question, as to which of the two alternatives just given is optimal, depends on the wage rate paid to public servants as compared to the opportunity costs facing citizens for spending their time in care, treatment and support.

Assume W_{pub} = \$10/hour and W_{prv} = \$20/hour, where W_{pub} is the public wage rate and W_{prv} is the private wage rate.[3] Assume TC = \$100. At the two 'extreme' cases, the public input will be ten hours and private input will be five hours. In Figure 10.10(a), AB is the relevant isocost line. Since inputs are perfectly substitutable, the isoquants, Q_1 and Q_2, are straight lines. The point of tangency between the isoquant Q_2 and the isocost line AB is at A, giving rise to a 'corner solution'. In this special case, the technically efficient arrangement for mental health care is government provision.

If the wage rates are reversed, such that W_{pub} = \$20/hour and W_{prv} = \$10/hour, then the isocost line would be CD as in Figure 10.10(b). In this alternative case, the 'corner solution' occurs at point D, and the technically efficient production of mental health care is to have treatment, care and support as a citizen-provided activity.

In both cases modelled above, it is not possible to combine inputs from the public and private sectors. That is, no synergy exists, to use Ostrom's (1996) term.

The Case Where Synergy Exists

Synergy is present where complementarity exists between the inputs from government and from citizens. Because the output is optimally produced by

---

3 Wage rates are just one type of measure of the input. The discussion of more sophisticated measures, or of other relevant measures, is not the focus here. Some of the problems encountered in measuring the contribution of household care-giving, for example, were raised in Chapter 8.

Figure 10.11 Complementary inputs from government and citizens for providing mental health care

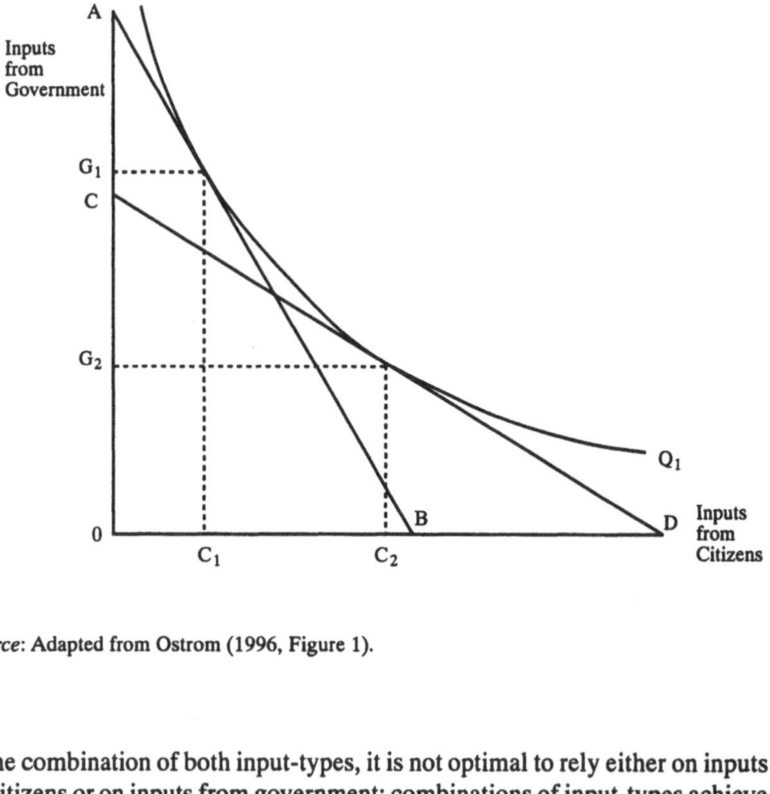

Source: Adapted from Ostrom (1996, Figure 1).

some combination of both input-types, it is not optimal to rely either on inputs of citizens or on inputs from government: combinations of input-types achieve the same level of output of the service. As in the previous analysis associated with Figure 10.7, the single isoquant, Q_1, in Figure 10.11 is downward sloping and convex to the origin.

Assume once again an instance where the public wage rate is less than the private wage rate, as depicted by the isocost line, AB. The amounts, OG_1 of government input and OC_1 of citizen input, achieve the level of output indicated by Q_1. If, on the other hand, the public wage rate is greater than the private wage rate and if the isocost line is CD, then the optimal combination of inputs to achieve Q_1 is OG_2 of government input and OC_2 of citizen input.

Having considered the conceptual matter of substitutability/ complementarity between citizen and government inputs in the context of mental health care, let us now address the matter of the degree to which synergy is present or absent between these inputs.

Synergy in Mental Health Care

The degree to which synergy does, or does not, exist between government and citizen inputs in mental health care is unknown. And yet, the deinstitutionalisation movement has been predicated on assumptions that synergy exists between these inputs.

By way of contrast to such assumptions about deinstitutionalisation, recall from Chapter 8 a brief statement about care-giving by households. This statement will now be considered in full, for several reasons. The first part of the statement reproduced below is important, as it provides a descriptive account of the multitudinous small tasks associated with care-giving in the household. The statement concludes with an anecdotal suggestion of a zero level of synergy between the household sector and the formal treatment system:

> Typical caregiving by households involved with mental illness is not thought to be like that of a relative with physical or developmental disabilities. For example, it normally does not involve nursing duties, as is the case with physically or developmentally delayed relatives. It can involve 'hours devoted to activities of daily living... [and] ... multiple expenditures of time and energy in trying to obtain timely services from mental health, welfare and medical systems, and interactions with legal and criminal justice systems. ... The emotional stress involved with dealing with behaviors that may be disruptive, assaultive, self-destructive, socially constraining and, above all, incomprehensible, *has been accompanied by a notable lack of information and help from the treatment system*' (Lefley, 1996, pp. 6-7) (emphasis added).

In the evaluation of deinstitutionalisation, a conceptual basis is crucial, as well as some empirical results that make quite clear the nature and magnitude of the effects of deinstitutionalisation. Towards this end, this Section has outlined an approach to co-production in mental health care, conceptualising the presence/absence of synergy between inputs from government and inputs from citizens. It is fundamentally important in the evaluation of change in mental health services, that evaluative analyses are based on appropriate empirical analysis: the presence or absence of synergy is **not** a matter of belief or assertion.

Motivation and Mental Health Care in the Community

The likely occurrence of compounding effects has been considered already in this Chapter in the example given by Ostrom (1996) of lowering expenditures on education. In this context here, formally applying Ostrom's approach once again to the case of motivation and mental health care is not necessary. However, it is an important qualification that poor motivation, compounded by decreased expenditure on mental health care, could well generate a downward spiral of lowered mental health output. As an aside, it should be noted that Myrdal (1957) does not regard a 'vicious downward spiral' as inevitable: a 'virtuous upward cycle' can occur and the objective is to create the pre-conditions for this latter cycle.

Some Notes on Empirical Estimation

The previous theoretical discussion leads to some empirically testable propositions that would enable us to determine if the outputs of mental health care were, or were not, increased by co-production between the public and private sectors. However, it is useful to make some comments on the issues associated with empirical estimation.

Generally, we are concerned with the 'ease' with which inputs can substitute for one another, i.e. we are concerned with the shape of the single isoquant rather than the shape of the whole isoquant map. It might be thought that the MRTS, or the slope of the isoquant, provides a measure of this responsiveness, but a little reflection indicates that the slope is not scale-free. Bringing together Marshall's concept of elasticity (Newman, 1987) and the long-standing concept of substitution, Hicks (1932) and Robinson (1933) provided the scale-free building block to the measuring rod we now know as the elasticity of substitution, for which the symbol is (commonly) σ.[4] Consequential to these early developments, share elasticities were introduced in the late 1960s and early 1970s (Samuelson, 1968; Christensen, Jorgenson and Lau, 1971, 1973).[5]

The importance of σ is that it enables the empirical specification of extreme, and other special, cases. The case of perfect substitutes is the case in which σ is equal to infinity, and in the fixed proportions (or perfect complements) case, $\sigma = 0$. The much-employed Cobb-Douglas functional form implies isoquants with a constant (and unitary) elasticity of substitution (Cobb and Douglas, 1928). Also, the constant elasticity of substitution (CES) production function is another special case, a case in which σ is a constant, but is data-determined (Arrow, Chenery, Minhas and Solow, 1961). Furthermore, Cobb-Douglas isoquants are asymptotic to both the X- and Y-axes, this precluding production with none of one input. See Nicholson (1992, pp. 309-14) and Debertin (1986, pp. 202-6) for details. More generally, see Connelly and Doessel (2000).

Given the centrality of the policy issues in mental health care, e.g. medication *vs* therapy and counselling, public *vs* private production and/or funding, it is crucial to estimate the extent of input substitution that is feasible in the production of mental health status. With the advent of duality theory,[6] it matters not whether production or cost functions are estimated (Fuss, 1987).

---

4 This pure number is always positive, i.e. it can take values from zero to infinity (Nicholson, 1992, p. 308).

5 For details, see Helm (1987) and Jorgenson (1987).

6 Cornes (1992) provides a neat exposition.

Furthermore, since the advent of flexible functional forms, estimation using, say, the transcendental logarithmic, or the translog, should typically be undertaken.

The significance of the discussion in this Chapter (albeit at an abstract level) of co-production is that it provides a conceptual framework for thinking about the economic dimension of the deinstitutionalisation phenomenon. It is recognised that deinstitutionalisation is a **process** that is now virtually completed in various countries. The relevant economic data necessary to analyse the phenomenon were not collected, thus precluding any economic analysis **then** or **now**. It is useful to observe that this is not unique to economic data and economic evaluation (Wyatt and De Renzio, 1986).

The point is to draw a moral from this tale of missed opportunities and missed analyses. The moral is that we should not repeat the pessimistic description of humanity's disposition not to learn, as indicated in the oft-quoted statement by Hegel in 1832 that '[w]hat experience and history teach is this – that peoples and governments never have learned anything from history, or acted on principles deduced from it' (quoted in Frank, 1999, p. 362). If another massive social experiment is undertaken, of the magnitude of the deinstitutionalisation movement, then the relevant data must be collected so that evaluation can take place.

Conclusion

In this Chapter a research agenda is outlined, suggesting an approach to the evaluation of deinstitutionalisation. This framework enables evaluative analysis that can be directed beyond anecdotal evidence. The analyses proposed here allow for a conceptual framework within which empirical work can be undertaken. Needless to say, empirical work on issues associated with mental health care need not be atheoretical.

The approach outlined in this Chapter actually involves conventional production and cost studies. In other words, an empirical study of change, such as deinstitutionalisation, would need first to consider the nature of the isoquants associated with the production function of mental health services, and the magnitude of the elasticity of substitution, the relevant concept that will specify the substitutability of inputs to the production process. Note that it is unlikely that isoquants would be entirely capricious, incomprehensible phenomena.

Next, the inputs, both for government and the private sector or community, would need to be identified and priced. The pricing of community inputs raises difficult problems, but such problems need to be addressed because the alternative, i.e. not pricing them, is to value them implicitly at zero.

Attention then would need to turn to the nature of the data required about the services provided. The key requirement for useful data in mental health care is to address the problem that the phenomenon, mental illness or disability, is highly heterogeneous and that 'mental health care' is a very imprecise term. If an empirical exercise is going to succeed in analysing 'like' with 'like', then disaggregated data need to be collected. More precisely, if the services provided in a home are going to be compared successfully with those provided in an institution, then data about such service provision need to be standardised for disability level. To illustrate this point, consider a brief example from another context. Just as it would be quite preposterous, for example, for an agricultural economist to estimate a single production function for wheat, bananas and milk, likewise, in the context here, estimating a single production function for mental health care would be just as ridiculous. To repeat, mental health care is a heterogeneous phenomenon. It varies with the differing disability levels associated with the severity of various illnesses/disorders. Data that are disaggregated by disability level are required.

By empirically estimating the production functions associated with each level of severity of the illness/disability, it would then be possible to determine the degree of substitutability/complementarity between government and citizen inputs for each disability level. Knowing these phenomena is the essence of the evaluation of the impact of deinstitutionalisation.

Deinstitutionalisation is a movement that has had critical implications for peoples' lives. Another perspective is that 'deinstitutionalisation' is a piece of jargon that refers to a sector that changed its technology drastically without exploring the empirical relationships between the level of the output, and the quantity and availability of the inputs. The deinstitutionalisation movement assumed that it could abstract from two quite important factors. First, fundamental empirical relationships behind deinstitutionalisation were assumed away. Second, deinstitutionalisation abstracted from the severity of illness, treating mental health care as a homogeneous product. This it is not. It is a heterogeneous product. Data that are disaggregated by disability level and illness type would enable an understanding of the diverse impacts of deinstitutionalisation.

11 Summary and Future Research

Introduction

How is an industry best studied and understood, and improved in its performance?[1] Casual empiricism indicates that the issues pertinent to mental health care are seldom encountered in economic studies of other industries.[2] For example, defining the outputs of an industry, a critical issue for the economics of mental health care, is not a central concern in Industrial Economics. Likewise, issues of public finance and public production, central also in this study, are typically encountered only in passing in Industrial Economics, and usually just in regard to particular problems, such as research and development.

Mental health care is different. It challenges an economist. Clearly, the contribution of this study is not in any advancement of economic theory, *per se*. Rather, developments from elsewhere in the literature have been used to shed light on the one industry, mental health care. Applications of several theoretical developments are to be found: Hicksian consumer demand theory; Lancaster's characteristics theory; the household production theory of Becker and Grossman; the economic rationale for the role of government; the 'contracting out' which has arisen with deinstitutionalisation (involving conceptions about public finance and/or production from Public Economics); and the notion of social capital which is used in conjunction with Ostrom's (1996) co-production theory.

The summary below specifies the major contributions of this book.

Summary

The traditional concern of economics is with the material well-being of the population, and of sub-sets of the population. At its broadest level, this book

---

1 Readers with limited background in economics may need to note that an industry-wide approach, which implies the focus is wide and is directed **across** individuals and phenomena, is a **common**, and usually necessary, procedure in economics.

2 The 'casual empiricism' referred to here is scanning Industrial Economics texts to sample the sorts of topics addressed by that literature (as in the Contents Pages of such texts as, for example, Carlton and Perloff, 1994; Martin, 1993; Clarke, 1985).

addresses some important issues affecting the standard of living of a sub-set of the population, people with mental illness. It also has implications for the standard of living of the care-givers.

The book commences with a discussion of some broad issues about mental illnesses, before turning to a review of the notion of the standard of living. Various definitions are considered, although providing the 'right' definition of the standard of living is not the purpose of Chapter 1. Rather, particular **relationships** underlying the notion of the standard of living are noted. These relationships are ones that exist between goods and services (which are the 'means' to a standard of living) and utility (or well-being) itself, thus leaving aside matters of definition of utility and well-being initially. Several points about these relationships are made. It is likely that intermediate links or connections exist between goods and utility. These links are not simple, but an understanding of such links is helpful when people with disabilities, in this case, psychiatric disabilities, are being considered. An approach to the relationships between goods and utility, that of Sen (1985, 1987b), is discussed. According to Sen, at least two intermediate links, 'functionings' and 'capabilities', appear to exist between goods (and services) and the utility derived from a set of goods (and services). The links between goods and utility for people with disabilities may not be as straightforward as they are for people without disabilities, and possibly even less straightforward for the sub-set of people with disabilities associated with mental illnesses. Having introduced the importance of the links between goods and utility, this book then addresses a far more precise matter affecting living standards, *viz.* the economic dimensions of the outputs of mental health care.

The next issue is the adequacy of the conventional framework for conceiving of economic welfare. The traditional framework used here is that of Welfare Economics, and Chapters 2 and 3 together form the next areas of contribution.

In Chapter 2, various issues of economic method associated with Welfare Economics are discussed. These issues include the rationality assumption, the distinction between positive and normative science, the individualistic framework of economics and the problem of 'consumer ignorance' in mental health care. The role of social investment appraisal is also discussed. Across all these issues, a particular contribution is the consideration given to the relevance of the rationality assumption: this book presents a study about a group of people traditionally ignored by economics because of their 'irrationality'.

After a brief overview in Chapter 2 of the rationality assumption in economics generally, the particular focus turns to considering the point at which this assumption is pertinent to economic studies of mental health care. A range of observations provided in Chapter 2 illustrates the significance of having an understanding of the multi-dimensionality of rationality. Sometimes highly distressed individuals choose rationally to admit themselves to hospital. This is because they can see that they would be better if they could have the care and treatment provided in hospital. In other instances, where a person's level of (clinical) irrationality slips below the societal threshold, standards of health or standards of behaviour are imposed upon such individuals. Another instance is considered. Some people with mental illnesses choose *not* to use mental health services. Sometimes this is partly due to the stigma of the illness, but it can also arise because people have worked out that ineffective mental health services provide them little utility. This is, of course, no different from people's economic behaviour with any other good or service in the economy, say, when consumers will not buy mouldy bread. Finally, the observation is made that people with mental illnesses live with a disability, just as is the case of people with physical disabilities or developmental disabilities.

Another contribution of Chapter 2 is the discussion of the complicated nature of mental illness and its treatment. A schematic approach to dealing with the complexities of the phenomena under study is suggested. The presence of heterogeneity is often hidden by such an all-embracing term as 'mental health care'. An approach that classifies important distinctions is useful. For example, there are wide variations in the severity of each type of illness/condition, i.e. the severity of each illness can be classified. The outputs of the mental health sector can also be classified functionally, that is, according to whether they are, say, 'diagnostic', 'treatment' or 'care' services. Given the existence of distinctions like these, then simple but useful cross-tabulations, such as those given in Table 2.1, are possible.

In Chapter 3, the conventional theorems of Welfare Economics are presented, and there is discussion of some of the factors thought to inhibit the attainment of Pareto optimality in mental health care. These factors include:

- the presence of uncertainty with respect to consumer preferences
- the difficulties associated with the existence of socially unacceptable preferences
- the occurrence of chronic illness which has effects upon both the demand for, and supply of, suitable services
- income as a factor in the demand for services provided by the mental health sector (which is not, of itself, a market failure)
- the presence of multilateral transactions which may complicate service provision
- the existence of under-consumption of both consumer aids and the services of aides in mental health care
- externalities in mental health care
- the complicated nature of the multi-product firm and service-provider, making regulation difficult
- missing information about the production function for mental health status.

The literature surveyed in Chapter 4 considers the range of contributions advancing the field of economics and mental health care. The survey reveals a new and growing, mainly North American, literature characterised by important cost studies and demand studies. Having surveyed these advances, Chapter 4 indicates fundamental conceptual issues that have not yet been addressed relating to the outputs of the mental health care sector.

Chapters 5, 6 and 7 together elaborate a conceptual framework for the economic analysis of the services provided by the mental health care sector, services which are both multiple and multi-dimensional. Also, a way forward is provided for empirical applications, a matter discussed further in a Sub-section of 'Future Research' below.

These Chapters present a key contribution in this book. The perspective on the outputs given here is new, in the sense of the applications here to mental health. Services are conceptualised as multi-dimensional and, in multi-dimensional space, preferences are expressed. Chapters 5 and 6 show that it is helpful to think of mental health care as entering a household production function as a commodity vector. Household production theory (Grossman 1972a, 1972b) is used in order to describe 'the outputs' of mental health care. The conceptual framework of the characteristics theory of consumer demand, associated with Lancaster (1966b, 1971) and Ironmonger (1972), is also employed, enabling the outputs of mental health care to be understood in terms of characteristics. Two characteristics, symptom alleviation and disability reduction, are used, by way of illustration. The use of indifference curves enables an explanation of the relationship between mental health care inputs and the outputs of the mental health care sector. The analysis then presents a theoretical problem: whether, or how, individual preferences can count with respect to mental health services. The indifference map is used to explain what it means in an economic sense where society 'draws the line' with individuals so that, with or without committal, some individuals are institutionalised. This explanation then enables an economic understanding of the deinstitutionalisation movement, *viz.* to conceive of it as a different 'drawing of the line', as shown in Chapter 6, i.e. a shift to the south-east of what is defined in that Chapter as the 'imposed indifference curve'.

Another contribution of this book is contained in Chapter 7. The characteristics theory of consumer demand is employed again, more broadly, to indicate that at least five characteristics exist in mental health care: treatment, accommodation, medical/nursing care, personal/familial support, and deprivation of liberty. In view of the relatively significant role of government in the financing and production of mental health care, some aspects of government involvement in the (joint) production of these characteristics are explained in Chapter 7. It is shown that the 'externality argument' clarifies the normative role of government better than does the 'public good argument'.

Some important distinctions are also drawn in Chapter 7 with respect to the role of government. Most individuals with mental disorders still have preferences, but often are unable to express them in the market places of life. This may arise because of an impaired preference capacity due to the nature of the illness, or because of (assumed) consumer ignorance, or because of the individual's wish for institutional care because it provides a time of sanctuary from the stress of making choices. On the other hand, socially unacceptable preferences have different implications for the role of government. If externality arguments are applied to explain market failure, then it is possible to know more clearly what it means, in an economic sense, when 'society' imposes preferences on individuals with mental disorders. Such imposed preferences may involve particular social or legal norms. They may also involve the preferences of specific interest groups, such as the medical profession or some other particularly powerful group.

The function of medical practitioners in acting as 'gatekeepers' to care is shown to have a specific economic role. It would appear to be an undesirable state of affairs that few medical practitioners are likely to be fully aware of the meaning of the economic role they perform; but this study does not investigate that possibility.

The final contribution is found in an approach, formalised in Chapter 10, to the evaluation of the current era of deinstitutionalisation and community-based care. The issue is introduced first in Chapter 8 with some descriptive and conceptual information about care being undertaken in households. Implicit in that Chapter are two simple economic observations about community-based care: first, the outputs of mental health care are derived from multiple inputs, flowing from both government and 'the community'; second, in an era of deinstitutionalisation, the implied objective of a policy of deinstitutionalisation is to secure a change in the input proportions between government and the community. Chapter 9 provides a theoretical foundation for the presence of inputs that flow from the community. This is achieved with the exposition in that Chapter of recent theories of social capital.

It is from these vantage points, given in the previous Chapters, that Chapter 10 reconsiders the jointness of inputs from government and the community. The Chapter approaches the issue through Ostrom's (1996) conceptual framework of co-production, and also via the 'synergy hypothesis'. The general theory of co-production (given in Chapter 10) represents inputs from government and inputs from citizens as the relevant dimensions of (co-production in) a production function framework. This approach enables an examination of the relationship between social capital and government, and it reveals a way of addressing a more specific question. A key question for the deinstitutionalisation issue is this: Is social capital from a government source a substitute for, or a complement to, social capital from non-government, or community, sources? Although the answer to that question is empirical, the conceptual foundation provided in that Chapter suggests a useful research agenda.

Essentially, the contributions of this book are in two areas. It contributes analysis and clarification of economic behaviour arising when mental illnesses and disorders are present. Also, it provides an approach to the policy debate over the increased policy emphasis on non-institutional or community-based care, that has come to the fore in this current era of deinstitutionalisation. Attention turns now to some areas in which future research can be directed.

Future Research

One of the predominant features of mental health care, from an economic perspective, is that it provides services. This study is concerned with several economic issues surrounding a service industry, but it does so at a time when service provision is currently not a central issue in Industrial Economics. Moreover, while 'the outputs' is an issue more or less taken for granted in Industrial Economics, mental health care is different: although it is a long-standing industry, its economic dimensions are difficult to conceptualise. This is paradoxical because 'mental health care' in everyday usage is like so many things: you seem to know it when you see it.

In this Section, four areas of useful future research that arise from this study are indicated: Baumol's cost disease and mental care health care; hedonic prices and heterogeneous services; the role of relative prices; and uncertainty and information in mental health care.

It is enlightening to turn our focus on the first Sub-Section to some of the non-traditional issues that confront economic analysis of other industries, in particular, the performing arts industry, which is another difficult industry (Throsby and Withers, 1979; Towse, 1997). For example, in both the performing arts industry and mental health care, a mix of funding exists from private industry; from foundations and other citizen sources; and from the public sector. Provision of capital infrastructure, which must be addressed in order for service provision to occur, is another significant characteristic in both industries. In the performing arts, for instance, the capital requirements often are major, involving the provision of theatres and concert halls. For mental health care, too, capital requirements involve complex issues of providing accommodation, for example, at times care has to be in institutional accommodation; at other times, care and accommodation in a non-institutional setting involve quite different capital requirements, not simply physical capital but also social capital.

In the next Sub-Section, a feature that predominates in mental health care and the performing arts will be examined.

Baumol's 'Cost Disease' and Mental Health Care

Early analysis In 1966, William Baumol, with William Bowen, published *Performing Arts – The Economic Dilemma* and provided an analysis of the rising real costs that are found in particular types of economic activities (Baumol and Bowen, 1966). This characteristic affecting the cost structure of such activities, first noted in regard to the performing arts, has subsequently been referred to as a 'cost disease', and 'Baumol's disease'. The cost disease occurs in industries to the degree that outputs are characterised by slow productivity growth relative to more progressive (mostly manufacturing) industries. Persistently rising average real production costs and rising prices result in the former group of industries.

The economic activities beset by the cost disease are the service industries (Baumol and Oates, 1972) and, thus, to the degree that mental health care involves personal services, then the cost structure of the mental health industry is subject to the cost disease. Of course, personal services characterise a diverse range of activities, for example, large parts of general health care, as well as the live performing arts, education, hairdressing, the hospitality sector, libraries, care for aged, disabled and indigent people, garbage collection, some postal services, police services, particular leisure services, motor vehicle repairs and so forth. Across the services sector, the 'human element' or 'the human touch' is crucial. Labour is the major input and labour services are the end product, and inputs of time are involved in fixed proportions with inputs of labour.[3] These attributes are present because of the essential feature of services which is that it is the producer's intervention, itself, which transforms a user's satisfaction, a point made by Hill (1977).

The general case It is important to note that, in spite of the initial focus on the performing arts, the cost disease is not confined to the live performing arts. In 1966, Baumol and Bowen argued the general case as follows. Their hypothesis is that some industries in the service sector cannot offset increasing costs of service provision, particularly labour costs in labour-intensive services, against gains from productivity improvements. By contrast, gains from both economies of scale and technological change accrue to the manufacturing sector. The industries that enjoy cumulative increases in productivity per hour can be grouped as the technologically 'progressive' sector, as opposed to the technologically 'non-progressive' or 'stagnant' sector. In the non-progressive sector, productivity gains from the substitution of capital for labour are relatively difficult to achieve. Also, productivity gains simply do not occur in the performing arts when Shakespearean performers gabble their lines. Likewise, concert revenues would plummet if the Woodwind section of an orchestra were laid off for a concert series in order to cut costs, and live performances involved the rest of the orchestra performing around a compact disc recording of the Woodwind parts. Baumol's (1987) illustration provides this perspective:

3 Becker (1965) makes these points also, in a somewhat different context.

> An illustration comparing the costs of watchmaking and of musical performance over the centuries shows the reason. There has been vast and continuing technical progress in watchmaking, but live performance benefits from no labour-saving innovations – it is still done in the old-fashioned way. Toward the end of the 17th century a Swiss craftsman could produce 12 watches per year. Three centuries later that same amount of labour produces over 1200 (non-quartz) watches. But a piece of music written three centuries ago by Purcell or Scarlatti takes exactly as many person hours to perform today as it did in 1685 and uses as much equipment (Baumol, 1987, p. 842).

The cost disease argument also implies a second hypothesis, as follows. Productivity gains occur in the technologically progressive sector and are matched by increases in the hourly wage rate. Real cost increases in industries in the non-progressive sector will result to the degree that wage rises are transferred, through time, across the economy. Baumol has also considered a third dimension of the cost disease, namely, its relevance to public services. He defines the urban crisis in the context of inescapable cost pressures faced by the **public sector** (Baumol, 1967). Baumol points out that no single economic influence can account for complex phenomena, and that non-economic influences (particularly sociological and political factors) are also likely factors in the cost pressures faced by government. However, his hypothesis is that, to the degree that low productivity growth characterises most personal services, and in so far as municipal governments provide or finance a range of services, then the cost disease is a key explanation for the persistent cost increases faced universally by government services. For another account of the cost disease in the public sector, see Brown and Jackson (1982, p. 113*ff.*).

It seems the 'stagnant' industries have escaped constant, major productivity growth for two reasons. As Baumol puts it, some service industries are 'inherently resistant to standardization [and] ... [a] second reason why it has been difficult to reduce the labour content of these services is the fact that in many of them the quality is, or is at least believed to be, inescapably correlated with the amount of labour expended on their production' (Baumol, 1996, p. 194).

Empirical evidence Empirical evidence from several sources, for example, in Baumol (1993, 1996) and Towse (1997), supports the case for the cost disease in the performing arts, as well as in other sectors, particularly health and education. The evidence indicates both the persistent and universal nature of the cost disease: persistent over the four decades in which it has been studied, after adjustments for inflation; universal in the range of countries and from across a spectrum of activities involving public/private funding and production; and present in varying approaches to output and productivity measurement. The importance of other factors that might instead explain rising real costs is also considered by Baumol, factors such as litigation in health care, lack of competitiveness, unscrupulous practices and so forth, but Baumol's argument is that none of these outweighs the overwhelming contribution of the cost disease.

In spite of strong *a priori* reasoning about the phenomenon, some authors, Tiongson (1997) for example, rightly argue that the empirical evidence for the cost disease remains inconclusive. Felton (1994), on the one hand, shows across a sample of 25 US orchestras over a 21-year period that the cost disease is present where productivity lags. On the other hand, Felton's study also reveals the productivity growth of orchestras in the sample, at a growth rate that outstripped the manufacturing sector. In a study of US government services over the period 1959-89, Ferris and West (1996) conclude that changes in real wages across sectors account for approximately one-third of the rise in the real cost of these government services, while slower productivity growth accounts for the remaining two-thirds.

It should be noted that statements about inconclusive evidence for the cost disease must be considered in the light of the conceptual and measurement problems that are present in the economics of services, rather than with concern that the phenomenon itself is unfounded. According to Tiongson (1997), the measurement of the cost disease in the performing arts presents difficulties that are largely of a conceptual or empirical nature regarding the outputs of services. For example, Tiongson argues that, to the extent that the performing arts are of a public good nature (and are thereby characterised by non-rivalry in consumption), then comparisons of the outputs and costs with those in the manufacture of private goods is not entirely satisfactory. Costs, revenues, inputs and outputs for services that are a public good nature require even more careful definition than these economic entities do for private goods. See also Ferris and West's (1996) argument that cost disease estimation, for government services, also requires an estimation of the deadweight loss associated with the taxation needed for the public funding of such services. Their study finds, as expected, rising deadweight loss. This means that the marginal welfare cost of these services is likely to rise over time; and the real cost increases of government-provided education and health services are only exacerbated.

Tiongson (1997) considers other particular measurement and conceptual difficulties in regard to the technology and diversification that have enabled productivity gains in service industries, and Cowan (1996) supports this in the following way. He argues that the empirical evidence for the cost disease is not yet clear because productivity measures are inaccurate, largely due to increases that have occurred in supposed 'stagnant' industries in both product quality and diversity of product range. To the extent that technological change has occurred, then '[w]hen the product is changing, cost-based productivity measurements are comparing apples and oranges' (Cowan, 1996, p. 211).

It has also been said of the cost disease phenomenon that Baumol overstates technological non-progressiveness in service industries. For example, in regard to the performing arts, Cowan (1996) points out that several innovations, of both the process type, such as the quality of reproduction enabled by compact disc technology, and the product type, such as expanding repertoire over time, have enhanced the productivity of that industry. See Blaug (1963) for a survey of process innovations. Cowan argues that, for cost disease to be present, the essential attribute of a service is that of a 'given, repetitive task performed with a fixed technology and with little prospect of future improvement' (Cowan, 1996, p. 211) such as men's hair cuts. While the case of the barber may well be quintessentially true, Baumol's position is that there is a matter of degree here. In regard to the issue of technological change, it is important to recall Baumol's (1987) examination of whether improved technology, for example in broadcasting, will necessarily alleviate the cost disease for the live performing arts:

> The explanation apparently lies in the structure of mass media production, which is made up of two basic components that are very different technologically. The first comprises preparation of material and the actual performance in front of cameras, while the second is transmission and filming.
>
> Television broadcasting of new material requires these two elements in relatively fixed physical proportions – one hour of programming (with some flexibility in rehearsal time) must be accompanied by one hour of transmission for every hour of broadcast. However, since the first component of television is virtually identical with live performance on a theatre stage, there is just as little scope for technical change in the one as in the other, while the second component, on the other hand, is electronic and 'high tech' in character and constantly benefits from innovation.
>
> Industries with this cost structure have been referred to as 'asymptotically stagnant'. ... If each year transmission costs decrease and programming expenses increase because of the cost disease that besets all live performance, eventually programming cost must begin to dominate the overall budget. Thereafter, total cost and programming cost must move closer and closer together until virtually the entire budget becomes a victim of the disease, with the stable technological costs too small a fragment of the whole to make a discernible difference (Baumol, 1987, p. 842).

The crucial point contained in the above quotation is that it is the **relative shares** of the progressive and stagnant components within an industry that require careful time series data collection. According to Baumol, the problem remains that 'the progressive component has a continually shrinking share of total costs, while the stagnant component has increased in real terms and as a share of total costs' (Baumol, 1996, p. 199).

Implications for public policy Before turning our attention to the cost disease in mental health care, let us address some general issues that the cost disease presents for public policy. Fiscal problems pervade government services, and it is well-established that the fiscal problems of health care and education in industrialised countries are multidimensional (Aaron, 1991; Weisbrod, 1991).

Baumol's argument is that the cost disease dominates a number of government functions. To the extent that this is so, some readers may now be concluding that the future for government services is exceedingly dismal. Baumol (1996) provides two reasons that a grim future is not at all inevitable. First, even the small productivity growth rates in stagnant services contribute to alleviating the cost disease. Second, productivity growth in the entire economy makes it possible for the relatively more expensive personal services to be affordable, on average. There are, however, several other factors which Baumol indicates need consideration, as those two factors just given indicate a rather simplistic scenario. First, there is the difficulty of financing the purchases by low-income groups of education and health services at ever-increasing prices. Second, Baumol recognises that it is unlikely the general public will understand easily that the rising prices of service industries are an illusion and that, really, the relative prices of those services are gradually declining. Third, the implication of the cost disease is that, in the absence of privatisation, the public sector share of GDP must increase. Even if such an increase were to occur, the consequences for economic efficiency and bureaucratic control of such an enormous increase in the public sector share are worrying. Fourth, Baumol points out that the popular approach to facing problems of such daunting proportions is to privatise government services. According to Baumol, privatisation is no panacea for the cost disease:

> The public's opposition to any threat to the survival of the public school system can hardly be dismissed as groundless, and similar remarks apply to a number of other services, such as police protection, currently supplied by government. In addition, any industry beset by the cost disease that is in private hands is sure to be suspected of greed and malfeasance. It is hard to believe that the calls for price controls to limit their cumulatively rising prices will not become irresistible politically. But if the rising costs are caused by unavoidably slow growth in productivity, price controls can confidently be expected to lead to deterioration in the quality of those services or to their partial or total disappearance (Baumol, 1996, p. 204).

See Ferris and West (1996, p. 48*ff*) for an opposing argument concerning the cost disease in education, namely, that privatisation is likely to bring significant changes to the structure of supply and thereby result in 'genuine' reductions in real costs.

The cost disease in service industries It is useful to provide a context for the above discussion and ask why the cost disease is applicable to the services sector. What unique elements in service industries create this problem? It should be noted that these industries have two characteristics that are not shared with the industries traditionally studied in Industrial Economics. These latter industries produce essentially standardised, mass-producible goods, such as cans of Coca-Cola. Such industries are characterised by a separation in time and place between consumption by consumers of the product and the production of the commodities by producers. Put otherwise, these goods share the characteristics of storability and portability. Service industries, on the other hand, cannot store their outputs in inventories, nor are they subject to gains from inter-regional trade, e.g. via transport services. Hence, service industries are unique in that they typically involve 'one-off' and localised production.

Implications for mental health services Our focus turns now to issues of the cost disease in mental health care, commencing with an illustration. It is helpful to ponder something about human behaviour: some of the things we own we throw out when they break down, and other things, we repair. It is undeniable that consumers do undertake repairs of some things, in the face of escalating repair prices. In the literature, discussions about the economic aspects of 'human repair' and 'car repair' are found in Baumol (1993) and Triplett (1999). Consider Baumol's (1993) account of the human element in repair services: 'Before one can undertake to cure a patient or repair a broken piece of machinery it is necessary to determine, case by case, just what is wrong, and then the treatment must be tailored to the individual case. The manufacture of thousands of identical automobiles can be carried out on an assembly line and much of the work done by industrial robots, but the repair of a car just hauled to a garage from the site of an accident cannot be entrusted to automated processes' (Baumol, 1993, p. 20). Some things, once broken, are thrown out. Other things undergo repair. What is the basis of the consumer's distinction? It is, of course, that the human being and a car share a common quality: each represents a significant capital investment, one being of the human capital kind, the other being of the physical capital kind. In spite of rising prices for the repair both of human beings and motor vehicles, outlays for repairs are small in comparison to the outlay required if replacement were undertaken (an uncomfortable, though not totally 'unheard of', thought in respect of human beings). The implication is that rising prices from the cost disease in some repair services are inescapable.

Consider productivity issues in mental health care. It can be argued that productivity gains have sometimes occurred in recent decades, due to improved medications, therapies, medical records management, evidence-based mental health care and data management systems, but the gain overall for mental health care is still very limited. This is predominantly because of the limits that exist in treatment. Limits exist, for example, as to how many patients a psychiatrist can treat properly per unit of time. Also, an effective therapy like Cognitive Behaviour Therapy (CBT) is undertaken over several sessions and it occurs (typically) on a one-on-one basis between patient and therapist. While additional input units of CBT can occur productively in a group, limits exist still as to the numbers in such a group. In other areas of mental health care, limits exist, for example, in regard to how many home visits a psychiatric nurse can make per morning or how much Home Help can be achieved in a day, and so on. People with mental illnesses, by the nature of their illnesses, require large inputs of personal service and human attention.

Empirical investigation of the cost disease in mental health care is a pressing need. Given that the cost disease explains increasing prices in the performing arts, in education and probably in haircuts too, it is likely to be present in mental health care.[4] Empirical work will not be easy. Few prices exist in mental health care because this is a sector that provides services with high degrees of public funding. Not unsurprisingly, we are unaware of any studies of the cost disease in mental health care, and it is worth noting that empirical investigation of the cost disease in this industry, while extremely important, is bound to be fraught with conceptual and estimation difficulties.

Lastly, there is a point to make about the role of public policy. Should it be found that public expenditure on mental health care persistently rises due to increasing labour costs in the presence of stagnant technological progress in these services, then an economic explanation of deinstitutionalisation is possible. The phenomenon of deinstitutionalisation may be understood best in terms of government shifting to the voluntary sector the burden of the cost disease arising with treating and caring for highly vulnerable people. Put bluntly, it has been politically feasible, indeed shockingly easy, over recent decades for government to shift its responsibility to pay for mental health care. Government achieved this action during a time when a relatively minor technological improvement, namely, some isolated advances in medications, generated just enough fog so as to cloud some crucial underlying economic forces.

Towards Application: Hedonic Prices and Heterogeneous Mental Health Services

The analysis of Chapters 5, 6 and 7 on the outputs of mental health care was theoretical and conceptual in nature, and little attention was directed to empirical or estimation issues. It is useful here to discuss how one could apply the concepts in these Chapters and 'push forward toward the concrete', to use an expression by Pigou (1929, p. 78).

An approach to empirical work on goods or services that have multiple attributes or characteristics, or heterogeneous goods or services, like mental health care, involves the calculation, and subsequent application, of hedonic prices. A concise definition of hedonic prices is as follows: '... the implicit prices of attributes [which] are revealed to economic agents from observed prices of differentiated products and the specific amounts of characteristics

---

[4] It is conceivable that the cost disease may exist in conjunction with falling prices for some inputs. Recent empirical work on price indexes for the treatment of depression (Frank, Busch and Berndt, 1998; Frank, Berndt and Busch, 1999; Berndt, Bir, Busch *et al.*, 2000) and on estimating real expenditures for mental illness (Triplett, 1999a; Triplett, 1999b) are relevant in this context.

associated with them' (Rosen, 1974, p. 34). For an overview, see Triplett (1987) and Streeting (1990), and for a comparison with survey techniques, Brookside *et al.* (1982).[5]

Essentially, hedonic pricing involves the application of statistical or econometric techniques to isolate the values that contribute to observed differences in product prices. The first step in applying the technique involves the estimation of the implicit price function. This function is based on the conception provided in Chapters 5 and 6 that a good or service is composed of a bundle of characteristics, and that the relative amounts of the characteristics embedded in the good or service contribute to the prices of particular varieties of the good or service. An undefined implicit price function is as follows:

$$P_i = f(c_1, c_2, \dots, c_n) \tag{11.1}$$

where P_i is the price of the *i* th good or service, and c_j is the *j* th embodied characteristic.

Econometrically, the process can be represented as follows, assuming an additive linear functional form:

$$P_i = \beta_0 + \beta_1 c_1 + \beta_2 c_2 + \beta_3 c_3 + \dots + \beta_n c_n \tag{11.2}$$

where β_j is the *j* th coefficient to be estimated, and P_i and c_j are as defined above.

This technique has been applied, *inter alia,* in labour markets to worker characteristics (Stewart and Jones, 1998), and goods markets such as live cattle (Williams, 1993), breakfast cereals (Stanley and Tschirhart, 1991), wine (Golan and Shalit, 1993), housing (Marks, 1984; and Benjamin and Lusht, 1993), environmental variables such as air pollution (Harrison and Rubinfeld, 1978; Blomquist and Worley, 1981; and Maani and Kask, 1991), environmental quality (Palmquist, 1991; Braden and Kolstad, 1991) and noise (Nelson, 1980, 1982), and other phenomena such as ethnic composition (Schnare, 1976). More recently, the technique has been applied to university courses (Gokcekus, 2000) and child care services (Hagy, 1998).

The above indicates a major concern of hedonic price analysis, i.e. the determination of the implicit prices of characteristics of goods or services. However, since Rosen (1974), a separate, and large, literature now exists which uses hedonic prices to estimate willingness-to-pay or, more generally, demand for characteristics, such as the quality of air. Additional steps are necessary to undertake such analysis.

---

5 Although the work by Griliches (1971) and Rosen (1974) are often considered to be the pioneering studies in this *genre*, there is reason to believe that the origins of the technique lie in a 1939 paper by Court on automobiles. See Goodman (1998). For a different view on the historical origins, see Berndt (1991), who emphasises an earlier (1928) analysis of vegetables (asparagus, tomatoes etc) in Boston.

First, the hedonic price function, equation (11.1), is estimated. Second, computation of each consumer's willingness-to-pay for a **marginal** change in the relevant characteristic is determined. In equilibrium, this is equal to the increased cost (say) incurred by purchasing or renting a different house with identical characteristics except for a marginal increase in the quality of air. This second step involves the calculation of the derivative of the hedonic price equation, as in equation (11.2). A third step, if there are 'lumpy', or non-marginal, changes to the characteristic, involves estimating a marginal willingness-to-pay **function**, a function that is analogous to a demand curve for the characteristic. This step involves regressing individuals' marginal valuations on the quantity of the characteristic and other variables (income, age, gender, etc.) that can be regarded as demand-shifters. To illustrate, Harrison and Rubinfeld (1978) calculated the own-price and income elasticities for clean air to be –1.2 and 1.2, respectively. A fourth step in the valuation process is to use the willingness-to-pay **function**, along with quantities of the characteristic (before and after a change), to calculate the benefits (where the term has its conventional economic meaning) of an economic change.

Needless to say, there are numerous theoretical and empirical problems associated with such work (Williams, 1993; Streeting, 1990). Some of the problems faced in the existing literature may pale into insignificance when compared with the challenges of applying this framework in the 'messy' context of the provision of mental health services. However, it should be recalled that Berndt, Bir, Busch *et al.*(2000) have calculated hedonic regression equations for price indices for the treatment of depression. Thus, this technique already exists in the economic literature on mental health.

A 'Big Question': The Role of Relative Prices [6]

A dilemma needs to be faced in regards to two issues discussed previously, *viz.*, the inexorable workings of the cost disease and an issue discussed in Chapter 5, the role of prices of pharmaceuticals. The previous sentence points to another underlying economic issue too. This is the relative price of labour (such as that of psychiatrists, clinical psychologists, social workers and psychiatric nurses) *vis-á-vis* the relative prices of pharmaceuticals for mental illness. It is clear that in the recent US health economics literature, some attention has been focussed on temporal price movements of pharmaceuticals. Relatively little attention has been devoted to the temporal prices of labour-intensive medical services which typically characterise mental health services. The major public policy issue that must be faced is the optimal combination of labour-intensive therapy and domestic support and low-priced pharmaceuticals. See Berndt, Cockburn and Griliches (1997, p. 136) for a brief discussion of

---

6 With apologies to Brinton (1950).

this larger context and Berndt, Frank and McGuire (1997) for some empirical evidence. The latter study shows that there was no support for the 'extreme patterns of substitution under managed care' that have been argued on the basis of anecdotal evidence. However, there was some evidence to indicate that consumers, subject to depression, would receive more antidepressant medication under Preferred Provider Organisations and 'carve-out' programs, than do consumers covered by indemnity plans. Clearly more research needs to be undertaken, taking account of different institutional arrangements.

This issue, about new anti-depressant medications being employed either with more, or with less, 'talk therapy', is a particular case of a more general issue, i.e. how societies react to, or use, new products or innovations. Clearly, these new pharmaceuticals could be employed as substitutes for existing treatments and therapies. Alternatively, they could be used as complements to those existing treatments and therapies. Institutional factors (e.g. government regulations and/or government subsidies, directives issued by managed care organisations, and so forth), and the underlying relative market prices, as well as the relative efficacy of the innovation compared to that of the existing treatments, are some of the important determinants of the outcome. For empirical studies of issues such as these in regard to innovations, see Levy and Pitcsh (1985) on the innovation of the video-cassette recorder (VCR) and Doessel (1992) for a study of fibre-optic endoscopy.

Uncertainty and Information in Mental Health Care

The economics of uncertainty and information is a vast area of study that is relevant in many industries, not just mental health care. Since a key focus of this study has been on the outputs, then it is useful here to address some uncertainty and information issues surrounding the outputs of mental health care.

Let us initially contrast the information issues of the outputs of another non-traditional industry, the performing arts. The issues there are different and less difficult. In the performing arts industry, consumers are relatively well-informed about the outputs, say, of theatre or a concert. First, it is possible to be well-acquainted with the theatrical script or the musical score prior to attending a performance. This is not the case in mental health care. Second, advertising about concerts and theatre informs audiences very well about what is available, when, where, the price and the marginal choices with which consumers concern themselves. Again, this is not so in mental health care. Third, information about performances in the performing arts is publicly available through critics' reviews found in the media. In mental health care, information about the personal efficacy of treatment is hard to find because treatment takes place behind a veil of confidentiality.

Since Arrow (1993a), economists have been keenly aware that various dimensions of uncertainty and/or lack of information characterise the health sector. For example, the information asymmetry between medical practitioners and consumers/patients is the keystone of the supplier-induced demand hypothesis, as formulated by Evans (1974). Although principal-agent problems are not unique to health, they are by no means trivial issues in various segments of the health sector. In fact, the literature on alternative theories of firm behaviour can be understood as descriptions of the principal-agent problem.[7] Needless to say, these general issues arise also in the theory of hospital behaviour, e.g. Newhouse (1970), Pauly and Redisch (1973) and Harris (1977). However, the issue to which attention is now directed is not associated with the principal-agent problem, but uncertainty associated with 'gaps' in medical knowledge.

Glover (1938) was first to observe that there were large geographical variations in rates for medical procedures: his interest was in the variations for tonsillectomy for school children in England and Wales. Since then, this 'infant industry' has developed and matured: there is now a huge literature on the problem, generally referred to as the small area variation (SAV) phenomenon, which has been documented for various regional aggregations, different countries, different time periods, etc. See Folland and Stano (1990) for a comprehensive review of this disparate literature.

The SAV literature is dominated by the work of epidemiologists and sociologists. Generally, it could be argued that the literature is mostly concerned with definitions and measures of SAVs, as well as attempts to find explanations for the existence of the phenomenon. However, contributions by economists are relatively few. One strand of the economics literature asks the following question: what are the welfare losses that may arise from differences in per capita utilisation (not explained by other variables, e.g. disease prevalence, income, etc)? A number of studies (Phelps and Parente, 1990; Phelps and Mooney, 1992) have applied traditional concepts of consumer surplus to answer this question. See also Dranove (1995) and Phelps (1995).

A second economic approach is relevant in this context. Consider Arrow's discussion of product uncertainty. His first sentence notes that '[u]ncertainty as to the quality of the product is perhaps more intense here than in any other important commodity' (Arrow, 1963a, p. 951). See also Phelps (1992). This issue has been taken up in the SAV literature, where it has been documented that particular medical or surgical procedures exhibit greater variation in utilisation rates than do other procedures. Wennberg, Barnes and Zubkoff (1982) have argued that different utilisation rates **between** procedures may be related to the degree of 'uncertainty' that the medical practitioner faces, when confronted with a decision to apply, or not to apply, a particular procedure. Particular procedures (for hip fractures, heart attacks and strokes) have low

7 The alternative theories of firm behaviour include theories about sales maximisation (Baumol, 1958); managerial discretion (Williamson, 1963); growth of the firm (Marris, 1963); and the behavioural theories of the firm (Simon, 1957, and Cyert and March, 1963).

variations whereas others (for knee and lower back injuries) have very high variations (Wennberg, 1987). Similar results were obtained in three countries (the US, England and Norway) where rates for some procedures (e.g. appendectomy) were relatively uniform, whereas rates for other procedures (haemorrhoidectomy, hysterectomy and prostatectomy) were extremely variable (McPherson *et al.*, 1982).

Phelps (1992) has pointed to some common characteristics in the groupings of these procedures, but the interesting question is whether particular 'beliefs' may arise in some regions and not in others and, if so, why this is so. This leads to the (regional) 'practice style hypothesis', as described by Phelps:

> Thus, local schools can emerge and persist that hold different beliefs about the efficacy of an intervention, and these schools can in turn lead to different recommendations from doctors to their patients, and hence to different patterns of practice in the aggregate (Phelps, 1992, p. 31).

Folland and Stano (1989, p. 86) define 'practice style' as 'a set of beliefs about the efficacy and appropriateness of alternative forms of care'. More specifically, it is argued that this 'set of beliefs' relates to the production function between medical inputs and some appropriate measure of health status. It must be emphasised that this set of beliefs is just that: it involves beliefs (or intuitive judgements), and is not based on an **empirical** relationship. Put otherwise, it involves an **assumption of fact** about an empirical relationship, a relationship that is, in principle, capable of being determined, but has not yet been determined. This can be illustrated in Figure 11.1 depicting members of a 'family' of production functions relating medical care to health status.

The X-axis of Figure 11.1 measures a composite of various inputs of medical care, and the Y-axis indicates an appropriate measure of health status. SB_1 and SB_2 represent two hypothesised relationships, *ceteris paribus*, held by two medical practitioners, concerning the efficacy of medical care for a specified medical condition, e.g. 'essential benign hypertension' or 'uterine leiomyomia'. Notice that Figure 11.1 indicates that the two medical practitioners even disagree on the person's health outcome given the natural history of the disease/condition. Also, these medical practitioners disagree on both the marginal and total product of medical care. There may, of course, be cases, such as inguinal hernia, 'for which beliefs about the production function are not widely dispersed ... suggesting that for some ailments physician uncertainty is not an important factor' (Folland and Stano, 1989, p. 89). The situation depicted in Figure 11.1 would give rise to varying utilisation rates if medical practitioners, holding different sets of beliefs, such as SB_1 and SB_2, are not uniformly distributed across geographical areas.

In terms of empirical estimation, Folland and Stano's conception of 'practice style' is such that it (practice style) becomes yet another explanatory variable, *inter alia*, in a multiple regression framework to explain utilisation rates, and its relative importance can be established empirically. It is important to observe that their conception involves a completely different epistemological approach from that of Wennberg and his colleagues, for whom practice style is the *deus ex machina* that enables them to answer a question such as 'What explains the variations across space?' Folland and Stano (1989) make this point as follows:

> [T]he practice style **hypothesis** has entered the literature through this back door. The Wennberg argument ... is that variations in utilization are not adequately explained by other variables and so may be due to the physician's style of practice (Folland and Stano, 1989, p. 92) (emphasis added).

It is not particularly relevant to describe in detail the empirical estimation procedures adopted, nor the results of their analysis. We are unaware of comparative studies comparing this dimension of mental health services and other medical services: how mental health compares to other services (in terms of this dimension of uncertainty) is an empirical issue to be determined.

Figure 11.1 Hypothesised production functions for medical care and health status

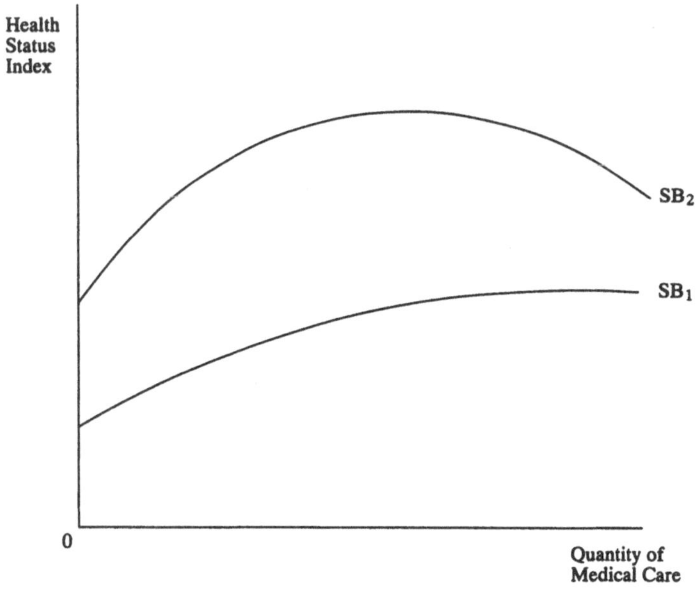

Source: Folland and Stano (1989).

In the above paragraphs, the question concerning health production functions, i.e. the empirical relationship between inputs (in the form of mental health services) and mental health outcome (in the form of mental health status) was raised. It is useful to note that there is now concern with health production functions in the health sector generally. Although this terminology (inputs, outputs etc.) is not employed by non-economists working in the health sector, there is an overlap between the economics literature and epidemiological/ sociological literatures on various issues of a health/medical kind. For example, the issues addressed in the health economics literature under the heading 'health production function' (Connelly and Doessel, 2000) are essentially the same as those addressed in the epidemiological and sociological literatures under the heading 'social determinants of health' (Wilkinson, 1996; and Marmot and Wilkinson, 1999). However, there is now a concordance between economic terminology and some recent health terminology, about to be discussed. The brief discussion following will show that most certainly it is no longer an 'unmentionable' to talk about empirical relationships between inputs and health outcomes.

Since the early arguments of Cochrane (1972), that many medical 'therapies', taught in medical schools and implemented by medical practitioners, have had no justification in terms of efficacy, the practice of 'evidence-based' medicine has arisen out of concern that a positive relationship between therapies (inputs) and outcomes (outputs) is achieved. Some of the characteristics of this 'movement' are captured in the following:

> Evidence-based medicine is the conscientious, explicit and judicious use of current best evidence in making decisions about care of individual patients. The practice of evidence-based medicine means integrating clinical expertise with the best available external evidence from systematic research (Sackett, Richardson, Rosenberg and Haynes, 1997, p. 2).

This concern is widespread (Lockett, 1997; and National Health and Medical Research Council, 2000) and arises in various aspects of medicine, e.g. primary care (Silagy and Haines, 1998) and the prevention of cardiovascular disease (Lawrence, 1996). Furthermore, a number of new journals have recently appeared, *viz. Clinical Evidence, Evidence Based Medicine, Evidence-based Nursing and Evidence-based Dentistry.* Yet further again, the Cochrane Collaboration (at McMaster University in Canada) and the National Health Service Centre for Reviews and Dissemination (at the University of York in England) are responsible for the Cochrane Library, which consists of four separate electronic databases.[8]

---

8 For *aficionados*, further information can be obtained, for example, at http://hiru.mcmaster.ca/cochrane/default.htm and http://www.york.ac.uk/inst/crd/ehrd.htm.

Like many treatments and technologies in general health care, reliable evidence on the effectiveness of treatments and other types of support/ interventions is lacking in mental health care. This *lacuna* can be explained by a range of factors, including econometrically challenging issues in regard to mental health production functions (e.g. Lu, 1999) as well as factors of a more philosophical nature (e.g. Mason, Eccles, *et al.*, 1999). What is without doubt, though, is that concern with evidence-based medicine in mental health care is growing. See Whiteford (1995). There is now a journal, *Evidence-Based Mental Health Care*. Also, Cochrane Reviews have been conducted for several aspects of mental health care inputs: treatment inputs such as medication and/or psychological therapy; and other input arrangements, like community mental health teams, case management and so forth.

In the US, the Agency for Healthcare Research and Quality (AHRQ) (formerly the Agency for Health Care Policy and Research), as part of the Department of Health and Human Services, functions as the research 'arm' for the private and public sectors to improve the quality and safety of health care. This Agency both undertakes and sponsors research that provides evidence-based information on key health care issues: outcomes, quality, cost, use and access. The information is directed to patients, medical practitioners, bureaucrats and policymakers to make more informed decisions about, and improve the quality of, health care. Through 12 Evidence-Based Practise (*sic*) Centers, evidence reports on treatments and technologies are developed. Mental health care is, thus, only a small fraction of the Agency's activities.

Many gaps exist in our knowledge, some of which relate to wide-reaching phenomena, such as the efficacy of institutionalised care compared to care outside of institutions. Such gaps in knowledge are a larger manifestation of finer gaps in knowledge. For example, the (now) AHRQ reports that it is not known if combinations of newer antidepressants (or new antidepressants plus another psychotropic, such as an anxiolytic) are more efficacious than a single antidepressant. Similarly, it is not known if combinations of newer antidepressants with 'talk therapy' is more or less efficacious than antidepressants alone (Agency for Health Care Policy and Research, 1999). One suspects that the knowledge gaps are larger in mental health care than they are in general health care.

Before closing, it is helpful to note two points about future research. The first point is to draw attention to three particular issues. Each in itself is important in its own right as a topic of further research. Those three dimensions of mental health care have been addressed in this Section and are as follows: labour intensity, price relativities of related goods (substitutes and complements) and uncertainty. The second point is a broader one. In undertaking any research, e.g. estimating demand equations on regional data, it is important that these three dimensions be incorporated in the analysis.

A Final Point

One of the roles of evidence-based medicine, discussed in the previous Subsection, is to identify gaps in our knowledge, and to proceed to fill them. Essentially, the purpose of this book is to expose the gaps in knowledge about various economic issues (both of an empirical and policy nature) in the provision of services of a mental health kind, and to provide the framework for filling some of those knowledge gaps.

References

Aaron, H.J. (1991), *Serious and Unstable Condition: Financing America's Health Care*, The Brookings Institution, Washington, DC.

Agency for Health Care Policy and Research (1999), 'Treatment of Depression – Newer Pharmacotherapies', Summary, Evidence Report/Technology Assessment, No. 7, March, Agency for Health Care Policy and Research, Rockville, MD, http://www.ahrq.gov/clinic/deprsumm.html.

Alter, C. and Hage, J. (1993), *Organisations Working Together*, Sage, Newbury Park.

American Psychiatric Association (1994), *Diagnostic and Statistical Manual of Mental Disorders*, 4th edn, American Psychiatric Association, Washington, DC.

Archibald, G.C. (1987), 'Theory of the Firm', in J. Eatwell, M. Milgate and P. Newman (eds)(1987), *The New Palgrave: A Dictionary of Economics*, Vol. 2, Macmillan, London, pp. 357-63.

Arden, R. (1979), 'A Second Look at Output Value Analysis: A Critique', *Administration in Mental Health*, Vol. 6, No. 3, Spring, pp. 251-64.

Arons, B. and Frank, R.G. (1993), 'Mental Health and Private Insurance Reform: How Broad Should the Benefit Be?', *Administration and Policy in Mental Health*, Vol. 20, No. 5, pp. 389-91.

Arrow, K.J. (1963a), 'Uncertainty and the Welfare Economics of Medical Care', *The American Economic Review*, Vol. 53, No. 5, December, pp. 941-73.

Arrow, K.J. (1963b), *Social Choice and Individual Values*, 2nd edn, John Wiley and Sons, New York.

Arrow, K.J. (1985), 'The Economics of Agency' in J.W. Pratt and R.W. Zeckhauser (eds)(1985), *Principals and Agents: The Structure of Business*, Harvard Business School Press, Boston, pp. 37-51.

Arrow, K.J. (1986), 'Economic Theory and the Hypothesis of Rationality', *Journal of Business*, Vol. 59, No. 4, Pt 2, in J. Eatwell, M. Milgate and P. Newman (eds)(1987), *The New Palgrave: A Dictionary of Economics*, Vol. 1, Macmillan, London, pp. 69-74.

Arrow, K.J., Chenery, H.B., Minhas, B.S. and Solow, R.M. (1961), 'Capital-Labor Substitution and Economic Efficiency', *The Review of Economics and Statistics*, Vol. XLIII, No. 3, pp. 225-50.

Auld, D.A.L. (1972), 'Imperfect Knowledge and the New Theory of Demand', *Journal of Political Economy*, Vol. 80, No.6, pp. 1287-94.

Auld, D.A.L. (1974), 'Advertising and the Theory of Consumer Choice', *Quarterly Journal of Economics*, Vol. 88, No. 3, pp. 480-87.

Auld, D.A.L. (1975), 'Advertising Strategy and the New Theory of Demand', *Southern Economic Journal*, Vol. 42, No. 2, pp. 225-30.

Auster, R.D., Leveson, I. and Saracheck, D. (1969), 'The Production of Health, an Exploratory Study', *Journal of Human Resources*, Vol. IV, No. 4, pp. 411-36.

Australian Bureau of Statistics (1998), *Mental Health and Wellbeing: Profile of Adults, Australia 1997*, ABS, Canberra, Cat. No. 4326.0.

Australian Bureau of Statistics (2000), *Unpaid Work and the Australian Economy 1997*, Occasional Paper, ABS, Canberra, Cat. No. 5240.0.

Bandelow, B. (1995), 'Assessing the Efficacy of Treatments for Panic Disorder and Agoraphobia. II. The Panic and Agoraphobia Scale', *International Clinical Psychopharmacology*, Vol. 10, No. 2, pp. 73-81.

Barham, P. (1992), *Closing the Asylum: the Mental Patient in Modern Society*, Penguin, Harmondsworth.

Barro, R.J. and Sala-I-Martin, X. (1995), *Economic Growth*, McGraw-Hill, New York.

Bates, E.M. (1979), 'Alternative Theories of Madness', in E.M. Bates and P.R. Wilson (eds)(1979), *Mental Disorder or Madness? Alternative Theories*, University of Queensland Press, Brisbane, pp. 20-32.

Bator, F. (1958), 'The Anatomy of Market Failure', *Quarterly Journal of Economics*, Vol. LXXII, No. 3, August, pp. 351-79.

Baumol, W.J. (1958), 'On the Theory of Oligopoly', *Economica*, n.s., Vol. 25, No. 99, pp. 187-98.

Baumol, W.J. (1967), 'Macroeconomics of Unbalanced Growth: The Anatomy of Urban Crisis', *The American Economic Review*, Vol. LVII, No. 3, June, pp. 415-26.

Baumol, W.J. (1987), 'Performing Arts', in J. Eatwell, M. Milgate and P. Newman (eds)(1987), *The New Palgrave: A Dictionary of Economics*, Vol. 3, Macmillan, London, pp. 841-43.

Baumol, W.J. (1993), 'Health Care, Education and the Cost Disease: A Looming Crisis for Public Choice', *Public Choice*, Vol. 77, No. 1, pp. 17-28.

Baumol, W.J. (1996) 'Children of Performing Arts, The Economic Dilemma', *Journal of Cultural Economics*, Vol. 20, No. 3, pp. 183-206.

Baumol, W.J. and Bowen, W.E. (1966), *Performing Arts – The Economic Dilemma: A Study of Problems Common to Theater, Opera and Dance*, The MIT Press, Cambridge, Mass.

Baumol, W.J. and Oates, W.E. (1972), 'The Cost Disease of the Personal Services and the Quality of Life', in R. Towse (ed.)(1997), *Baumol's Cost Disease: The Arts and Other Victims*, Edward Elgar, Cheltenham, pp. 82-92.

Baumol, W.J., Panzar, J.C. and Willig, R.D. (1982), *Contestable Markets and the Theory of Industry Structure*, Harcourt Brace Jovanovich, New York.

Bazzoli, G., Stein, R., Alexander, J.A., Conrad, D.A., Sofaer, S. and Shortell, S.M. (1997), 'Public-Private Collaboration in Health and Human Service Delivery: Evidence from Community Partnerships', *The Milbank Quarterly*, Vol. 75, No. 4, pp. 533-61.

Becker, G.S. (1965), 'A Theory of the Allocation of Time', *The Economic Journal*, Vol. LXXV, No. 299, September, pp. 493-517.

Becker, G.S. (1974), 'A Theory of Social Interactions', in G.S. Becker (1996), *Accounting for Tastes*, Harvard University Press, Cambridge, MA, pp. 162-94.

Becker, G.S. (1996), *Accounting for Tastes*, Harvard University Press, Cambridge, MA.

Beer, M.D. (1990), 'The Dichotomies: Psychosis/Neurosis and Functional/Organic: A Historical Perspective', *History of Psychiatry*, Vol. 6, October, pp. 231-55.

Benjamin, J.D. and Lusht, K.M. (1993), 'Search Costs and Apartment Rents,' *Journal of Real Estate Finance and Economics*, Vol. 6, No. 2, March, pp. 189-97.

Bentham, J. (1789), *Principles of Morals and Legislation*, Clarendon, Oxford.

Berk, A.A. (1982), 'Overview of Cost Studies of Hospitalization', in Z. Taintor, P. Widem and S.A. Barett. (eds)(1982), *Cost Considerations in Mental Health Treatment: Settings, Modalities, and Providers*, National Institute of Mental Health, Bethesda, pp. 19-23.

Berk, R.A. (1987), 'Household Production', in J. Eatwell, M. Milgate and P. Newman (eds)(1987), *The New Palgrave: A Dictionary of Economics*, Vol. 2, Macmillan, London, pp. 676-78.

Berndt, E.R. (1991), *The Practice of Econometrics: Classic and Contemporary*, Addison Wesley, Reading, Mass.

Berndt, E.R., Bir, A., Busch, S.H., Frank, R.G., Normand, S.T. (2000), 'The Medical Treatment of Depression, 1991-1996: Productive Inefficiency, Expected Outcome Variations, and Price Indexes', *NBER Working Paper*, No. W7816.

Berndt, E.R., Cockburn, I.M. and Griliches, Z. (1997), 'Pharmaceutical Innovations and Market Dynamics: Tracking Effects on Price Indexes for Antidepressant Drug', *Brookings Papers on Economic Activity: Microeconomics 1996*, pp. 133-88.

Berndt, E.R., Frank, R.G. and McGuire, T.G. (1997), 'Alternative Insurance Arrangements and the Treatment of Depression: What are the Facts?' *American Journal of Managed Care*, Vol. 3, No. 2, pp. 243-50.

Berndt, E.R., and Greenberg, P. (1995), 'An Updated and Extended Study of the Price Growth of Prescription Pharmaceutical Preparations', in R.B. Helms (ed.)(1995), *Competitive Strategies in the Pharmaceutical Industry*, The AEI Press, Washington, DC, pp. 35-48.

Berndt, E.R., Griliches, Z. and Rosett, J.G. (1993), 'Auditing the Producer Price Index: Micro Evidence from Prescription Pharmaceutical Preparations', *Journal of Business and Economic Statistics*, Vol. 11, No. 3, pp. 251-64.

Bishai, D. (1996), 'Quality Time: How Parent Schooling Affects Child Health through its Interaction with Childcare Time in Bangladesh", *Health Economics*, Vol. 5, No. 5, pp. 383-407.

Blaug, M. (1963), 'A Survey of the Theory of Process Innovations', *Economica*, Vol. 30, No. 1, pp. 13-32.

Blinder, A.S. (1987), *Hard Heads, Soft Hearts: Tough-Minded Economics for a Just Society*, Addison Wesley, Reading, MA.

Blomquist, G. and Worley, L. (1981), 'Hedonic Prices for Urban Amenities, and Benefit Estimates', *Journal of Urban Economics*, Vol. 9, No. 2, March, pp. 212-21.

Bourdieu, P. (1986), 'The Forms of Capital', in J.G. Richardson (1986)(ed.), *Handbook of Theory and Research for the Sociology of Education*, Greenwood Press, New York, pp. 241-58.

Bowles, S. (1998), 'Endogenous Preferences: The Cultural Consequences of Markets and Other Economic Institutions', *Journal of Economic Literature*, Vol. 36, No. 1, May, pp. 75-111.

Braden, J.B. and Kolstad, C.D. (eds)(1991), *Measuring the Demand for Environmental Quality*, Elsevier, Amsterdam.

Brinton, C. (1950), *Ideas and Men: The Story of Western Thought*, Prentice Hall, Englewood Cliffs.

Brookside, D.S. *et al.* (1982), 'Valuing Public Goods: A Comparison of Survey and Hedonic Approaches', *The American Economic Review*, Vol. 72, No. 1, March, pp. 165-77.

Brown, C.V. and Jackson, P.M. (1982), *Public Sector Economics*, 2nd edn, Martin Robertson, Oxford.

Brown, C. and Preece, A. (1987), 'Housework', in J. Eatwell, M. Milgate and P. Newman (eds)(1987), *The New Palgrave: A Dictionary of Economics*, Vol. 2, Macmillan, London, pp. 678-80.

Buchanan, J. and Tullock, G. (1967), *The Calculus of Consent*, University of Michigan Press, Ann Arbor.

Burkhead, J. and Miner, J. (1971), *Public Expenditure*, Macmillan, New York.

Butler, J.R.G. (1995), *Hospital Cost Analysis*, Klewer, Dordrecht.

Carling, P.J. (1995), *Return to Community: Building Support Systems for People with Psychiatric Disabilities*, Guildford, New York.

Carlton, D.W. and Perloff, J.M. (1994), *Modern Industrial Organization*, 2nd edn, Harper Collins, New York.

Christensen, L.R., Jorgenson, D.W. and Lau, L.J. (1971), 'Conjugate Duality and the Transcendental Logarithmic Production Function', *Econometrica*, Vol. 39, No. 3, July, pp. 255-56.

Christensen, L.R., Jorgenson, D.W. and Lau, L.J. (1973), 'Transcendental Logarithmic Production Frontiers', *Review of Economics and Statistics*, Vol. 55, No. 1, February, pp. 28-45.

Clark, A.E. and Oswald, A.J. (1994), 'Unhappiness and Unemployment', *The Economic Journal*, Vol. 104, No. 424, May, pp. 648-59.

Clarke, R. (1985), *Industrial Economics*, Basil Blackwell, Oxford.

Coase, R.H. (1960), 'The Problem of Social Cost', *Journal of Law and Economics*, Vol. 3, October, pp. 1-44.

Cobb, C.W. and Douglas, P.H. (1928), 'The Theory of Production', *The American Economic Review*, Vol. XVIII, No. 1, Supplement, pp. 139-65.

Cochrane, A.L. (1972), *Effectiveness and Efficiency: Random Reflections on Health Services*, Nuffield Provincial Hospitals Trust, London.

Cocks, E. (1995), 'The Relationship between Social Role Valorisation and Safeguards Concepts, and the Quality of Outcomes in Major Human Service Agency Change', unpublished PhD thesis (Education), The University of Queensland, Brisbane.

Cohen, J.W. and Spector, W.D. (1996), 'The Effect of Medicaid Reimbursement on Quality of Care in Nursing Homes', *Journal of Health Economics*, Vol. 15, No. 1, pp. 23-48.

Coleman, J.S. (1988), 'Social Capital in the Creation of Human Capital', *American Journal of Sociology*, Vol. 94, Supplement, S95-S120.

Coleman, J.S. (1990), *Foundations of Social Theory*, Harvard University Press, Cambridge, MA.

Colm, G. (1955), *Essays in Public Finance and Fiscal Policy*, Oxford University Press, New York.

Commons, M., McGuire, T.G. and Riordan, M.H. (1997), 'Performance Contracting for Substance Abuse Treatment', *Health Services Research*, Vol. 32, No. 5, December, pp. 631-50.

Conley, R.W., Conwell, M. and Arrill, M.B. (1967), 'An Approach to Measuring the Cost of Mental Illness', *American Journal of Psychiatry*, Vol. 124, No. 12, December, pp. 63-70.

Connelly, L. and Doessel, D.P. (2000), 'A Survey of the Health Production Literature', in Baldry, J.C. (ed.)(2000), *Economics and Health: 1999 Proceedings of the Twenty-First Australian Conference of Health Economists*, School of Health Services Management, Sydney, pp. 31-58.

Cooper, D. (1970), *Psychiatry and Anti-psychiatry*, Paladin, London.

Cooper, J. and Bennett, C. (1984), 'The Development of a Program Classification of Health Services for the South Australian Health Commission – Reflections of The First Three Years', in Butler, J.R.G. and Doessel, D.P. (eds)(1989), *Health Economics: Australian Readings*, Australian Professional Publications, Sydney, pp. 266-77.

Corman, H., Joyce, T. J. and Grossman, M. (1987), 'Birth Outcome Production Functions in the United States', *Journal of Human Resources*, Vol. 15, No. 2, pp. 200-18.

Cornes, R. (1992), *Duality and Modern Economics*, Cambridge University Press, Cambridge.

Cousens, P. and Crawford, J. (1988), 'Moving the Mentally Ill into the Community: The Problem of Acceptance and the Effect of Contact', *Australian Journal of Social Issues*, Vol. 23, No. 3, August, pp. 196-207.

Cowen, T. (1996), 'Why I Do Not Believe in the Cost-Disease', *Journal of Cultural Economics*, Vol. 20, No. 3, pp. 207-14.

Cullis, J.G. and Jones, P.R. (1985), 'National Health Service Waiting Lists: A Discussion of Competing Explanations and a Policy Proposal', *Journal of Health Economics*, Vol. 4, No. 2, pp. 119-35.

Culyer, A.J. (1975), 'Health: The Social Cost of Doctors' Discretion', *New Society*, 27 February, pp. 517-19.

Culyer, A.J. (1976), *Need and the National Health Service: Economics and Social Choice*, Martin Robertson, London.

Culyer, A.J. (1980), *The Political Economy of Social Policy*, Martin Robertson, Oxford.

Cutler, D.M. and Berndt, E.R. (eds)(forthcoming), *Medical Output and Productivity*, University of Chicago Press for the National Bureau of Economic Research, Chicago.

Cutler, D.M., McClellan, M. and Newhouse, J.P. (1998), 'What Has Increased Medical-Care Spending Bought?', *The American Economic Review*, Vol. 88, No. 2, May, pp. 132-36.

Cutler, D.M., McClellan, M. and Newhouse, J.P. (1999), 'The Costs and Benefits of Intensive Treatment for Cardiovascular Disease', in J.E. Triplett (ed.)(1999), *Measuring the Prices of Medical Treatments*, Brookings Institution Press, Washington, DC, pp. 34-71.

Cutler, D.M., McClellan, M., Newhouse, J.P. and Remler, D. (1998), 'Are Medical Prices Declining?' *Quarterly Journal of Economics*, Vol. CXIII, No. 4, November, pp. 991-1024.

Cutler, D. and Zeckhauser, R. (1998), 'The Anatomy of Health Insurance', in J.P. Newhouse and A.J. Culyer (eds)(1998), *Handbook of Health Economics*, North-Holland, Amsterdam.

Cyert, R.M. and March, J.G. (1963), *A Behavioural Theory of the Firm*, Prentice Hall, Englewood Cliffs.

D'Arcy, C., Bold, G. and Schmitz, J.A. (1981), 'Psychiatric Health Care and Costs Under Comprehensive Public Health Insurance: Experience in a Canadian Province', *Medical Care*, Vol. 19, No. 9, September, pp. 881-94.

Dasgupta, A.K. and Pearce, D.W. (1972), *Cost-Benefit Analysis: Theory and Practice*, Macmillan, Basingstoke.

Deaton, A. and Muellbauer, J. (1980), *Economics and Consumer Behavior*, Cambridge University Press, Cambridge.

Deb, P. and Holmes, A.M. (1998), 'Substitution of Physicians and Other Providers in Outpatient Mental Health Care', *Health Economics*, Vol. 7, No. 4, June, pp. 347-61.

Debertin, D.L. (1986), *Agricultural Production Economics*, Macmillan, New York.

Dickey, B. and Cohen, M.D. (1993), 'Changing the Financing of State Mental Health Programs: Using Carrots, Not Sticks, to Improve Care', *Administration and Policy in Mental Health*, Vol. 20, No. 5, pp. 343-56.

Dickey, B., McGuire, T.G., Cannon, N.L. and Gudeman, J. (1986), 'Mental Health Cost Models: Refinements and Applications', *Medical Care*, Vol. 24, No. 9, pp. 857-67.

Diewert, W.E. and Fox, K.J. (1999), 'Can Measurement Error Explain the Productivity Paradox?' *Canadian Journal of Economics*, Vol. 32, No. 2, April, pp. 251-80.

Diewert, W.E., Nakamura, A.O. and Sharpe, A. (1999), 'Introduction and Overview', *Canadian Journal of Economics*, Vol. 32, No. 2, April, pp. v-xv.

Dixon, L. (1999), 'Providing Services to Families of Persons with Schizophrenia: Present and Future', *The Journal of Mental Health Policy and Economics*, Vol. 2, No. 1, pp. 3-8.

Doessel, D.P. (1986), 'Medical Diagnosis as a Problem in the Economics of Information', *Information Economics and Policy*, Vol. 2, No. 1, pp. 49-68.

Doessel, D.P. (1987), 'Health Outcome and Higher Medical Qualifications: An Economic Conception and Notes on Implementation', *Social Science and Medicine*, Vol. 24, No. 11, pp. 897-910.

Doessel, D.P. (1988), 'A Note on Nutrition and Economics', *Health Policy*, Vol. 10, No. 1, pp. 33-39.

Doessel, D.P. (1992), *The Economics of Medical Diagnosis: Technological Change and Health Expenditure*, Avebury, Aldershot.

Doessel, D.P. (1994), 'Cost-Utility Analysis and All That: Some Issues in Social Investment Appraisal', *mimeo.*, General Practice Evaluation Program Conference, The Australian National University, 5-7 May.

Doessel, D.P. and Gargett, S. (2001), 'The Small Area Variation (SAV) Phenomenon in the Health Sector: Economic Issues', in *Economics and Health: 2000 Proceedings of Twentieth-Second Australian Conference of Health Economists*, School of Health Services Management, Sydney (forthcoming).

Doessel, D.P. and Marshall, J. (1983), 'An Economic Approach to the Care of the Handicapped', in P.M. Tatchell (ed.)(1983), *Economics and Health 1982: Proceedings of the Fourth Australian Conference of Health Economists*, Health Economics Research Unit, Canberra, pp. 107-61.

Doessel, D.P. and Marshall, J. (1985), 'A Rehabilitation of Health Outcome in Quality Assessment', *Social Science and Medicine*, Vol. 21, No.12, pp. 1319-28.

Dorwart, R.A., Rodriguez, E. and Causino, N. (1993), 'The RBRVS for Psychiatry', in T-W. Hu and A. Rupp (eds)(1993), *Advances in Health Economics and Health Services Research: Vol. 14 Research into the Economics of Mental Health*, JAI Press, Greenwich, pp. 139-58.

Dranove, D. (1995), 'A Problem with Consumer Surplus Measures of the Cost of Practice Variations', *Journal of Health Economics*, Vol. 14, No. 2, pp. 243-51.

Drummond, M.F., O'Brien, B., Stoddart, G.L. and Torrance, G.W. (1997), *Methods for Economic Evaluation of Health Care Programmes*, 2nd edn, Oxford University Press, Oxford.

Easterly, W. and Levine, R. (1997), 'Africa's Growth Tragedy: Policies and Ethnic Divisions', *Quarterly Journal of Economics*, Vol. CXII, No. 4, Nov., pp. 1203-50.

Eisen, P. and Wolfenden, K. (1988), 'A National Mental Health Services Policy. A Report of the Consultancy to Advise Commonwealth, State and Territory Health Ministers', *mimeo.*, Department of Community Services and Health, Canberra.

Eisenberg, L. (1992), 'Treating Depression and Anxiety in Primary Care', *New England Journal of Medicine*, Vol. 376, No. 16, pp. 1080-84.

el-Guebaly, N., Bebchuk, W. and Prosen, H. (1985), 'Payment for Psychiatric Services Under Canada's Insurance System', *Hospital and Community Psychiatry*, Vol. 36, No. 6, June, pp. 628-32.

Ellis, R.P. and McGuire, T.G. (1986), 'Cost Sharing and Patterns of Mental Health Care Utilization', *The Journal of Human Resources*, Vol. 21, No. 3, Summer, pp. 359-79.

Ellison, S.F. and Hellerstein, J.K. (1999), 'The Economics of Antibiotics: An Exploratory Study', in J.E. Triplett (ed.)(1999), *Measuring the Prices of Medical Treatments*, Brookings Institution Press, Washington, DC, pp. 118-43.

English, J.T. and McCarrick, R.G. (1989), 'The Economics of Psychiatry', in H.I. Kaplan and B.J. Sadock (eds)(1989), *Comprehensive Textbook of Psychiatry*, 5th edn, Vol. 2, Williams and Wilkins, Washington, DC, pp. 2074-83.

Enthoven, A.C. (1981), 'The Behaviour of Health Care Agents: Provider Behaviour', in J. van der Gaag and M. Perlman (eds)(1981), *Health, Economics, and Health Economics*, North-Holland, Amsterdam, pp. 173-88.

Enthoven, A.C. (1988), *Theory and Practice of Managed Competition in Health Care Finance*, North-Holland, Amsterdam.

Ettner, S.L. (1996), 'New Evidence of the Relationship Between Income and Health', *Journal of Health Economics*, Vol. 15, No. 1, pp. 67-85.

Evans, R. (1969), 'Charitable Institutions of the Queensland Government to 1919', unpublished MA thesis, Department of History, University of Queensland, Brisbane.

Evans, R.G. (1974), 'Supplier-Induced Demand: Some Empirical Evidence and Implications', in M. Perlman (ed.)(1974), *The Economics of Health and Medical Care*, Macmillan, London, pp. 162-73.

Evans, R.G. (1984), *Strained Mercy: The Economics of Canadian Health Care*, Butterworth and Co., Toronto.

Evers, S.M.A.A., van Wijk, A.S. and Ament, A.J.H.A. (1997), 'Economic Evaluations of Mental Health Care Interventions: A Review', *Health Economics*, Vol. 6, No. 2, pp. 161-77.

Fein, R. (1958), *Economics of Mental Illness*, Basic Books, New York.

Feldman, A.M. (1987), 'Welfare Economics', in J. Eatwell, M. Milgate and P. Newman (eds)(1987), *The New Palgrave: A Dictionary of Economics*, Vol. 4, Macmillan, London, pp. 889-95.

Feldstein, M.S. (1965), 'Hospital Cost Variation and Case-Mix Differences', *Medical Care*, Vol. 3, pp. 95-103.

Feldstein, P.J. (1983), *Health Care Economics*, 2nd edn, Wiley, New York.

Felton, M.V. (1994), 'Evidence of the Existence of the Cost Disease in the Performing Arts', *Journal of Cultural Economics*, Vol. 18, No. 4, pp. 301-12.

Ferris, J.S. and West, E.G. (1996), 'The Cost Disease and Government Growth', *Public Choice*, Vol. 89, No. 2, October, pp. 35-52.

Fetter, R.B. (ed.)(1991), *DRGs: Their Design and Development*, Health Administration Press, Ann Arbor.
Fetter, R.B. (1999), 'Casemix Classification Systems', *Australian Health Review*, Vol. 22, No. 2, pp. 16-34.
Fetter, R.B., Thompson, J.D. and Mills, R.E. (1976), 'A System for Cost and Reimbursement Controls in Hospitals', *Yale Journal of Biology and Medicine*, Vol. 49, pp. 123-36.
Fetter, R.B., Shin, Y., Freeman, J.L. *et al.*, (1980), 'Case-Mix Definition by Diagnosis Related Groups', *Medical Care*, Vol. 18, No. 2, Supplement, pp. 1-53.
Fine, M. and Thompson, C. (1995), *Factors Affecting the Outcome of Community Care Service Interventions: A Literature Review*, AGPS, Canberra.
Fixler, D.J. (1999), 'Comments' in J.E Triplett (ed.)(1999), *Measuring the Prices of Medical Treatments*, Brookings Institution Press, Washington, DC, pp. 103-8.
Flatau, P., Galea, J. and Petridis, R. (1998), 'Mental Health and Unemployment: Results from the 1995 National Health Survey', *Centre for Labour Market Research Discussion Paper No. 98/7*, Murdoch University, Western Australia.
Folland, S., Goodman, A.C. and Stano, M. (1997), *The Economics of Health and Health Care*, 2nd edn, Prentice Hall, Upper Saddle River.
Folland, S. and Stano, M. (1989), 'Sources of Small Area Variations in the Use of Medical Care', *Journal of Health Economics*, Vol. 8, No. 1, pp. 85-107.
Folland, S. and Stano, M. (1990), Small Area Variations: A Critical Review of Propositions, Methods and Evidence', *Medical Care Review*, Vol. 47, No. 4, pp. 419-65.
Foucault, M. (1967), *Madness and Civilisation: A History of Insanity in the Age of Reason*, New American Library, New York.
Frank, L.R. (1999), *Random House Webster's Quotationary*, Random House, New York.
Frank, R.G. (1981), 'Cost-Benefit Analysis in Mental Health Services: A Review of the Literature', *Administration in Mental Health*, Vol. 8, No. 3, Spring, pp. 161-76.
Frank, R.G. (1985a), 'Pricing and Location of Physician Services in Mental Health', *Economic Inquiry*, Vol. 23, No. 1, pp. 115-33.
Frank, R.G. (1985b), 'Rationing of Mental Health Services: Simple Observations on the Current Approach and Future Prospects', *Administration in Mental Health*, Vol. 13, No. 1, Fall, pp. 22-29.
Frank, R.G. (1990), 'Mental Health Economics', *Administration and Policy in Mental Health*, Vol. 17, No. 3, Spring, pp. 189-91.
Frank, R.G. (1993), 'Cost-Benefit Evaluations in Mental Health: Implications for Financing Policy', in T-W. Hu and A. Rupp (Guest eds)(1993), *Advances in Health Economics and Health Services Research: Research into the Economics of Mental Health*, Vol. 14, JAI Press, Greenwich, pp. 1-16.
Frank, R.G., Busch, S.H. and Berndt, E.R. (1998), 'Measuring Prices and Quantities of Treatment for Depression', *The American Economic Review*, Vol. 88, No. 2, May, pp. 106-12.
Frank, R.G., Berndt, E.R. and Busch, S.H. (1999), 'Price Indices for the Treatment of Depression', in J.E. Triplett (ed.)(1999), *Measuring the Prices of Medical Treatments*, Brookings Institution Press, Washington, DC, pp. 34-71.
Frank, R.G., Goldman, H.H. and McGuire, T.G. (1992), 'A Model Mental Health Benefit in Private Hospital Insurance', *Health Affairs*, Vol. 11, No. 3, pp. 98-117.
Frank, R.G., Huskampf, H.A., McGuire, T.G. and Newhouse, J.P. (1997), 'Some Economics of Mental Health "Carve-Outs" ', *Archives of General Psychiatry*, Vol. 53, No.10, pp. 933-37.
Frank, R.G. and Lave, J.R. (1986), 'The Effect of Benefit Design on the Length of Stay of Medicaid Psychiatric Patients', *The Journal of Human Resources*, Vol. 21, No. 3, Summer, pp. 321-37.

Frank, R.G. and McGuire, T.G. (1986), 'Review of Studies of the Impact of Insurance on the Demand and Utilization of Specialty Mental Health Services', *Health Services Research*, Vol. 21, No. 2, Part II, June, pp. 241-66.

Frank, R.G. and McGuire, T.G. (1995), 'Estimating Costs of Mental Health and Substance Abuse Coverage', *Health Affairs*, Vol. 14, No. 3, pp. 102-15.

Frank, R.G. and McGuire, T.G. (1997), 'Guest Editors' Introduction, Special Issue: Mental Health Economics', *Administration and Policy in Mental Health*, Vol. 24, No. 4, March, pp. 275-77.

Frank, R.G. and McGuire, T.G. (1998), 'Parity for Mental Health and Substance Abuse Care under Managed Care', *Journal of Mental Health Policy and Economics*, Vol. 1, No. 4, November, pp. 153-59.

Frank, R.G. and McGuire, T.G. (1999), 'Economics and Mental Health', *National Bureau of Economic Research Working Paper*, No. 7052, March, National Bureau of Economic Research, Cambridge, Mass., http://www.nber.org/papers/w7052.

Frank, R.G., McGuire, T.G. and Newhouse, J.P. (1995), 'Risk Contracts in Managed Mental Health Care,' *Health Affairs*, Vol. 14, No. 3, pp. 102-15.

Frank, R.G. and Salkever, D.S. (1992), 'Do Public Mental Health Hospitals Crowd Out Care for Indigent Psychiatric Patients in Nonprofit General Hospitals?', in R.G. Frank and W.G. Manning (eds)(1992), *Economics and Mental Health*, The Johns Hopkins University Press, Baltimore, pp. 68-86.

Franks, D.D. (1990), 'Economic Contribution of Families Caring for Persons with Severe and Persistent Mental Illness', *Administration and Policy in Mental Health*, Vol. 18, No.1, September, pp. 9-18.

Freedman, R.I. and Moran, A.E. (1984a), 'A Case Vignette of a Chronically Mentally Ill Person', *Medical Care*, Vol. 22, No. 12, December, Supplement, pp. S4-7.

Freedman, R.I. and Moran, A.E. (1984b), 'Who Are the Chronically Mentally Ill?', *Medical Care*, Vol. 22, No. 12, December, Supplement, pp. S8-13.

Freeman, H.L. (1995), 'The General Hospital and Mental Health Care: A British Perspective', *The Milbank Quarterly*, Vol. 73, No. 4, pp. 653-76.

Frey, B.S. (1997), *Not Just for the Money: An Economic Theory of Personal Motivation*, Edward Elgar, Cheltenham.

Fuchs, V. (1983), *Who Shall Live? Health, Economics and Social Choice*, Basic Books, New York.

Fukuyama, F. (1995), *Trust: The Social Virtues and the Creation of Prosperity*, Hamish Hamilton, London.

Fuss, M.A. (1987), 'Production and Cost Functions', in J. Eatwell, M. Milgate and P. Newman (eds)(1987), *The New Palgrave: A Dictionary of Economics*, Vol. 3, Macmillan, London, pp. 995-1000.

Geneen, H. (1997), *The Synergy Myth: And Other Ailments of Business Today*, St Martins Press, New York.

Gerdtham, U.-G., Löthgren, M., Tambour, M. and Rehnberg, C. (1999), 'Internal Markets and Health Care Efficiency: A Multiple- Output Stochastic Frontier Analysis', *Health Economics*, Vol. 8, No. 2, March, pp. 151-64.

Gill, D. (1980), *Quest: The Life of Elizabeth Kubler-Ross*, Harper and Row, London.

Glick, I.D., Klar, H.M. and Braff, D.L. (1984), 'Guidelines for Hospitalisation of Chronic Psychiatric Patients', *Hospital and Community Psychiatry*, Vol. 35, No. 9, September, pp. 934-5.

Glover, J.A. (1938), 'The Incidence of Tonsillectomy in School Children', *Proceedings of the Royal Society of Medicine*, Vol. 31, May, pp. 1219-36.

Goffman, E. (1963), *Stigma: Notes on the Management of Spoiled Identity*, Penguin, Harmondsworth.

Gokcekus, O. (2000), 'How Do University Students Value Economics Courses? A Hedonic Approach', *Applied Economics Letters*, Vol. 7, No. 8, August, pp. 493-96.

Golan, A. and Shalit, H. (1993), 'Wine Quality Differentials in Hedonic Grape Pricing', *Journal of Agricultural Economics*, Vol. 44, No. 2, May, pp. 311-21.

Goldman, H.H. (1983), 'Mental Illness and the Family Burden', *Hospital and Community Psychiatry*, Vol. 33, No. 7, July, pp. 557-60.

Goldman, H.H., Morrisey, J.P. and Ridgely, M.S.(1992), 'Lessons from the Program on Chronic Mental Illness', *Health Affairs*, Vol. 11, No. 3, pp. 51-68.

Goldman, H.H. and Regier, D.A. (1983), 'The Multiple Functions of the State Mental Hospital', *American Journal of Psychiatry*, Vol. 140, No. 3, pp. 296-300.

Goldman, H.H., Scheffler, R.M. and Cheadle, R. (1987), 'Demand for Psychiatric Services: A Clinical Episode Model for Specifying "The Product" ', in T.G. McGuire and R.M. Scheffler (Guest eds)(1987), in *Advances in Health Economics and Health Services Research: The Economics of Mental Health Services*, Vol. 8, JAI Press, Greenwich, Conn., pp. 255-74.

Goodman, A.C. (1998), 'Andrew Court and the Invention of Hedonic Price Analysis', *Journal of Urban Economics*, Vol. 44, No. 2, September, pp. 291-98.

Goodman, A.C. (1989), 'Estimation of Offset and Income Effects on the Demand for Mental Health Treatment', *Inquiry*, Vol. 26, No. 2, Summer, pp. 235-48.

Green, H.A.J. (1971), *Consumer Theory*, Penguin, Harmondsworth.

Greene, W.H. (1997), 'Frontier Production Functions', in M.H. Pesaran and P. Schmidt (eds)(1997), *Handbook of Applied Econometrics Volume II: Microeconomics*, Blackwell, Oxford, pp. 81-166.

Griliches, Z. (ed.)(1971), *Price Indexes and Quality Change: Studies in New Methods of Measurement*, Harvard University Press, Cambridge, Mass.

Griliches, Z. and Cockburn, I. (1994), 'Generics and New Goods in Pharmaceutical Price Indexes', *The American Economic Review*, Vol. 84, No. 5, December, pp. 1213-32.

Grossman, M. (1972a), 'On the Concept of Health Capital and the Demand for Health', *Journal of Political Economy*, Vol. 80, No. 2, April, pp. 223-55.

Grossman, M. (1972b), *The Demand for Health: A Theoretical and Empirical Investigation*, Columbia University Press, New York.

Grusky, O., Tierney, K. and Holstein, J. (1985), 'Models of Local Mental Health Delivery Systems', *American Behavioral Scientist*, Vol. 28, pp. 685-703.

Gulbinat, W., Manderscheid, R.W. and Beigel, J-A. (1996), 'A Multinational Strategy on Mental Health Policy and Care. A WHO Collaborative Initiative and Consultative Strategy', in M. Moscarelli, A. Rupp and N. Sartorious (eds)(1996), *Handbook of Mental Health Economics and Health Policy, Volume 1: Schizophrenia*, John Wiley & Sons, Chichester, pp. 531-36.

Hadley, J. (1982), *More Medical Care, Better Health? An Economic Analysis of Mortality Rates*, Urban Institute, Washington DC.

Hadley, J. (1988), 'Medicare Spending and Mortality Rates of the Elderly', *Inquiry*, Vol. 25, No. 4, pp. 485-93.

Hagy, A.P. (1998), 'The Demand for Child Care Quality: An Hedonic Price Theory Approach', *The Journal of Human Resources*, Vol. XXXIII, No. 3, Summer, pp. 683-710.

Halpern, J. and Binner, P.R. (1972), 'A Model for an Output Value Analysis of Mental Health Programs', *Administration in Mental Health*, Vol.1, No. 2, Winter, pp. 40-51.

Hanson, K.W. (1998), 'Public Opinion and the Mental Health Parity Debate: Lessons from the Survey Literature', *Psychiatric Services*, Vol. 49, No. 8, pp. 1059-66.

Harris, J. (1977), 'The Internal Organization of Hospitals: Some Economic Implications', *Bell Journal of Economics*, Vol. 8, No. 2, pp. 467-82.

Harrison, D. and Rubinfeld, D.L. (1978), 'The Air Pollution and Property Value Debate: Some Empirical Evidence', *Review of Economics and Statistics*, Vol. LX, No. 4, November, pp. 635-38.

Harriss, J. and De Renzio, P. (1997), ' "Missing Link" or Analytically Missing? The Concept of Social Capital: An Introductory Bibliographic Essay', *Journal of International Development*, Vol. 9, No. 7, pp. 919-37.

Harrow, B.S. and Ellis, R.P. (1992), 'Mental Health Providers' Response to the Reimbursement System', in R.G. Frank and W.G. Manning (eds)(1992), *Economics and Mental Health*, The Johns Hopkins University Press, Baltimore, pp. 19-39.

Hart, R.F.G. (1989), 'Economics and Mental Health Care: Outputs and Implications for Government', unpublished MEconSt thesis, The University of Queensland, Brisbane.

Hawthorn, G. (1987), 'Introduction', in G. Hawthorn (ed.), *The Standard of Living: The Tanner Lectures, Clare Hall, Cambridge, 1985*, Cambridge University Press, Cambridge, pp. vii-xiv.

Head, J.G. (1966), 'On Merit Goods', *Finanzarchiv*, Vol. 25, No. 1, March, pp. 1-29.

Healey, A., Mirandola, M., Amaddeo, F. *et al.* (2000), 'Using Health Production Functions to Evaluate Treatment Effectiveness: An Application to a Community Mental Health Service', *Health Economics*, Vol. 9, No. 5, pp. 373-83.

Helm, D.R. (1987), 'Elasticity of Substitution', in J. Eatwell, M. Milgate and P. Newman (eds)(1987), *The New Palgrave: A Dictionary of Economics*, Vol. 3, Macmillan, London, pp. 1002-07.

Hicks, J.R. (1932), *The Theory of Wages*, Macmillan, London.

Hicks, J.R. (1946), *Value and Capital: An Inquiry into Some Fundamental Principles of Economic Theory*, Clarendon Press, Oxford.

Hill, T.P. (1977), 'On Goods and Services', *Review of Income and Wealth*, Vol. 23, No. 4, December, pp. 315-38.

Hitch, C.J. (1965), *Decision Making for Defense*, University of California Press, Berkeley.

Hitch, C.J. and McKean, R.H. (1960), *The Economics of Defense in the Nuclear Age*, Harvard University Press, Cambridge, MA.

Hodgson, G.M. (1998), 'The Approach of Institutional Economics', *Journal of Economic Literature*, Vol. 36, No. 1, March, pp. 166-92.

Holmes, A.M. and Deb, P. (1998), 'Factors Influencing Informal Care-Giving', *The Journal of Mental Health Policy and Economics*, Vol. 1, No. 2, pp. 77-87.

Horgan, C.M. (1986), 'The Demand for Ambulatory Mental Health Services from Specialty Providers', *Health Services Research*, Vol. 21, No. 2, Part II, June, Supplement, pp. 291-319.

Horgan, C.M. and Jencks, S. (1987), 'Research on Psychiatric Classification and Payment Systems', *Medical Care*, Vol. 25, No. 9, pp. 522-36.

Horsfall, J. (1987), 'Psychiatric Non-Institutionalisation: Whose Needs are Served?', *Australian Journal of Social Issues*, Vol. 22, No. 3, August, pp. 530-41.

Howells, J.G. (ed.)(1976), *World History of Psychiatry*, Balliere Tindall, London.

Human Rights and Equal Opportunity Commission (1993), *Human Rights and Mental Illness: Report of the National Inquiry into the Human Rights of People with Mental Illness*, AGPS, Canberra.

Illich, I. (1976), *Limits to Medicine. Medical Nemesis: The Expropriation of Health Care*, Calder and Boyars, London.

Ironmonger, D.S. (1972), *New Commodities and Consumer Behaviour*, Cambridge University Press, Cambridge.

Ironmonger, D.S. (1994), 'The Value of Care and Nurture Provided by Unpaid Household Work', *Family Matters*, No. 37, April, pp. 46-51.

Jablensky, A., McGrath, J., Herrman, H., Castle, D., Gureje, O., Morgan, V. and Korten, A. (1999), *People Living with Psychotic Illness: An Australian Study 1997-98, National Survey of Mental Health and Wellbeing Report 4*, National Mental Health Strategy, Commonwealth Department of Health and Aged Care, Canberra.

Jackson, J., McIver, R. and McConnell, C. (1994), *Macroeconomics*, 4th edn, McGraw-Hill, Sydney.

Jacobs, J. (1962), *The Death and Life of Great American Cities*, Cape, London.

Jencks, C. (1994), *The Homeless*, Harvard University Press, Cambridge, MA.
Joint, S.A. (1996), 'Implementation of Disability Services: Deinstitutionalisation and Contractual Arrangements, Is There a Conflict?' unpublished Master of Public Administration thesis, The University of Queensland, Brisbane.
Jönsson, B. and Rosenbaum, J. (eds)(1993), *Health Economics of Depression*, John Wiley & Sons, Chichester.
Jorgenson, D.W. (1987), 'Production Functions', in J. Eatwell, M. Milgate and P. Newman (eds)(1987), *The New Palgrave: A Dictionary of Economics*, Vol. 3, Macmillan, London, pp. 1002-07.
Kafka, F. (1925), *The Trial*, Penguin, Harmondsworth.
Keeler, E.B., Manning, W.G. and Wells, K.B. (1988), 'The Demand for Episodes of Mental Health Services', *Journal of Health Economics*, Vol. 7, No. 4, pp. 369-92.
Kelly, G.G. (1997), 'Improving the PPI Samples for Prescription Pharmaceuticals', *Monthly Labour Review*, Vol. 120, No. 10, pp. 10-17.
Kenny, B. and Whitehead, T. (1973), *Insight: A Guide to Psychiatry and Psychiatric Services*, Croom Helm, London.
Kessler, L.G., Steinwachs, D.M. and Hankin, J.R. (1982), 'Episodes of Psychiatric Care and Medical Utilization', *Medical Care*, Vol. 20, No. 12, December, pp. 1209-21.
Kirby, M.D. (1983), 'Law Reform, Politics and Mental Health', *Australian and New Zealand Journal of Psychiatry*, Vol. 17, No. 1, pp. 39-47.
Kitwood, T. (1997), *Dementia Reconsidered: The Person Comes First*, Open University Press, Buckingham.
Klamer, A. (1989), 'A Conversation with Amartya Sen', *Journal of Economic Perspectives*, Vol. 3, No. 1, Winter, pp. 135-50.
Klerman, G. and Schechter, G. (1981), 'Ethical Aspects of Drug Treatment', in S. Bloch and P. Chodoff (eds)(1981), *Psychiatric Ethics*, Oxford University Press, Oxford, pp. 117-30.
Knack, S. and Keefer, P. (1997), 'Does Social Capital have an Economic Payoff? A Cross-Country Investigation', *The Quarterly Journal of Economics*, Vol. 112, No. 4, November, pp. 1251-88.
Knapp, M. (1999), 'Economic Evaluation and Mental Health: Sparse Past ... Fertile Future?', *The Journal of Mental Health Policy and Economics*, Vol. 2, No. 4, pp. 163-67.
Knapp, M., Beecham, J., Koutsogeorgopoulou, V., Hallam, A., Fenyo, A., *et al.*, (1994), 'Service Use and Costs of Home-Based versus Hospital-Based Care for People with Serious Mental Illness', *British Journal of Psychiatry*, Vol. 165, No. 2, pp. 195-203.
Knesper, D.J., Belcher, B.E. and Cross, J.G. (1989), 'A Market Analysis Comparing the Practices of Psychiatrists and Psychologists', *Archives of General Psychiatry*, Vol. 46, No. 4, April, pp. 305-14.
Koestler, A. (1968), *The Sleepwalkers*, The Danube Edition, Hutchinson & Co., London.
Kolsen, H.M. (1968), *The Economics of Road Rail Competition*, Sydney University Press, Sydney.
Krupinski, J. and Stoller, A. (1962), 'Survey of Institutionalised Mental Patients in Victoria, Australia, 1882-1959', *The Medical Journal of Australia*, Vol. 1, No. 8, February 24, pp. 269-76; March 3, pp. 314-20; March 10, pp. 359-67.
Krupinski, J. and Stoller, A. (1975), 'Changing Patterns of Psychiatric Hospitalisation in the Past Fifty Years: A Cohort Study', *Australian and New Zealand Journal of Psychiatry*, Vol. 9, No. 4, December, pp. 231-39.
Kubler-Ross, E. (ed.)(1975), *Death: The Final Stage of Growth*, Prentice Hall, Englewood Cliffs.
Kubler-Ross, E. (1981), *Living with Death and Dying*, Souvenir Press, London.
Laing, R.D. (1965), *The Divided Self: An Existential Study in Sanity and Madness*, Penguin, Harmondsworth.

Lamb, H.R. (1984), 'Keeping the Mentally Ill Out of Jail,' *Hospital and Community Psychiatry*, Vol. 35, No. 6, p. 529.

Lancaster, K.J. (1966a), 'A New Approach to Consumer Theory', *Journal of Political Economy*, Vol. 74, No. 2, April, pp. 132-57.

Lancaster, K.J. (1966b), 'Change and Innovation in the Technology of Consumption', *The American Economic Review*, Vol. 56, No. 2, May, pp. 14-23.

Lancaster, K.J. (1971), *Consumer Demand: A New Approach*, Columbia University Press, New York.

Lancaster, K.J. (1972), 'Operationally Relevant Characteristics in the Theory of Consumer Behaviour', in M. Peston and B. Corry (eds)(1972), *Essays in Honour of Lord Robbins*, Weidenfeld and Nicolson, London, pp. 43-62.

Lapsley, H. and Cass, Y. (1982), 'The Economics of Institutional and Non-institutional Care for Psychiatric Patients', in P.M. Tatchell (ed.)(1982), *Economics and Health 1981: Proceedings of the Third Australian Conference of Health Economists*, Health Economics Research Unit, Canberra, pp. 105-24.

Lawrence, M. (ed.)(1996), *Prevention of Cardiovascular Disease: An Evidence-Based Approach*, Oxford University Press, Oxford.

Ledyard, J.O. (1987), 'Market Failure', in J. Eatwell, M. Milgate and P. Newman (eds)(1987), *The New Palgrave: A Dictionary of Economics*, Vol. 3, Macmillan, London, pp. 326-29.

Leff, J. (1996), 'Working with Families of Schizophrenic Patients: Effects on Clinical and Social Outcomes', in M. Moscarelli, A. Rupp and N. Sartorious (eds)(1996), *Handbook of Mental Health Economics and Health Policy, Volume 1: Schizophrenia*, John Wiley & Sons, Chichester.

Lefley, H.P. (1996), *Family Caregiving in Mental Illness*, Sage, Thousand Oaks.

Lefley, H.P. (1997), 'An Alliance of Care', Proceedings of the Twentieth Anniversary National Conference of the Association of Relatives and Friends of the Mentally Ill (Brisbane Inc.), Brisbane, 7-9 August.

Leibenstein, H. (1966), 'Allocative Efficiency *vs* X-efficiency', *The American Economic Review*, Vol. 56, No. 3, June, pp. 392-415.

Levy, J.D. and Pitsch, P.K. (1985), 'Statistical Evidence of Substitutability among Video Delivery Systems', in E.M. Noam (ed.)(1985) *Video Media Competition: Regulation, Economics and Technology*, Columbia University Press, New York, pp. 56-92.

Lewis, M.J. (1988), *Managing Madness*, Australian Institute of Health, Canberra.

Lipton, G.L. (1983), 'Politics of Mental Health: Circles or Spirals', *Australian and New Zealand Journal of Psychiatry*, Vol. 17, No. 1, March, pp. 50-56.

Little, I.M.D. (1957), *A Critique of Welfare Economics*, 2nd edn, Oxford University Press, Oxford.

Lloyd, P.J. (1983), 'Why Do Firms Produce Multiple Outputs?', *Journal of Economic Behaviour and Organisation*, Vol. 4, No. 1, March, pp. 41-51.

Lockett, T. (1997), *Evidence-based and Cost-effective Medicine for the Uninitiated*, Radcliffe Medical Press, Oxford.

Lu, M. (1999), 'The Productivity of Mental Health Care: An Instrumental Variable Approach', *The Journal of Mental Health Policy and Economics*, Vol. 2, No. 2, pp. 59-71.

Ma, C-T. A. and McGuire, T.G. (1997), 'Optimal Health Insurance and Provider Payment', *The American Economic Review*, Vol. 87, No. 4, September, pp. 685-704.

Maani, S.A. and Kask, S.B. (1991), 'Risk and Information: A Hedonic Price Study of the New Zealand Housing Market', *The Economic Record*, Vol. 67, No. 198, September, pp. 227-36.

Maddison, F.D. (1998), 'Disability, Institutional Reform and De-institutionalisation: the Queensland Experience', unpublished Master of Social Planning and Development thesis, The University of Queensland, Brisbane.

Malin, N.A. (ed.)(1994), *Implementing Community Care*, Open University Press, Buckingham.

Manning, W.G. Jnr and Frank, R.G. (1992), 'Econometric Issues in the Demand for Mental Health Care Under Insurance', in R. Frank and W. Manning Jnr (eds)(1992), *Economics and Mental Health*, Johns Hopkins University Press, Baltimore, pp. 197-217.

Manning, W.G. Jnr, Newhouse, J.P., Duan, N., Keeler, E.B., Leibowitz, A. and Marquis, S. (1987), 'Health Insurance and the Demand for Medical Care', *The American Economic Review*, Vol. 77, No. 3, June, pp. 251-77.

Manning, W.G. Jnr, Wells, K.B., Buchanan, J.L., Keeler, E.B., Valdez, E.B. and Newhouse, J.P. (1989), 'Effects of Mental Health Insurance: Evidence from the Health Insurance Experiment', RAND R-3015-NIMH/HCFA.

Mansell, J. and Ericsson, K. (eds). (1996), *Deinstitutionalization and Community Living: Intellectual Disability Services in Britain, Scandinavia and the USA*, Chapman and Hall, London.

Marks, D. (1984), 'The Effect of Rental Control on the Price of Rental Housing: A Hedonic Approach', *Land Economics*, Vol. 60, No. 1, February, pp. 81-94.

Marmot, M.G. and Wilkinson, R.G. (eds)(1999), *Social Determinants of Health*, Oxford University Press, Oxford.

Marris, R. (1963), 'A Model of the Managerial Enterprise', *Quarterly Journal of Economics*, Vol. 77, No. 2, pp. 185-209.

Martin, S. (1993), *Advanced Industrial Economics*, Blackwell, Oxford.

Mason, J., Eccles, M., Freemantle, N. and Drummond, M. (1999), 'Incorporating Economic Analysis in Evidence-Based Guidelines for Mental Health: The Profile Approach', *The Journal of Mental Health Policy and Economics*, Vol. 2, No. 1, pp. 13-19.

Maynard, A. (1993), 'Are Mental Health Services Efficient', *International Journal of Mental Health*, Vol. 22, No. 3, pp. 3-32.

McClellan, M. and Newhouse, J.P. (1997), 'The Marginal Cost-Effectiveness of Medical Technology: A Panel Instrumental Variables Approach', *Journal of Econometrics*, Vol. 77, No. 1, pp. 39-64.

McCoombs, J.S., Nichol, M.B., Stimmel, G.L., Sclar, D.A., Beasley Jnr, C.M. and Gross, L.F. (1990), 'The Cost of Antidepressant Drug Therapy Failure: A Study of Antidepressant Drug Use Patterns in a Medicaid Population', *Journal of Clinical Psychiatry*, Vol. 51, No. 6, Supplement, pp. 60-69.

McGuire, A., Henderson, J. and Mooney, G. (1988), *The Economics of Health Care: An Introductory Text*, Routledge and Kegan Paul, London.

McGuire, T.G. (1981), *Financing Psychotherapy: Costs, Effects and Public Policy*, Ballinger Press, Cambridge, MA.

McGuire, T.G. (1985), 'Economics of Mental Health', in *Psychiatry*, Vol. 3, Basic Books, New York.

McGuire, T.G. (1989a), 'Combining Demand- and Supply-Side Cost Sharing: The Case of Inpatient Mental Health Care', *Inquiry*, Vol. 26, No. 2, Summer, pp. 292-303.

McGuire, T.G. (1989b), 'Financing and Reimbursement for Mental Health Services', in C. Taube, D. Mechanic and A. Hohmann (eds)(1989), *The Future of Mental Health Services*, US Government Printing Office, Washington, DC.

McGuire, T.G. (1990), 'Growth of a Field in Policy Research: The Economics of Mental Health', *Administration and Policy in Mental Health*, Vol. 17, No. 3, Spring, pp. 165-175.

McGuire, T.G. (1992), 'Research on Economics and Mental Health: The Past and Future Prospects', in R.G. Frank and W.G. Manning Jnr (eds)(1992), *Economics and Mental Health*, The Johns Hopkins University Press, Baltimore, pp. 1-14.

McGuire, T.G. and Riordan, M.H. (1993), 'Contracting for Community-Based Public Mental Health Services', *Advances in Health Economics and Health Services Research: Research into the Economics of Mental Health*, Vol. 14, JAI Press, Greenwich, pp. 55-70.

McKeown, T. (1979), *The Role of Medicine: Dream, Mirage or Nemesis?*, Rev. edn, Basil Blackwell, Oxford.

McPherson, K., Wennberg, J.E., Hovind, O.B. and Clifford, P. (1982), 'Small-Area Variations in the Use of Common Surgical Procedures: An International Comparison of New England, England and Norway', *The New England Journal of Medicine*, Vol. 307, No. 21, pp. 1310-14.

McTaggart, D., Findlay, C. and Parkin, M. (1999), *Economics*, 3rd edn, Addison Wesley Longman, South Melbourne.

Meade, J. (1952), 'External Economies and Diseconomies in a Competitive Situation', *The Economic Journal*, Vol. LXII, No. 245, pp. 54-67.

Means, R. and Smith, R. (1998), *Community Care: Policy and Practice*, 2nd edn, Macmillan, Houndmills.

Mechanic, D. (1998), 'Emerging Trends in Mental Health Policy and Practice', *Health Affairs*, Vol. 17, No. 6, pp. 82-98.

Medicare Benefits Review Committee (1985), *Second Report*, AGPS, Canberra.

Mental Health Branch, Commonwealth Department of Health and Aged Care (1998), *National Mental Health Report 1997: Fifth Annual Report, Changes in Australia's Mental Health Services under the National Mental Health Strategy 1996-97*, Commonwealth Department of Health and Aged Care, Canberra.

Mental Health Branch, Commonwealth Department of Health and Family Services (1997), *National Mental Health Report 1996: Fourth Annual Report, Changes in Australia's Mental Health Services under the National Mental Health Strategy 1995-96*, Commonwealth Department of Health and Family Services, Canberra.

Mills, E.S. (1968), 'Comment', in H.E. Klarman (ed.)(1968), *Empirical Studies in Health Economics, Proceedings of the Second Conference on the Economics of Health*, The Johns Hopkins University Press, Baltimore, pp. 249-51.

Mishan, E.J. (1960), 'Survey of Welfare Economics 1939-1959', *The Economic Journal*, Vol. LXX, No. 278, pp. 197-265.

Mishan, E.J. (1981), *Introduction to Normative Economics*, Oxford University Press, Oxford.

Mishan, E.J. (1982), *Introduction to Political Economy*, Hutchinson, London.

Mooney, G.H. (1986), *Economics, Medicine and Health Care*, Wheatsheaf Books, Brighton.

Moroney, R. (1980), *Families, Social Services, and Social Policy: The Issue of Shared Responsibility*, U.S. Government Printing Office, Washington DC, DHHS Publication No. ADM 80-846.

Morrissey, J.P. and Goldman, H.H. (1984), 'Cycles of Reform in the Care of the Chronically Mentally Ill', *Hospital and Community Psychiatry*, Vol. 35, No. 8, August, pp. 785-93.

Morrissey, J.P., Tausig, M. and Lindsey, M.L. (1991), 'Network Analysis Methods for Mental Health Service Systems Research: A Comparison of Two Community Support Systems', National Institute of Mental Health, Bethesda, MD, Pub. No. (ADM) 85-1383.

Moscarelli, M., Rupp, A. and Sartorious, N. (eds)(1996), *Handbook of Mental Health Economics and Health Policy, Volume 1: Schizophrenia*, John Wiley & Sons, Chichester.

Moulton, B.R. and Moses, K.E. (1997), 'Addressing the Quality Change Issue in the Consumer Price Index', *Brookings Papers on Economic Activity*, No. 1, Brookings Institution, Washington D.C., pp. 305-49.

Muellbauer, J. (1987), 'Professor Sen on the Standard of Living', in G. Hawthorn (ed.), *The Standard of Living: The Tanner Lectures, Clare Hall, Cambridge, 1985*, Cambridge University Press, Cambridge, pp. 39-58.

Muller, C.F. and Caton, L.M. (1983), 'Economic Costs of Schizophrenia', *Medical Care*, Vol. 21, No. 1, January, pp. 92-101.

Musgrave, R.A. (1959), *The Theory of Public Finance*, McGraw-Hill, New York.

Musgrave, R.A. (1987), 'Merit Goods', in J. Eatwell, M. Milgate and P. Newman (eds)(1987), *The New Palgrave: A Dictionary of Economics*, Vol. 3, Macmillan, London, pp. 452-53.

Musgrave, R.A. and Musgrave, P.B. (1984), *Public Finance in Theory and Practice*, 4th edn, McGraw-Hill, New York.

Myrdal, G. (1944), *An American Dilemma: The Negro Problem and Modern Democracy*, Harper, New York.
Myrdal, G. (1957), *Economic Theory and Underdeveloped Regions*, Duckworth, London.
National Health and Medical Research Council (2000), *How to Use the Evidence: Assessment and Application of Scientific Evidence*, NHMRC, Canberra.
Nelson, J.P. (1980), 'Airports and Property Values: a Survey of Recent Evidence', *Journal of Transport Economics and Policy*, Vol. XIV, No. 1, January, pp. 37-52.
Nelson, J.P. (1982), 'Highway Noise and Property Values: A Survey of Recent Evidence', *Journal of Transport Economics and Policy*, Vol. XVI, No. 2, May, pp. 117-30.
Newhouse, J.P. (1970), 'Towards a Theory of Nonprofit Institutions: An Economic Model of the Hospital', *The American Economic Review*, Vol. LX, No. 1, March, pp. 64-74.
Newhouse, J.P. and Friedlander, L.J. (1980), 'The Relationship Between Medical Resources and Measures of Health: Some Additional Evidence', *Journal of Human Resources*, Vol. 15, No. 2, pp. 200-18.
Newhouse, J.P. and The Health Insurance Experiment Group (1994), *Free for All? Lessons from the RAND Health Insurance Experiment*, Harvard University Press, Cambridge, MA.
Newman, P. (1987), 'Elasticity', in J. Eatwell, M. Milgate and P. Newman (eds)(1987), *The New Palgrave: A Dictionary of Economics*, Vol. 2, Macmillan, London, pp. 125-27.
Nicholson, W. (1992), *Microeconomic Theory: Basic Principles and Extensions*, 5th edn, The Dryden Press, Fort Worth.
Nirje, B. (1969), 'The Normalisation Principle', in R.B. Kugel and A. Shearer (eds)(1975), *Changing Patterns in Residential Services for the Mentally Retarded*, Presidential Committee on Mental Retardation, Washington DC, pp. 231-40.
Nirje, B. (1980), 'The Normalisation Principle', in R.J. Flynn and K.E. Nitsch (eds)(1980), *Normalisation, Social Integration and Community Services*, Pro-Ed, Austin, pp. 31-50.
Niskanen, W.A. (1968), 'The Peculiar Economics of Bureaucracy', *The American Economic Review*, Vol. LVIII, No. 2, May, pp. 293-305.
North, D. (1990), *Institutions, Institutional Change and Economic Performance*, Cambridge University Press, Cambridge.
North, D. (1995), 'The New Institutional Economics and Third World Development', in J. Harriss, J. Hunter and C. Lewis (eds)(1995), *The New Institutional Economics and Third World Development*, Routledge, London, pp. 17-26.
Nugent, J.B. (1993), 'Between State, Market and Households: A Neoinstitutional Analysis of Local Organisations and Institutions', *World Development*, Vol. 21, No. 4, pp. 623-32.
Nussbaum, M. and Sen, A. (1993), 'Introduction', in M. Nussbaum and A. Sen (eds)(1993), *The Quality of Life*, Clarendon Press, Oxford, pp. 1-8.
O'Donnell, O., Maynard, A. and Wright, K. (1988), 'The Economic Evaluation of Mental Health Care: A Review', *Centre for Health Economics Discussion Paper*, No. 15, University of York, York.
O'Flaherty, B. (1996), *Making Room: The Economics of Homelessness*, Harvard University Press, Cambridge, MA.
Okun, A.M. (1975), *Equality and Efficiency: The Big Tradeoff*, Brookings Institution, Washington, DC.
Olson, M. (1982), *The Rise and Decline of Nations*, Yale University Press, New Haven.
Olson, M. (1996), 'Big Bills Left on the Sidewalk: Why Some Nations are Rich and Others Poor', *Journal of Economic Perspectives*, Vol. 10, No. 2, pp. 3-24.
Olson, M. and Kähkönen, S. (2000), 'Introduction: The Broader View,' in M. Olson and S. Kähkönen (eds)(2000), *A Not-So-Dismal Science: A Broader View of Economics and Societies*, Oxford University Press, Oxford, pp. 1-36.
Organization for Economic Cooperation and Development (2000), *OECD Health Data: A Comparative Analysis of 29 OECD Countries*, OECD, Paris.

Ostrom, E. (1996), 'Crossing the Great Divide: Coproduction, Synergy, and Development', *World Development*, Vol. 24, No. 6, pp. 1073-87.

Palmer, G.R. and Short, S.D. (1994), *Health Care and Public Policy: An Australian Analysis*, 2nd edn, Macmillan, South Melbourne.

Palmquist, R.B. (1991), 'Hedonic Methods', in J.B. Braden and C.D. Kolstad (1991)(eds), *Measuring the Demand for Environmental Quality*, Elsevier, Amsterdam.

Patrick, R. (1987), *A History of Health and Medicine in Queensland 1824-1960*, University of Queensland Press, Brisbane.

Payne, M. (1995), *Social Work and Community Care*, Macmillan, London.

Pauly, M.V. (1968), 'The Economics of Moral Hazard: Comment', *The American Economic Review*, Vol. LVIII, No. 3, June, pp. 531-37.

Pauly, M.V. (1981), 'Paying the Piper and Calling the Tune: The Relationship between Public Financing and Public Regulation of Health Care', in M. Olson (1981)(ed.), *A New Approach to the Economics of Health Care*, American Enterprise Institute for Public Policy Research, Washington, DC, pp. 67-86.

Pauly, M.V. (1983), 'More on Moral Hazard', *Journal of Health Economics*, Vol. 2, No.1, pp. 81-85.

Pauly, M.V. (1986), 'Taxation, Health Insurance, and Market Failure in the Medical Economy', *Journal of Economic Literature*, Vol. 24, No. 2, June, pp. 629-75.

Pauly, M.V. and Redisch, M. (1973), 'The Not-for-profit Hospital as a Physician's Cooperative', *The American Economic Review*, Vol. 63, No. 1, March, pp. 87-100.

Pearce, D.W. (ed.)(1986), *Macmillan Dictionary of Modern Economics*, 3rd edn, Macmillan, Basingstoke.

Peele, R. and Chodoff, P. (1999), 'The Ethics of Involuntary Treatment and Deinstitutionalization', in S. Bloch, P. Chodoff and S.A. Green (eds)(1999), *Psychiatric Ethics*, 3rd edn, Oxford University Press, New York, pp. 423-40.

Pepper, B. and Ryglewicz, H. (1985), 'The Role of the State Hospital: A New Mandate for a New Era', *Psychiatric Quarterly*, Vol. 57, Nos 3 & 4, Fall/Winter, pp. 230-51.

Peterson, R. (1982), 'What Are the Needs of Chronic Mental Patients?', *Schizophrenia Bulletin*, Vol. 8, No. 4, pp. 610-6.

Phelps, C.E. (1992), 'Diffusion of Information in Medical Care', *Journal of Economic Perspectives*, Vol. 6, No. 3, pp. 23-42.

Phelps, C.E. (1995), 'Welfare Loss from Variations: Further Considerations', *Journal of Health Economics*, Vol. 14, No. 2, pp. 253-60.

Phelps, C.E. (1999), 'Comment', in J.E. Triplett, (ed)(1999), *Measuring Prices of Medical Treatments*, Bookings Institution Press, Washington, DC, pp. 108-17.

Phelps, C.E. and Mooney, C. (1992), 'Correction and Update on "Priority Setting in Medical Technology and Medical Practice Assessment" ', *Medical Care*, Vol. 30, No. 8, pp. 744-51.

Phelps, C.E. and Parente, S.T. (1990), 'Priority Setting in Medical Technology and Medical Practice Assessment', *Medical Care*, Vol. 28, No. 8, pp. 703-23.

Phillips, K.A. and Rosenblatt, A. (1992), 'Speaking in Tongues: Integrating Economics and Psychology into Health and Mental Health Services Outcomes Research', *Medical Care Review*, Vol. 49, No. 2, Summer, pp. 191-230.

Pigou, A.C. (1929), *A Study of Public Finance*, 2nd edn, Macmillan, London.

Pigou, A.C. (1932), *The Economics of Welfare*, 4th edn, Macmillan, London.

Pindyck, R.S. and Rubinfeld, D.L. (1992), *Microeconomics*, 2nd edn, Macmillan, New York.

Pindyck, R.S. and Rubinfeld, D.L. (1998), *Microeconomics*, 4th edn, Prentice Hall, Upper Saddle River.

Pink, A. and Connelly, L.B. (1999), 'Economic and Financial Analyses of Alternative Plasma Collection Technologies: "Whole Blood" Collection *Versus* "Erythroplasmaphresis" ', in J. Baldry (ed.)(1999), *Economics and Health 1998: Proceedings of the Twentieth Conference of Health Economists*, School of Health Services Management, Sydney, pp. 219-57.

Pollak, R.A. and Wachter, M.L. (1975), 'The Relevance of the Household Production Function and Its Implications for the Allocation of Time', *Journal of Political Economy*, Vol. 88, No. 2, pp. 255-77.

Posnett, J.S. (1996), 'Indirect Cost in Economic Evaluation: The Opportunity Cost of Unpaid Inputs', *Health Economics*, Vol. 5, No.1, pp. 13-23.

Power, R. (1989), 'A World Apart', *New Statesman and Society*, Vol. 2, No. 54, 16 June, pp. 23-24.

Prior, L. (1993), *The Social Organization of Mental Illness*, Sage, London.

Putnam, R.D. (with Leonardi, R. and Nanetti, R.Y.)(1993a), *Making Democracy Work: Civic Traditions in Modern Italy*, Princeton University Press, Princeton.

Putnam, R.D. (1993b), 'The Prosperous Community: Social Capital and Public Life', *The American Prospect*, No. 13, Spring, http://epn.org/prospect/13/13putn.html.

Putnam, R.D. (1995), 'Bowling Alone: America's Declining Social Capital', *Journal of Democracy*, Vol. 6, No.1, pp. 65-78.

Putnam, R.D. (1996), 'The Strange Disappearance of Civil America', *The American Prospect*, No. 24, Winter, http://epn.org/prospect/24/24putn.html.

Putterman, L. and Krosner, K.J. (1996)(eds), *The Economic Nature of the Firm: A Reader*, 2nd edn, Cambridge University Press, Cambridge.

Racino, J.A. (1993), *Housing, Support, and Community*, P.H. Brooks, Baltimore.

Rawls, J. (1971), *A Theory of Justice*, Oxford University Press, London.

Reder, M.W. (1969), 'Some Problems in the Measurement of Productivity in the Medical Care Industry', in V.R. Fuchs (ed.)(1969), *Production and Productivity in the Service Industries*, National Bureau of Economic Research Studies in Income and Wealth, Vol. 34, Columbia University Press, New York, pp. 95-131.

Reich, W. (1981), 'Psychiatric Diagnosis as an Ethical Problem', in S. Bloch and P. Chodoff, P. (eds)(1981), *Psychiatric Ethics*, Oxford University Press, Oxford, pp. 61-88.

Reinhardt, U. (1972), 'A Production Function for Physician Services', *The Review of Economics and Statistics*, Vol. LIV, No. 1, pp. 55-65.

Rice, D.P. and Kelman, S. (1989), 'Measuring Comorbidity and Overlap in the Cost of Hospitalization for Alcohol and Drug Abuse and Mental Illness', *Inquiry*, Vol. 26, No. 2, Summer, pp. 249-60.

Rice, D.P. and Miller, L.S. (1993), 'The Economic Burden of Affective Disorders', in T-W. Hu and A. Rupp (Guest eds)(1993), *Advances in Health Economics and Health Services Research: Research into the Economics of Mental Health*, Vol. 14, JAI Press, Greenwich, pp. 37-54.

Rice, D.P. and Miller, L.S. (1996), 'The Economic Burden of Schizophrenia: Conceptual and Methodological Issues, and Cost Estimates', in M. Moscarelli, A. Rupp and N. Sartorious (eds)(1996), *Handbook of Mental Health Economics and Health Policy, Volume 1: Schizophrenia*, John Wiley & Sons, Chichester, pp. 321-34.

Rice, T.H. (1992), 'An Alternative Framework for Evaluating Welfare Losses in the Health Care Market', *Journal of Health Economics*, Vol. 11, No. 1, pp. 86-92.

Ritschl, H. (1931), 'Communal Economy and Market Economy', reprinted in R. A. Musgrave and A.T. Peacock (eds)(1967), *Classics in the Theory of Public Finance*, Macmillan, London, pp. 233-41.

Robinson, J. (1933), *The Economics of Imperfect Competition*, Macmillan, London.

Rosen, S. (1974), 'Hedonic Prices and Implicit Markets: Product Differentiation in Pure Competition', *Journal of Political Economy*, Vol. 82, No. 1, January/February, pp. 34-55.

Rosenblatt, A. (1984), 'Concepts of the Asylum in the Care of the Mentally Ill', *Hospital and Community Psychiatry*, Vol. 35, No. 3, March, pp. 244-50.

Rosenhan, D. and Seligman, M.E.P. (1984), *Abnormal Psychology*, Norton, New York.

Rosenheck, R., Cramer, J., Xu, W., Grabowski, J. *et al.* (1998), 'Multiple Outcome Assessment in a Study of the Cost-Effectiveness of Clozapine in the Treatment of Refractory Schizophrenia', *Health Services Research*, Vol. 33, No. 5, Part I, December, pp. 1237-61.

Rubin, J. (1982), 'Cost Measurement and Cost Data in Mental Health Settings', *Hospital and Community Psychiatry*, Vol. 33, No. 9, September, pp. 750-54.

Rutherford, M. (1994), *Institutions in Economics: The Old and the New Institutionalism*, Cambridge University Press, Cambridge.

Sackett, D.L., Richardson, W.S., Rosenberg, W. and Haynes, R.B. (1997), *Evidence-based Medicine: How to Practise and Teach Evidence-based Medicine*, Churchill Livingstone, London.

Sacks, O. (1995), *An Anthropologist from Mars*, Picador, Sydney.

Salzer, M. (1999), 'The Outcomes Measurement Movement and Mental Health Services Research: A Review of Three Books', *Mental Health Services Research*, Vol. 1, No.1, pp. 59-63.

Samuelson, P.A. (1954), 'The Pure Theory of Public Expenditure', *Review of Economics and Statistics*, Vol. 36, No. 4, November, pp. 387-89.

Samuelson, P.A. (1955), 'Diagrammatic Exposition of a Theory of Public Expenditure', *Review of Economics and Statistics*, Vol. 37, No. 4, November, pp. 350-56.

Samuelson, P.A. (1968), 'Two Generalizations of the Elasticity of Substitution', in J.N. Wolfe (ed.)(1968), *Value, Capital and Growth: Essays in Honour of Sir John Hicks*, Edinburgh University Press, Edinburgh, pp. 467-80.

Samuelson, P.A. (1969), 'Pure Theory of Public Expenditure and Taxation', in J. Margolis and H. Guitton (eds), *Public Economics: An Analysis of Public Production and Consumption and Their Relations to the Private Sectors*, Macmillan, London, pp. 98-123.

SANE Australia (1999), *Senior Service: A National Survey of Services for Older Australians with a Mental Illness 1999*, SANE Australia, South Melbourne.

Sax, S. (1984), *A Strife of Interests: Politics and Policies in Australian Health Services*, Allen and Unwin, Sydney.

Schanding, D., Siomopoulos, V., Godbole, A. and Smith, M. (1984), 'Readmissions to a General Hospital's Psychiatric Unit', *Hospital and Community Psychiatry*, Vol. 35, No. 2, February, pp. 170-1.

Scheffler, R.M. and Watts, C.A. (1986), 'Determinants of Inpatient Mental Health Use in a Heavily Insured Population', *The Journal of Human Resources*, Vol. 21, No. 3, Summer, pp. 338-58.

Scheper-Hughes, N. and Lovell, A.M. (1986), 'Breaking the Circuit of Social Control: Lessons in Public Psychiatry', *Social Science and Medicine*, Vol. 23, No. 2, pp. 159-78.

Schnare, A. (1976), 'Racial and Ethnic Price Differentials in an Urban Housing Market', *Urban Studies*, Vol. 13, No. 2, June, pp. 107-20.

Schwartz, S. and Griffin, T. (1986), *Medical Thinking: The Psychology of Medical Judgement and Decision Making*, Springer-Verlag, New York.

Schwartz, S.R. and Goldfinger, S.M. (1981), 'The New Chronic Patient: Clinical Characteristics of an Emerging Subgroup', *Hospital and Community Psychiatry*, Vol. 32, No. 7, 7 July, pp. 470-81.

Scitovsky, A.A. (1964), 'An Index of the Cost of Medical Care: A Proposed New Approach', in S.J. Axelrod (ed.)(1964), *The Economics of Health and Medical Care*, University of Michigan Press, Ann Arbor, pp. 128-47.

Scitovsky, A.A. (1967), 'Changes in the Costs of Treatment of Selected Illnesses, 1951-1965', *The American Economic Review*, Vol. 57, No. 5, December, pp. 1182-95.

Scitovsky, A.A. (1979), 'Changes in the Use of Ancillary Services for "Common Illnesses" ', in S.H. Altman and R. Blendon (eds)(1979), *Medical Technology: The Culprit Behind Health Care Costs?*, National Centre for Health Services Research, Washington, DC, pp. 39-56.

Scitovsky, A.A. (1985), 'Changes in the Costs of Treatment of Selected Illnesses, 1971-1981', *Medical Care*, Vol. 23, No. 12, pp. 1245-57.

Scitovsky, A.A. and McCall, N. (1980), 'Use of Hospital Services under Two Prepaid Plans', *Medical Care*, Vol. 18, No. 1, pp. 30-43.

Scitovsky, T. (1966), 'Discussion', *The American Economic Review*, Vol. LVI, No. 2, May, pp. 47-9.
Scotton, R.B. and Macdonald, C.R. (1993), *The Making of Medibank*, School of Health Services Management, Kensington.
Scotton, R.B. and Macdonald, C.R. (1995), *Medibank Sources: Unpublished Documents Relating to the Establishment of National Health Insurance in Australia*, Centre for Health Program Evaluation, West Heidelberg.
Sen, A. (1985), *Commodities and Capabilities*, North-Holland, Amsterdam.
Sen, A. (1987a), 'The Standard of Living: Lecture I, Concepts and Critiques', in G. Hawthorn (ed.), *The Standard of Living: The Tanner Lectures, Clare Hall, Cambridge, 1985*, Cambridge University Press, Cambridge, pp. 1-19.
Sen, A. (1987b), 'The Standard of Living: Lecture II, Lives and Capabilities', in G. Hawthorn (ed.), *The Standard of Living: The Tanner Lectures, Clare Hall, Cambridge, 1985*, Cambridge University Press, Cambridge, pp. 20-38.
Sen, A. (1987c), 'Rational Behaviour', in J. Eatwell, M. Milgate and P. Newman (eds)(1987), *The New Palgrave: A Dictionary of Economics*, Vol. 4, Macmillan, London, pp. 68-76.
Shapiro, M.P. and Wilcox, D.W. (1996), 'Mismeasurement in the Consumer Price Index: An Evaluation', *NBER Macroeconomics Annual*, Vol. 11, pp. 93-142.
Sharfstein, S.S. and Taube, C.A. (1982), 'Reductions in Insurance for Mental Disorders: Adverse Selection, Moral Hazard, and Consumer Demand', *American Journal of Psychiatry*, Vol. 139, No. 11, November, pp. 1425-30.
Shiell, A. (1997), 'Health Outcomes are About Choices and Values: An Economic Perspective on the Health Outcomes Movement', *Health Policy*, Vol. 39, pp. 5-15.
Silagy, C. and Haines, A. (eds)(1998), *Evidence-based Practice in Primary Care*, BMJ Books, London.
Simon, H.A. (1957), *Models of Man: Social and Rational*, Wiley, New York.
Sloan, F.A. (1971), *Planning Public Expenditures on Mental Health Service Delivery*, Rand Institute, New York.
Small, W. (1996), 'Emotion Work', in C. Grbich (ed.)(1996), *Health in Australia: Sociological Concepts and Issues*, Prentice Hall, Sydney, pp. 263-87.
Smith, J.P. (1999), 'Healthy Bodies and Thick Wallets: The Dual Relation Between Health and Economic Status', *The Journal of Economic Perspectives*, Vol. 13, No. 2, pp. 145-66.
Smith, W. and Wenham, M. (2000), 'Monitor', *The Courier Mail*, 1 April, p. 26.
Solzhenitsyn, A. (1978), *The Gulag Archipelago, 1918-1956*, translated by H. T. Willetts, Collins and Harrill, London.
Spitzer, R.L. and Klein, D.F. (1978), *Critical Issues in Psychiatric Diagnosis*, Raven Press, New York.
Stanley, L.R. and Tschirhart, J. (1991), 'Hedonic Prices for a Non-durable Good: the Case of Breakfast Cereals', *Review of Economics and Statistics*, Vol. LXXIII, No. 3, August, pp. 537-41.
Stevens, C.M. (1968), 'Hospital Market Efficiency: The Anatomy of the Supply Response', in H. E. Klarman (ed.)(1968), *Empirical Studies in Health Economics, Proceedings of the Second Conference on the Economics of Health*, The Johns Hopkins University Press, Baltimore, pp. 229-48.
Stewart, R.G. and Jones, J.C.H. (1998), 'Hedonics and Demand Analysis: The Implicit Demand for Player Attributes', *Economic Inquiry*, Vol. XXXVI, No. 2, April, pp. 192-202.
Stigler, G.J. and Kindahl, J.K. (1970), *Behavior of Industrial Prices*, National Bureau of Economic Research, New York.
Stoller, A. and Arscott, K.W. (1955), *Report on Mental Health Facilities and Needs of Australia*, Government Printing Office, Canberra.
Stonecash, R.E., Gans, J.S., King, S.P. and Mankiw, N.G. (1999), *Principles of Macroeconomics*, Harcourt, Sydney.

Streeting, M.C. (1990), *A Survey of the Hedonic Price Technique*, AGPS, Canberra.

Szasz, T.S. (1961), *The Myth of Mental Illness: Foundations of a Theory of Personal Conduct*, Hoeber-Harper, New York.

Szasz, T.S. (1998), 'Parity for Mental Illness, Disparity for the Mental Patient', *Lancet*, Vol. 352, No. 9135, 10 October, pp. 1213-15.

Taube, C.A. and Burns, B.J. (1988), 'Mental Health Services System Research: The National Institute of Mental Health Program', *Health Services Research*, Vol. 22, No. 6, February, pp. 837-55.

Taube, C.A., Kessler, L.G. and Burns, B.J. (1986), 'Estimating the Probability and Level of Ambulatory Mental Health Services', *Health Services Research*, Vol. 21, No. 2, Part II, June, Supplement, pp. 321-40.

Taube, C.A., Lee, E.S., and Forthofer, R.N. (1984), 'DRGs in Psychiatry: An Empirical Evaluation', *Medical Care*, Vol. 22, No. 7, pp. 597-610.

Taylor, S.J., Bogdan, R. and Racino, J.A. (eds)(1991), *Life in the Community: Case Studies of Organizations Supporting People with Disabilities*, P.H. Brooks, Baltimore.

Tessler, R. and Gamache, G. (1994), 'Continuity of Care, Residence, and Family Burden in Ohio', *The Milbank Quarterly*, Vol. 72, No. 1, pp. 149-69.

Throsby, C.D. and Withers, G.A. (1979), *The Economics of the Performing Arts*, Edward Arnold, Melbourne.

Throsby, D. (1999), 'Cultural Capital', *Journal of Cultural Economics*, Vol. 23, No. 1, pp. 3-12.

Tiongson, E.R. (1997), 'Baumol's Cost Disease Reconsidered', *Challenge*, Vol. 10, No. 6, Nov.-Dec., pp. 117-21.

Torrey, E.F. (1994), 'Violent Behaviour by Individuals with Serious Mental Illness', *Hospital and Community Psychiatry*, Vol. 45, No. 7, pp. 653-62.

Towse, R. (ed)(1997), *Baumol's Cost Disease: The Arts and Other Victims*, Edward Elgar, Cheltenham.

Triplett, J.E. (1987), 'Hedonic Functions and Hedonic Indexes', in J. Eatwell, M. Milgate and P. Newman (eds)(1987), *The New Palgrave: A Dictionary of Economics*, Vol. 2, Macmillan, London, pp. 630-34.

Triplett, J.E. (1999a), 'Accounting for Health Care: Integrating Price Index and Cost-Effectiveness Research', in J.E. Triplett (ed.)(1999), *Measuring the Prices of Medical Treatment*, Brookings Institution Press, Washington DC, pp. 220-50.

Triplett, J.E. (1999b), 'What's Different About Health? Human Repair and Car Repair in National Accounts and in National Health Accounts', paper presented at the NBER-CRIW Conference on Medical Output and Productivity, June 12-13, 1998. Forthcoming in D. Cutler and E.R. Berndt (eds), *Medical Output and Productivity*, University of Chicago Press for the National Bureau of Economic Research, Chicago.

Triplett, J.E. (ed.)(1999c), *Measuring the Prices of Medical Treatment*, Brookings Institution Press, Washington DC.

Triplett, J.E. and Berndt, E.R. (1999), 'Introduction: New Developments in Measuring Medical Care', in J.E. Triplett (ed.)(1999), *Measuring the Prices of Medical Treatment*, Brookings Institution Press, Washington DC, pp. 1-33.

Tullock, G. (1967), 'The Welfare Costs of Tariffs, Monopolies and Theft', *Western Economic Journal*, Vol. 5, No. 3, pp. 224-32.

Varian, H.R. (1984), *Microeconomic Analysis*, 2nd edn, Norton, New York.

Wagstaff, A. (1986), 'The Demand for Health: Theory and Applications', *Journal of Epidemiology and Community Health*, Vol. 40, No. 1, pp. 1-11.

Wallen, J. (1987), 'Resource Use by Psychiatric Patients in Community Hospitals: The Influence of Illness Severity, Physician Specialty, and Presence of a Psychiatric Unit', in T-W Hu and A. Rupp (1993)(Guest eds), *Advances in Health Economics and Health Services Research: Research in the Economics of Mental Health*, Vol. 8, JAI Press, Greenwich, CT, pp. 103-26.

Wallen, J., Roddy, P. and Meyers, S.M. (1986), 'Male-Female Differences in Mental Health Visits Under Cost-Sharing', *Health Services Research,* Vol. 21, No. 2, Part II, June, Supplement, pp. 341-52.

Ware, J.E., Snow, K.K., Kosinski, M. and Gandek, B. (1993), *SF36 Health Survey Manual and Interpretation Guide*, The Health Institute, New England Medical Center, Boston, MA.

Watts, C.A., Scheffler, R.M. and Jewell, N.P. (1986), 'Demand for Outpatient Mental Health Services in a Heavily Insured Population: The Case of the Blue Cross and Blue Shield Association's Federal Employees Health Benefits Program', *Health Services Research,* Vol. 21, No. 2, Part II, June, Supplement, pp. 267-90.

Waud, R.N., Maxwell, P., Hocking, A., Bonnici, J. and Ward, I. (1996), *Macroeconomics,* 3rd Austn edn, Longman, South Melbourne.

Weisbrod, B.A. (1964), 'Collective-Consumption Services of Individual-Consumption Goods', *Quarterly Journal of Economics*, Vol. LXXVIII, No.3, August, pp. 471-77.

Weisbrod, B.A. (1991), 'The Health Care Quadrilemma: An Essay on Technological Change, Insurance, Quality of Care, and Cost Containment', *Journal of Economic Literature*, Vol. XXIX, No. 2, pp. 523-52.

Weisbrod, B.A., Test, M.A. and Stein, L.I. (1980), 'Alternative to Mental Hospital Treatment: II. Economic Benefit-Cost Analysis', *Archives of General Psychiatry,* Vol. 37, No. 4, April, pp. 400-5.

Wells, K.B. and Sturm, R. (1995), 'Care for Depression in a Changing Environment', *Health Affairs*, Vol. 14, No. 3, pp. 78-89.

Wennberg, J.E. (1987), 'Population Illness Rates Do Not Explain Population Hospitalization Rates', *Medical Care*, Vol. 25, No. 4, pp. 354-59.

Wennberg, J.E., Barnes, B.A. and Zubkoff, M. (1982), 'Professional Uncertainty and the Problem of Supplier-Induced Demand', *Social Science and Medicine*, Vol. 68, No. 1, pp. 811-24.

White, W.D. and Dada, M. (1993), 'Financial Risk and Behavioral Implications of Prospective Payment for Psychiatric Services', in T-W Hu and A. Rupp (1993)(Guest eds), *Advances in Health Economics and Health Services Research: Research in the Economics of Mental Health*, Vol. 14, JAI Press, Greenwich, CT, pp. 105-21.

Whiteford, H. (1995), 'Economic Thinking About Mental Health Resource Allocation', *Australasian Psychiatry*, Vol. 3, No. 1, February, pp. 17-18.

Whiteford, H., Thompson, I. and Casey, D. (2000), 'The Australian Mental Health System', *International Journal of Law and Psychiatry*, Vol. 23, No. 3-4, pp. 403-17.

Wilkinson, R.G. (1996), *Unhealthy Societies: The Afflictions of Inequality*, Routledge, London.

Williams, A. (1978), 'The Budget as a (Mis-)Information System', in A. J. Culyer and K. G. Wright, K.G. (eds)(1978), *Economic Aspects of Health Services*, Martin Robertson, Oxford, pp. 84-91.

Williams, C.H. (1993), 'Price Discovery at Queensland Cattle Auctions' unpublished Doctor of Philosophy thesis presented to The University of Queensland, Brisbane.

Williamson, O.E. (1963), 'Managerial Discretion and Business Behaviour', *The American Economic Review*, Vol. LIII, No. 5, December, pp. 1032-57.

Windle, C. (1991), 'What Mental Health Services Research Does NIMH Support?' *Administration and Policy in Mental Health*, Vol. 18, No. 3, pp. 199-203.

Winefield, H.R. and Harvey, E.J. (1994), 'Needs of Family Caregivers in Chronic Schizophrenia', *Schizophrenia Bulletin*, Vol. 20, No. 4, Sept. pp. 557-66.

Wolfensberger, W. (1983), 'Social Role Valorization: A Proposed New Term for the Principle of Normalisation', *Mental Retardation*, Vol. 21, No. 6, pp. 234-39.

Wolfensberger, W. (1998), *A Brief Introduction to Social Role Valorization: A High-Order Concept for Addressing the Plight of Socially Devalued People, and for Structuring Human Services*, Training Institute for Human Service Planning, Toronto.

Wolfensberger, W. and Nirje, B. (1972), *The Principle of Normalisation in Human Services*, National Institute on Mental Retardation, Toronto.

Wolff, N. and Helminiak, T.W. (1993), 'The Anatomy of Cost Estimates – The Other Outcome', in T-W. Hu and A. Rupp (Guest eds)(1993), *Advances in Health Economics and Health Services Research: Research into the Economics of Mental Health*, Vol. 14, JAI Press, Greenwich, pp. 159-80.

World Health Organization (1992), *The ICD-10 Classification of Mental and Behavioural Disorders Clinical Descriptions and Diagnostic Guidelines*, WHO, Geneva.

Wyatt, R.J. and De Renzio, E.G. (1986), 'Scienceless to Homeless', *Science*, Vol. 234, No. 4782, 12 December, p. 1309.

Young, L., Sigafoos, J., Suttie, J., Ashman, A. and Grevell, P. (1998), 'Deinstitutionalisation of Persons with Intellectual Disabilities: A Review of Australian Studies', *Journal of Intellectual and Developmental Disability*, Vol. 23, No. 2, pp. 155-70.

Zeckhauser, R. (1970), 'Medical Insurance: A Case Study of the Tradeoff between Risk Spreading and Appropriate Incentives', *Journal of Economic Theory*, Vol. 2, No. 1, March, pp. 10-26.

Zupan, M.A. (1998), 'Conference on Economics and Sociology', *Economic Inquiry*, Vol. XXXVI, No. 3, July, pp. 333-34.

Name Index

Subject Index